Mastering the Hidden Curriculum

Medical students and residents are immersed in a busy world with unspoken expectations, invisible challenges, and other influences that comprise a hidden curriculum. This book provides a deeper understanding of this complex system, unique "insider" perspectives, and practical advice. To do this, it provides a platform built on applied sociology, history, organizational psychology, and science that reimagines how to manage medical training. This book seeks to level the playing field by demystifying the hidden curriculum, enabling medical trainees to achieve their full potential using well-defined effective strategies.

Key Features:

- Unravels the many unspokens—the hidden curriculum—of medical training
- Provides basic background material and strategies to succeed in medical training, focusing on information left out of the formal curriculum and often not conveyed to trainees
- Features a balanced, evidence-based discussion on many areas of misinformation and controversy, such as statistical testing, the gender pay gap in medicine, the replication crisis, generational trends and biases, and more

Mastering the Hidden Curriculum

Unlocking Success in Medical Training

Vance T. Lehman, MD

CRC Press
Taylor & Francis Group
Boca Raton London New York

CRC Press is an imprint of the
Taylor & Francis Group, an **informa** business

First edition published 2026
by CRC Press
2385 NW Executive Center Drive, Suite 320, Boca Raton FL 33431

and by CRC Press
4 Park Square, Milton Park, Abingdon, Oxon, OX14 4RN

CRC Press is an imprint of Taylor & Francis Group, LLC

© 2026 Vance T. Lehman

This book contains information obtained from authentic and highly regarded sources. While all reasonable efforts have been made to publish reliable data and information, neither the author[s] nor the publisher can accept any legal responsibility or liability for any errors or omissions that may be made. The publishers wish to make clear that any views or opinions expressed in this book by individual editors, authors or contributors are personal to them and do not necessarily reflect the views/opinions of the publishers. The information or guidance contained in this book is intended for use by medical, scientific or health-care professionals and is provided strictly as a supplement to the medical or other professional's own judgement, their knowledge of the patient's medical history, relevant manufacturer's instructions and the appropriate best practice guidelines. Because of the rapid advances in medical science, any information or advice on dosages, procedures or diagnoses should be independently verified. The reader is strongly urged to consult the relevant national drug formulary and the drug companies' and device or material manufacturers' printed instructions, and their websites, before administering or utilizing any of the drugs, devices or materials mentioned in this book. This book does not indicate whether a particular treatment is appropriate or suitable for a particular individual. Ultimately it is the sole responsibility of the medical professional to make his or her own professional judgements, so as to advise and treat patients appropriately. The authors and publishers have also attempted to trace the copyright holders of all material reproduced in this publication and apologize to copyright holders if permission to publish in this form has not been obtained. If any copyright material has not been acknowledged please write and let us know so we may rectify in any future reprint.

For Product Safety Concerns and Information please contact our EU representative GPSR@taylorandfrancis.com. Taylor & Francis Verlag GmbH, Kaufingerstraße 24, 80331 München, Germany.

Trademark notice: Product or corporate names may be trademarks or registered trademarks and are used only for identification and explanation without intent to infringe.

ISBN: 978-1-041-05998-1 (hbk)
ISBN: 978-1-041-05988-2 (pbk)
ISBN: 978-1-003-63338-9 (ebk)

DOI: 10.1201/9781003633389

Typeset in Minion
by SPi Technologies India Pvt Ltd (Straive)

Contents

Contents

Preface

Why do medical trainees with similar motivation and aptitude experience widely divergent professional outcomes? For some, success seems to come effortlessly, because the forces making the difference are unseen. These occult factors, including unspoken expectations, invisible challenges, and stealth influences, culminate into the *hidden curriculum*. Unlike the formal curriculum, which is explicitly taught, the hidden curriculum is usually learned through observation, subconscious associations, and trial and error. What I've learned along the way, though, is that these forces can be recognized, managed, and (with dedication) even mastered.

Taking a step back, when I was younger, I thought that only those from the higher echelons of society—*other people*—could become physicians. Indeed, it is true that formidable psychological, social, and economic barriers to entering the profession of medicine do exist, barriers that are significantly easier to overcome with the right information. Despite not having insider information at the time, it was through a combination of hard work, good strategy, and a healthy dose of luck that I had the opportunity to complete my radiology residency and neuroradiology fellowship at Mayo Clinic in Rochester Minnesota, where I received an outstanding medical education and where I am still proud to practice as a neuroradiologist to this day.

Perhaps the most striking pattern I have observed in training and beyond in my career in medicine is that even if a medical trainee has encyclopedic book knowledge (which is undoubtedly valuable), there is far more to learn to be a truly successful doctor. It is the complete package of know-how, preparation, problem-solving skills, intuition, ability to seek help when needed, and, above all, capacity to focus intently on the task at hand. The typical classroom does not prepare anyone for this. Instead, we learn through imitation and deliberate practice. Our basic medical education falls short in preparing us not only for a career in medicine but also for the workplace and personal concerns that accompany it. These latter factors are certainly relevant, because if these go awry, so too will professional performance.

While serving various roles in medical education, staff recruitment, research, clinical practice and procedures, and professional societies, I've had the opportunity to work with colleagues from around the world. Regardless of background or work setting, no one is exempt from the powerful influences of the hidden curriculum. The ideas for this book emerged naturally when I connected the dots between my own experiences in medical education and those of others.

Knowing what I know now as a tenured attending, I wish trainees understood the significant impact their approach to learning and professionalism has on their reputation, how easily they can undermine their own success, and how these factors can create significant downstream effects, both positive and negative. They may not fully grasp how much these unspoken expectations influence trainee feedback and outcomes.

I also believe that trainees do not realize how much of an impact the system can have on them personally. The system sets trainees up for challenges arising from powerful real and perceived generational differences. Furthermore, the formal curriculum omits many useful topics and shields trainees from controversies that are necessary to understand in real-world practice.

I've been in practice long enough to observe several classes of new physicians complete their training, yet I'm still close enough to my own experience to remember the challenges firsthand. This gives me (and others in my cohort) a unique perspective, relating to the different generational viewpoints of both current senior faculty and junior trainees. In doing so, I've concluded that navigating the hidden curriculum is a major factor that sets successful trainees apart. Unfortunately, there are not enough high-quality resources available to help novices do so, which is where this book comes in. *In this book, you will learn what the hidden curriculum is, where it comes from, and how to manage it.*

Specifically, insights for this book come from a combination of my personal experience as a medical doctor, the medical education literature, and information from many other disciplines on related subjects, such as organizational psychology, sociology, philosophy, and complexity. In training, I knew little about these disciplines; it was only when I stumbled upon them later did a light bulb go off for me. That is, while these other bodies of knowledge explain much behind the daily work experience, most physicians are unfamiliar with them, and so the influences remain largely out of sight.

Because the hidden curriculum is so complex and multifaceted, I needed to develop a conceptual scheme to understand how all the pieces fit together for this book. This effort culminated into recognition of broader **themes** (such as professionalism, medical culture, history of human nature and medicine, and well-being) and **special topics** (such as failure, negotiation, feedback, mentorship, and social media use) that commonly emerge when exploring the hidden curriculum.

Divided into five parts, this book starts with essential background material and progresses to practical advice for clinical rotations and beyond:

Part I. Foundations. Introduces the hidden curriculum as well as the basic concepts of medical learning, medical vocabulary, and problem-solving—all areas where the formal and null curricula present their own challenges.

Part II. Themes. Presents 12 themes that commonly arise when considering the hidden curriculum.

Part III. Special Topics. Explores additional special topics that are critical for addressing the hidden curriculum.

Part IV. Clinical Rotations. Applies the concepts directly to clinical practice, providing practical strategies for daily training scenarios.

Part V. Mastery. Synthesizes the main book objectives and extends them to a discussion of becoming an expert and comprehending complexity in the hidden curriculum and medicine at large.

As we elucidate components of the hidden curriculum, we'll uncover **six central strategies** to turn the hidden curriculum to your advantage, which are integrated throughout the book: (1) get the easy things right, (2) use effective learning methods, (3) be proactive, (4) understand how others think, (5) identify influences, and (6) embrace challenges.

Before proceeding, we should establish our expectations. This is a general book with principles that apply broadly. Thus, it is beyond the scope of this book to provide an exhaustive exploration of each topic or detailed tips for each core rotation in medical school. You will need to supplement your education with other resources. I have strived to distill this book down to the most essential information – the knowledge I wish I had possessed earlier in my training. This information is quite different than what I thought was important going into training 20 some years ago.

As a fair warning, the information is essential, but not superficial; if you are only looking for educational hacks and shortcuts, then this book is not for you. However, if you are interested in digging deeper into important topics to fully grasp what it takes to become an effective physician, then read on. After investing over two years researching this book, I can confidently say that you can't learn this information from any other single source. Though this work primarily addresses the hidden curriculum as it pertains to careers in medicine, the concepts are useful for anyone needing to adapt to complex areas of learning, teaching, work, and life.

So... now that we are familiar with the essential reasons why I wrote this book, and a framework of how this book came together, I invite you to read on with self-reflection and an open mind.

Acknowledgments

Manuscript Preparation: Desiree Lanzino, PhD, PT

Content review and Input: Rushna Ali, MD; Timothy J. Kaufmann, MD; Karen L. Shanton, PhD; and Marysia S. Tweet, MD

Author Biography

Dr. Vance T. Lehman obtained a Bachelor of Science in biochemistry and completed medical school at the University of Wisconsin-Madison. He then completed a radiology residency and neuroradiology fellowship at Mayo Clinic, Rochester, Minnesota. Dr. Lehman has been a consultant neuroradiologist at Mayo Clinic since 2012. He is currently an Associate Professor of Radiology, having authored or co-authored over 120 peer-reviewed academic research and educational articles. He has served as head of neuroradiology education (which oversees greater than 50 residents and 6–7 fellows per year, and medical students) at Mayo Clinic and has been a long-term member of the neuroradiology physician recruitment committee, among many other appointments. He recently received the 2024 Carman Excellence in Education Award from Mayo Clinic. Dr. Lehman's clinical practice focuses on innovative advanced imaging techniques and interventions, including minimally invasive MRI-guided neurointerventional/neurosurgical procedures in the brain, including MRI-guided focused ultrasound and laser interstitial thermal ablation. For these procedures, he works side-by-side with the Mayo Clinic neurosurgical faculty and trainees. On the innovation side, he spearheaded the first focused ultrasound program for refractory facet joint pain in the Unites States and established the intracranial vessel wall imaging program at Mayo Clinic. He is active in several radiology and interventional pain management professional societies, including serving frequently on key committees (educational, research, evidence-based medicine, and meeting planning). He is frequently invited to speak at national and international venues. In his personal life, he is the proud spouse of an accomplished Mayo Clinic physician in dermatology/dermatopathology and enjoys raising their two daughters. He has a strong interest in personal health and fitness (frequently participating in half and full marathons) and other aspects of well-being.

Contributors

John C. Benson, MD
Department of Radiology,
Mayo Clinic
Rochester, MN, USA

Michael W. Cullen, MD
Department of Cardiovascular Medicine,
Mayo Clinic
Rochester, MN, USA

Amy L. Kotsenas, MD
Department of Radiology,
Mayo Clinic
Rochester, MN, USA

Julia S. Lehman, MD
Departments of Dermatology and
Laboratory Medicine and Pathology,
Mayo Clinic College of Medicine
Rochester, MN, USA

Vance T. Lehman, MD
Department of Radiology,
Mayo Clinic
Rochester, MN, USA

Ajay Madhavan, MD
Department of Radiology,
Mayo Clinic
Rochester, MN, USA

Ariela Marshall, MD
University of Minnesota Hematology
Minneapolis, MN, USA

Kai Miller, MD, PhD
Department of Neurological Surgery,
Mayo Clinic
Rochester, MN, USA

Kendal Weger, MD
Department of Radiology,
Mayo Clinic
Rochester, MN, USA

Mark L. Wieland, MD, MPH
Department of Medicine, Division of
Community Internal Medicine,
Mayo Clinic
Rochester, MN, USA

Abbreviations *

AI	Artificial Intelligence	**LP**	Lumbar Puncture
AMA	American Medical Association	**MCAT**	Medical College Admission Test
BATNA	Best Alternative to Negotiated Agreement	**MSPE**	Medical Student Performance Evaluation
BT-RADS	Brain Tumor Reporting and Data System	**NBME**	National Board of Medical Examiners
CDC	Centers for Disease Control and Prevention	**NEJM**	New England Journal of Medicine
CMS	Centers for Medicare and Medicaid Services	**NHST**	Null Hypothesis Statistical Testing
CV	Curriculum Vitae	**NIH**	National Institutes of Health
DCIS	Ductal Carcinoma In Situ	**NRMP**	National Resident Matching Program
DSM	Diagnostic and Statistical Manual of Mental Disorders	**OR**	Operating Room
EBM	Evidence-Based Medicine	**OSCE**	Observed Structured Clinical Examination
EC	Emotional Competence		
EQ	Emotional Intelligence	**PD**	Program Director
EMR	Electronic Medical Record	**P/F**	Pass/Fail
ESP	Extrasensory Perception	**PMID**	PubMed ID
FDA	U.S. Food and Drug Administration	**RCT**	Randomized Controlled Trial
		SDOH	Social Determinants of Health
GRADE	Grading of Recommendations, Assessment, Development, and Evaluations	**STARD**	Standards for Reporting of Diagnostic Accuracy
H&E	Hematoxylin and Eosin	**TSA**	Transportation Security Association
HIPAA	Health Insurance Portability and Accountability Act	**USMLE**	U.S. Medical Licensing Examination
IQ	Intelligence Quotient	**WHO**	World Health Organization
MBTI	Myers–Briggs Type Indicator		

---

* Excludes commonly known abbreviations like MRI, common healthcare professional credential abbreviations (e.g., MD, RN), and clinical trial abbreviations

Part I

Foundations

Introduction

Vance T. Lehman

Introduction

As was written by Professor Frank Bruni of Duke University journalism and public policy in a recent *New York Times* op-ed on the virtue of humility, "The most important thing I teach my students isn't on the syllabus."[1]

Many new medical students don't realize that admission to medical school (or any other professional school) and simply following the curriculum isn't enough to reach their full potential. This common misunderstanding of success in medical school can be represented by a simple equation:

Premedical Student + Formal Medical Curriculum = Full Potential Physician.

But this model is wrong—or at least incomplete. True, following the formal curriculum will get you to the finish line but perhaps not with the performance you had hoped for. Something is missing from the left-hand side of the equation, something that is not necessarily mentioned during our education: the hidden curriculum.

Nevertheless, understanding the hidden curriculum is critical to being able to achieve your greatest potential. For now, we'll introduce the amplifying effects of being clued into the hidden curriculum (or consequence of not) with the following scenario.

The Insider Butterfly Effect

Meet Claire, a college undergraduate with nearly identical paper credentials and personal characteristics as you. Imagine that the two of you arrive at an airport simultaneously. Both of you are over an hour late due to the same traffic jam. Both of you are scheduled for the same flight to interview at your first-choice medical school. The only difference between you and Claire is that Claire was clued into the advantages of obtaining the Transportation Security Administration (TSA) precheck status for this airport, while you were not.

Claire breezes through security with time to spare, arrives at the interview, and ultimately secures a position, while you stand anxiously in the agonizingly slow security line for over an hour only to miss the flight. Through no fault of your own, you miss the interview and lose the opportunity to be considered for your first-choice medical school.

Not unique to airport security, the amplifying impact of relatively small advantages or liabilities can compound to have drastic enduring effects, the so-called *butterfly effect*. This type of scenario is assuredly common in everyday life, and the ultimate effect can be based more on

DOI: 10.1201/9781003633389-2

insider preparation than on ability, diligence, character, or any other personal attribute. The seemingly minor advantage that Claire had over you highlights the significant impact of insider knowledge—a key component of the hidden curriculum we'll explore in this book.

Introducing the Hidden Curriculum

Given various definitions in the literature, the term *hidden curriculum* risks becoming a catch-all phrase or merely a buzzword.[2,3] For this book, I believe the hidden curriculum is best conceptualized as being comprised of **three pervasive forces**: (1) unspoken expectations, (2) invisible challenges, and (3) stealth influences. When examining these forces, several broader **themes**, or common threads in the hidden curriculum, emerge (Table 1.1). Beyond these themes, several **special topics**, that are more specific in scope, provide a more complete picture of the hidden curriculum. While some topics relate predominantly to a single theme, others are complex and can span multiple themes.

Though not formally taught or often even acknowledged, hidden forces infiltrate nearly every aspect of medical training. Unearthing these subterraneous expectations, challenges, and influences is a key task. Unfortunately, we might not recognize hidden factors until downstream effects materialize. Only then are we able to understand their impact and make a causal connection. Too often, we are ignorant of, or we flat-out ignore, the hidden things that are hard to perceive but have a true effect.

In the upcoming chapters, we'll see that savvy navigation of these forces lies at the heart of trainee success. What's more, even a minor incremental edge made through understanding these hidden challenges can be leveraged to reap big downstream gains—a butterfly effect. Trainees with the right insight can be clear-eyed in an otherwise bewilderingly complex system.

Table 1.1 Twelve Themes of the Hidden Curriculum

History
Culture
Hierarchy
Conflict
Change
Psychology
Gender-Related Topics
Generational Trends
Expectations
Communication
Professionalism
Well-Being

Road Map

Part I introduces the hidden curriculum, as well as the basic concepts of medical learning, medical vocabulary, and problem-solving; as we'll see in the next chapter, these are areas where the formal and null curricula present their own challenges. This paves the way to a discussion of 12 themes in Part II, special topics in Part III, and applications to clinical practice in Part IV. Part V synthesizes the book's highlights, focusing on becoming an expert and on complexity in medicine. In the next chapter, we'll introduce the types of curricula found in a training program, with an emphasis on arguably the most impactful for your career: the hidden curriculum.

The Hidden Curriculum

Vance T. Lehman

Types of Curricula

Success Often Comes from Experiences Outside the Formal Curriculum

It was widely acknowledged that Warren Buffett, the founder and long-time leader of the immensely successful investment group Berkshire Hathaway, was an expert investor. However, in his daily work, people (particularly shareholders) also expected him to be a good speaker. So much so that Buffett says that an on-the-side $100 Dale Carnegie public speaking course he took after he spotted it in a newspaper ad was his most important education (take note: we'll encounter this interpersonal skills guru several times in this book). Exaggeration or not, this story shows how some of our most important skills in the real world come from sources outside our formal diploma-oriented curriculum. This principle holds true in medicine as well.

Two Similar Trainees with Different Outcomes

Imagine it is your first day of medical school, and you meet your new classmate, Joe. Joe is not so different from you in academic ability, energy, or ambition. As you progress through your first two years though, he always seems to be one step ahead of you and is gaining steam. He performs well on his tests and always has the most important information from prior classes on the tip of his tongue. What's more, he maintains a healthy lifestyle, exercises most days, gets adequate sleep, and usually seems in a positive mood.

By the third year, Joe's advantage had become undeniable. You feel that if you were chasing him on a track, he would have pulled away and been nearly out of sight. Come graduation day, he has out lapped you and many of your classmates. He seems to have a sixth sense for what to know and what to do. Attendings notice this and grant him more responsibility and opportunities in turn.

Your experience is different. During the first two years, the volume of information to learn seems overwhelming. You do everything you can think of to follow the formal curriculum and the stated learning objectives. While you do get through the tests, you have trouble recalling much of the information—even the important things—just a few months after a class is done.

Furthermore, the rigorous academic requirements and life's other chores have conspired to erode your old exercise routines and sleep. On clinical rotations, you diligently follow the learning objectives but often feel like a passive observer and are unsure how to be more involved. By the end of medical school, you get to the finish line and earn your diploma,

DOI: 10.1201/9781003633389-3

but you feel as if Joe performed at a different level and, when it came to matching into residency programs, had so many more opportunities available to him. You have come to believe Joe must have some superhuman ability that you lack.

But it turns out that Joe does not have superhuman ability. No one does. Instead, his key insight was this: dutifully following the formal curriculum is simply not enough.

Four Types of Curricula

Let's break this story down to see why we need to consider factors beyond the formal curriculum. In general, a curriculum has four main components: formal, informal, null, and hidden.[4,5] In common parlance, the term *curriculum* is usually meant to refer to the *formal curriculum*, which includes the stated learning objectives, structured lectures and activities, tests, and other explicit expectations.

Beyond the formal curriculum lies the *informal curriculum*, which includes expected but unstructured interactions with attendings and peers. A prime example is *ad hoc* teaching about topics directly relevant to a patient's care during rounds. In our hypothetical scenario, you tried to harness as much information from both the formal and informal curricula as you could, but you still did not achieve peak performance.

One reason for this is that you did not recognize the full impact of the *null curriculum*. The null curriculum describes topics intentionally omitted from the formal curriculum due to time constraints and/or deprioritization. Still, the null curriculum offers a world of useful information like how to address cognitive biases, negotiate well, understand emotions, perform literature appraisals, and much more. Behind the scenes, Joe had recognized that some of the information omitted from the curriculum was still useful and took a few extra measures to integrate learning this material alongside the formal curriculum. This helped him gain incremental advantages along the way.

However, even mastering the formal, informal, and null curricula isn't sufficient; success also hinges on understanding the *hidden curriculum* of unspoken expectations, invisible challenges, and stealth influences—which is where Joe had his edge. We'll see that, for several reasons, it is often mastery of the hidden curriculum that is the tiebreaker for access to opportunities and the key to success.

The Blurry Boundaries of Curricula

The boundaries between the different types of curricula can get murky and understanding how they interact is crucial for success in medical training.

For example, understanding how to manage information in both the formal and the null curriculum is an often-unmentioned challenge in medical training and so is included as a major topic in this book, particularly in the remainder of Part I. As we've seen from the fictional scenario with Joe, excluding too many topics (null curriculum) creates challenges, because it limits trainees' abilities to manage common and important situations. Therefore, proactively integrating these topics into your training becomes part of navigating the hidden curriculum and an important step toward achieving the self-directed education needed to be a professional.

There are also various ways the formal curriculum blurs with the hidden curriculum. Many trainees have difficulty learning the large volume of information included in the formal curriculum and then sorting out what is most important to remember and how to use it to solve problems. In our example, it seems that Joe had gained some insight into using effective learning methods and optimized his productivity so he could make best use of the formal curriculum.

Another part of the hidden curriculum is to identify and resolve mixed messages, such as times when the wording and tone of formal curricular content conflict with what is formally taught. For example, a formal lecture could promote paternalistic approach to clinical decision-making with statements such as, "How should clinicians determine which treatment to prescribe for condition X?"[6] Although subtle, such statements can imply the lack of need for shared decision-making, an outdated style that is no longer considered best practice.

Origin and Evolution of the Hidden Curriculum Concept

Discovering the Hidden Curriculum

The idea of the hidden curriculum was first explored in the mid-20th century by researchers such as Emile Durkheim, a pioneer in sociology who studied the nature of unstated socialization in school.[7] In recent decades, this concept of the hidden curriculum has expanded to various descriptions and settings, including college campus culture for incoming students—especially first-generation students.[8]

In 2011, the *New York Times* published an article entitled "What They Don't Teach Law Students: Lawyering."[9] The implication is that the very *essence* of being a lawyer lies outside the formal syllabus. Similarly, the socialization aspect of the hidden curriculum was once described as "what students learn instead of what they are formally taught."[10]

Samuel Shem's legendary 1978 satire *House of God* described aspects of the hidden curriculum including conformity, pain, debauchery, and unofficial "laws" during medical internship.[4,11-13] Formal recognition of the hidden curriculum in medicine took a foothold in the 1980s and 1990s and has since amplified.[14-17] With few exceptions, direct academic publications on this topic remain descriptive, interview-based, or survey-based studies, with scant observational data.[18] Thus, the perspectives here depend in part on anecdotal and experiential evidence.

Basic Expectations

What are the unspoken expectations in medical school that comprise an important part of the hidden curriculum? First, let's consider the century-old observations of Durkheim,[7] who concluded that the basic purpose of general education is to instill discipline and responsibility. We can summarize these as follows:

- Being reliable
- Being punctual
- Maintaining a positive attitude
- Avoiding misbehavior or disrespect
- Studying diligently at home to master material

We'll call these the *basic expectations*, and surprisingly, these simple tacitly expected behaviors are where medical trainees often stumble. You might think these expectations are obvious for anyone entering medical school, but experience indicates otherwise. There are many plausible explanations for why trainees fall short, but I think it is largely because medical rotations are often the first real professional step out of the classroom.

I also think that many trainees underestimate how impactful following these basic expectations is. There will be more to say on this later, but this topic is so important that we should take a few moments to get a few things out of the way right now. If you are even five minutes late to clinic (for example), and other people have started working, they will notice. Asking to leave early for the day for anything unexceptional is even worse than arriving late. This can make some attendings quite upset and, as we will see, can reinforce intergenerational perceptions of professionalism problems. These examples are directly related to the concept that you must get the easy things right to master the hidden curriculum, which we'll explore in more detail shortly.

Failing to meet these basic expectations in medical training can have more significant consequences than you might imagine. These lapses could be discussed among other staff who interact with trainees and lead to magnified hidden penalties, such as an unrealized fellowship or job offer. Unprofessional behavior in medical school is also a strong predictor of future disciplinary action by medical boards.[19] These basic expectations are always important but especially are early on in clinical training when there is little else by which to judge you. Additionally, these simple everyday interactions amplify into large downstream effects through mechanisms like labeling.

Labeling arises from teacher-trainee interactions and helps to explain why your first impressions matter so much. Such labeling, which can be fast and subconscious, can become explicit when trainees are described as *highly motivated* or *undermotivated*. In fact, teachers often unknowingly label trainees' abilities early on based on insufficient information.[20]

This labeling can propagate a cycle of *self-fulfilling prophecy* of providing more teaching to a subset of "promising" trainees who then enjoy long-lasting benefit from this attention. Trainees may also internalize these perceptions, even if inaccurate or dogmatic. In medicine, once an attending labels a student, this label can disseminate among staff and can be difficult to shake.

Still, staff and students have starkly divergent viewpoints on basic expectations. One study evaluating attitudes of in-person class attendance by trainees found that attendings viewed it as a professionalism issue while students viewed it as a learning issue.[21] Specifically, staff viewed skipping class as a substantial detriment to student learning while students thought online videos are an acceptable substitution and rationalized skipping out to do other worthwhile activities.[21] There is admittedly merit to the student viewpoint here in that adult learners are ultimately responsible for their own education and may learn best by other methods and venues.

Nevertheless, realize that if you do not show up to a lecture, attendings may perceive this as lack of interest, seriousness, or work ethic and may even be less motivated to invest time into teaching you in the future. This also means that in-person attendance is usually preferred over the video-conference method when possible. Understanding these dynamics is important for navigating the hidden curriculum effectively.

There will be more to say about the origins of the hidden curriculum later. For now, the message is that understanding the historical roots of the hidden curriculum and prioritizing these basic expectations can help you lay a solid foundation for success in training and beyond. Before moving on though, we should take a moment to acknowledge a few critiques of the hidden curriculum concept.

Is the Hidden Curriculum a Helpful Concept or Unhelpful Hype?

The concept of the medical hidden curriculum has been rightfully critiqued on multiple grounds; in particular, it has been noted that the term is overused, too variable, and nonspecific.[22] The idea of a hidden curriculum is so pervasive that it is sensationalized in the popular press and depicted on the television series *ER*, *Scrubs*, and *Grey's Anatomy*.[23,24] A 2009 *New York Times* article cited cynical or fixed mindset axioms encountered during training, such as "keep them alive until 6:05" as part of the hidden curriculum.[23] I agree that the term *hidden curriculum* is becoming a bit cliché, but it is mostly used in a narrow academic sense. However, despite these critiques, the need for a comprehensive guide to navigate this unspoken curriculum remains.

Indeed, there is ample published and anecdotal evidence to make a strong case that navigating the hidden curriculum is critical for success in many environments. Remarkably, the hidden curriculum in medicine is a widespread phenomenon described around the world.[3,25-41] The hidden curriculum transcends cultures and locations, showing the general applicability of the concepts in this book. This book, however, focuses on the U.S. medical system to offer concrete examples of historical, social, and policy influences.

Where Does the Hidden Curriculum Come From?

Thinking in broad terms, the hidden curriculum has far-reaching origins from the human condition to the current state of human affairs. A rigorous analysis would require a dissertation on history, evolution, psychology, politics, and much more. Since this would be beyond our scope, we'll distill this down to the essentials. Specifically, in this book, we'll consider several *fundamental factors*, such as the following:

- Commoditization of education
- Development of medical training norms and culture
- Historical purposes of education
- Historical under-recognition of well-being fundamentals
- Increasing complexity and knowledge in medicine
- Increasing societal demands on citizens at large
- Lingering effects from controversies in the scientific method and statistics
- Rise of humanism and spirituality of immanence in medicine
- Roles of careerism, self-promotion, and the rise of the extrovert ideal
- Self-esteem movement and decreasing resilience
- Shift from a culture of character to a culture of personality
- Tectonic shift of gender roles during the past century
- Tensions between evolutionary forces and modern society

Many of these sources represent far-reaching and deeply ingrained forces in society, but, as we'll see, a few have been heavily influenced by a relatively small group of historical influencers like Francis Galton, William Halsted, and Emile Durheim.

Practically speaking, however, what you will notice in everyday life if you know where to look are the *downstream effects*. Examples include the following:

- Awards and rewards
- Discordant verbal and written performance evaluations

- Exercise facility accessibility
- Food offerings in healthcare facility cafeterias
- Institutional and regulatory policies
- Labels
- Medical appointment lengths
- Offhand comments/crisis/praise by senior residents and attendings
- Oaths and ceremonies
- Prioritization of formal curriculum content
- Productivity metrics
- Role modeling
- Word choices (like slang)

How to Master the Hidden Curriculum

Once you understand the nature and origins of the hidden curriculum, the following **six central strategies**, integrated throughout the book, will help you navigate it:

1. **Get the easy things right**. While medicine is complex, the lion's share of success is often as simple as being polite, preparing for the day, asking for feedback, responding to feedback, being (and looking!) interested, and showing appreciation. This also means excelling at the collection of clinical information, patient presentations, and follow-through on routine clinical tasks.

   Why is this so important? Not only does this show basic competency, but early on there is not much else you can contribute. Paradoxically, it can be more difficult for attendings to give you constructive feedback about easy things (that they think should be obvious) than glaring mistakes. It also means avoiding major mistakes like engaging in gossip, being a poor team player, taking credit for others' work, or projecting unprofessionalism on social media.

2. **Use effective learning methods**. This means developing effective learning strategies, applying knowledge to clinical problem-solving, and understanding how basic science fits into the larger picture. In the next chapter, we'll explore specific learning techniques and strategies for organizing the vast amount of information you'll encounter in medical training and expand on this in Part IV.

3. **Be proactive**. This means staying one step ahead of the formal curriculum by being organized, productive, and proactive. A proactive approach is needed to execute many tactics we will discuss, such as determining expectations, seeking feedback, forming relationships, making stellar first impressions, and negotiating clinical task involvement.[42] We'll also see the benefit of arriving equipped with useful knowledge and skills that are de-emphasized in the formal curriculum.

   Just as professional athletes use the off-season to prepare for the next season, you should use your time outside of classes and rotations (your "off-season") to define your values, set goals, and establish healthy habits.

4. **Understand how others think**. Or, in technical jargon, develop a *theory of mind* for people around you. In medicine, you can't assume to know what an attending or anyone else wants or expects. Instead, you need to observe carefully, ask questions, and actively listen to their feedback. This also involves developing empathy, understanding personality types, working on emotional competency, and considering generational viewpoints or biases.

5. **Identify influences**. This means recognizing the subtle influences that shape your perceptions, behaviors, and self-image. Medical training is filled with influences, from the culture of the institution to the attitudes and behaviors of your peers and attendings. In fact, the effects of those around us (our in-groups) are so powerful that they create a social identity, making individual identity part illusion.[43] By recognizing these influences, you can choose which ones to welcome and which ones to resist.

6. **Embrace challenges**. Remember that the medical curriculum is designed to serve all medical trainees but is not entirely tailored to your specific goals or necessarily to push you to your highest potential. We'll see how to apply the principles of deliberate practice, finding ways to challenge yourself to meet personal goals. By appropriately embracing challenges and committing to lifelong learning, you can work toward your full career potential.

Key Takeaways

Now that we've introduced the hidden curriculum and the six central strategies for mastering it, let's start putting it into action. First, thinking back to our opening story, notice how Buffett was not only a talented investor but also someone who recognized expectations, valued communication, took initiative, and embraced challenge. These concepts apply broadly in work, life, and in medicine because the roots are related to the human condition.

In addition, we'll briefly revisit Joe's approach in Part IV to see how he gained insight into the hidden curriculum. But in the next chapter, we will turn to strategies for learning medicine, a topic that directly addresses the central strategy of using effective learning methods and incorporates the virtues of being proactive and embracing challenges.

3

Learning Medicine

Vance T. Lehman

Learning Styles and Senses

Overview

This chapter introduces one of the principal skills needed in medical training: mastering a vast amount of material in both classroom and clinical settings. This task requires a blend of effective learning methods and can be viewed as an art form encompassing problem-solving, applied knowledge, observation, and skill. In general, our educational system does a better job delivering information than teaching effective learning methods.

Medical practice uses tactile, motor, auditory, visual, and even olfactory functions. It is usually most effective to learn via the most relevant mode to a task. Many medical tasks are visual, and it is much better to learn with visual resources instead of purely written descriptions, for example. That is, you cannot learn to interpret an x-ray, diagnose a skin rash, evaluate a hematoxylin and eosin (H&E)–stained slide, or characterize a heart murmur merely by reading textbook descriptions. Task-specific learning is even important when it seems to contradict a person's preferred learning style. In fact, evidence refutes the notion that people are "auditory," "visual," or "book" learners.[44]

The Power of Pictures

Humans evolved without reading and writing. Thus, our brains are well-equipped with specialized neural pathways for language, vision, auditory, and motor tasks but lack these for reading and writing. Instead, these tasks rely mostly on indirect synthesis and integration of information within unspecialized association areas. Some believe that the (often-maligned) image-rich, "reading-lite" digital era is actually a return to our more natural state of learning.[45]

Generally, we learn more effectively from pictures than words alone.[44] This is why no one learns anatomy only by reading *Gray's Anatomy*, which despite high-quality illustrations, has a high text-to-image ratio. Therefore, use books with high-quality figures, but remember that experiential, image-rich learning is often best. This helps us visualize the full range of normal and learn countless anatomic (or other) nuances. This is not to say that reading lacks power; in fact, it allows us to access the thoughts of great minds. The key is to use high-quality reading as one resource, complementing it with other active learning strategies.

Overall, this preference for visual learning is rooted in our evolutionary history and has significant implications for how we approach medical education.

DOI: 10.1201/9781003633389-4

Types of Intelligence

The topic of intelligence is closely related to general concepts of learning. Traditional intelligence can be measured with an intelligence quotient (IQ) test and has crystalized and fluid components.[44] The concept of multiple other types of intelligence emerged in the 1980s, and the notion of emotional intelligence (EQ) soon followed.[46,47]

While the concept of multiple intelligences is debatable,[48,49] practically speaking, this means that you probably have strengths that you can leverage that are not fully captured with traditional measures or tests. You should realize that your test-taking skills, while useful, are insufficient for success and that you should also work on other areas like EQ. Understanding these different forms of intelligence helps us identify our strengths or growth areas and tailor our learning approaches accordingly.

Learning Strategies

Effective Versus Ineffective Strategies

Most people, for various reasons, favor low-effective learning styles.[50] Despite their success, I think this is true for many medical trainees, and it matters because their performance has been linked to learning strategy effectiveness.[51-57] Even those who adopted highly effective strategies in college can revert to ineffective ones under the pressure of medical coursework. Fortunately, extensive literature offers insights on this topic. [45,58-62] We'll focus on key points, leaving a deeper discussion to the references.

The principles of effective learning are grounded in our understanding of how the brain acquires and retains information.[44,50,58] Unlike computers, we learn by connecting new information to existing knowledge. Though our working and short-term memory are limited, our capacity for long-term knowledge is vast, and every time we learn something new it makes it easier to make more connections and acquire additional knowledge.[50] Synaptic connections strengthen with use, especially through active information retrieval. However, information retrieval depends on context and knowledge may be inaccessible if not practiced in the relevant setting.

Effective Learning Is Effortful

Highly effective learning is effortful and active.[44,50,58] Low-effective learning strategies such as rereading text, highlighting, or passive didactics require low effort but yield low long-term retention.[44,50,58] One problem with didactic learning and rereading is that these foster an *illusion of understanding*.[63,64] There is also a special type of this illusion called the *illusion of explanatory depth* in which we believe we know a topic by superficial familiarity—like using internet searches or AI prompts to learn—but are ill-equipped to explain it to others.[65,66]

For making connections and active retrieval, effortful activities to apply and teach information are best.[44,58] The amount of learning versus arousal (stress) follows an *inverted U-curve*, with highest learning occurring at intermediate levels of arousal, and low learning at both the extremes (Figure 3.1).[67]

For these reasons, effective teachers let you struggle (safely) for a time at level-appropriate tasks, and effective training will be uncomfortable at times (though never abusive or excessively anxiety-provoking). While it's natural to avoid discomfort, and learners may dislike well-intentioned, effective teachers at times, it's best to embrace challenges.

The Inverted U Curve of Learning and Stress

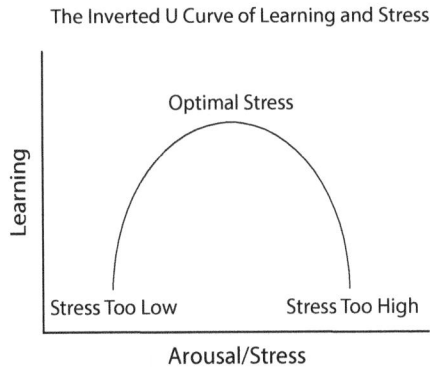

Figure 3.1 The inverted U-curve of learning. Optimal learning typically occurs with a moderate level of stress. Insufficient stress leads to complacency, a lack of challenge, and low stimulation of cognitive engagement, while excessive stress is counterproductive and impairs cognitive function.

Table 3.1 Components of Deliberate Practice, According to Anders Ericsson

1. Setting well-defined goals
2. Keeping focus
3. Incorporating feedback
4. Leaving one's comfort zone

One framework for understanding effortful learning is the concept of *deliberate practice* proposed by Anders Ericsson.[68] Deliberate practice has four main components (Table 3.1). This concept acknowledges that repetition is a vital component of task mastery, as experts have often performed a task 10,000 or more times (a concept that was popularized by Malcolm Gladwell but originally developed from a study of musicians by Anders Ericsson).

However, how it is done matters too.[68] Deliberate practice is task-specific, active, and pushes you to the limits of your abilities rather than just observing, going through the motions, or taking it easy. It also requires consistent, high-quality feedback. As an important counterexample to deliberate practice, *cramming* is effortful but lacks consistency. While it is often criticized, this method can help exam performance and is sufficient for some students to pass some classes; however, it results in poor long-term retention if used as a primary learning method.[50]

Effective Learning Considers Timing

Effective learning also involves strategic timing and spacing of study sessions. For example, application of knowledge to unknown problems after a short washout period to "forget" some information facilitates long-term retention.[44] *Spaced repetition* with increasing intervals (and ideally varied context) between study sessions is far more effective than bursts of mass learning or cramming.[44] It turns out that we forget most details within the first 24 hours, so ideally, new information is reviewed for the first time the next day. After that, it is effective and efficient to use increasing intervals a variable learning environment, schedule, and subject context.[69]

15

Another counterintuitive technique is *interleaving* topics—that is, by alternating them instead of learning them consecutively. This may result in slower learning at first but is more effective over time.[44] Interleaving is most effective when the topics are related on a higher level (think biochemistry, physiology, and anatomy) than entirely unrelated (think economics and art history).[70] It helps to struggle through a problem before the answer has been revealed.

Effective Learning Creates Meaning

Creating meaning and actively engaging with the material also promote effective learning. *Elaboration*, creating new meaning in our own words for why new information is true, is an effective learning technique that helps us create meaning and practice retrieval.[44,50] *Self-explanation*, creating connections to information we already know or explaining steps in a process, is an active process that is in sync with how we learn.[58] We elaborate and apply self-explanation naturally when we prepare to *teach*.

Effective Learning Takes Planning and Reflection

Effective learning also requires planning and reflection. *Previewing* the contents of a lecture or a chapter, noting the major learning objectives, overall organization, sub-headings, and definitions of major key words a day or two before you formally tackle a topic improves comprehension, creating a mental roadmap and providing context—this is an easy way to stay one step ahead of the formal curriculum.[71]

Additionally, *reflection* on your cases, patients, and experiences helps you learn medicine.[44] A wise physician and teacher of mine in medical school shared that he had made it a practice to read something—anything—about his patients every day after work. Though he had been so busy during his clinical rotations that he had not had time to officially study for his board examinations, he passed them without difficulty. While this approach may not be sufficient for all trainees, this anecdote illustrates the value of putting new information in the context of patient scenarios and the cumulative benefit to steady and consistent effort. In radiology, one of the most effective learning tools I use is a simple Excel spreadsheet that I use to revisit and follow-up cases I see.

The comparison of effective and ineffective learning approaches shown in Table 3.2 helps explain why trainees who favor ineffective learning strategies struggle to learn medicine. These differences in learning approaches also explain why the pass/fail (P/F) multiple-choice

Table 3.2 Comparison of Ineffective and Effective Learning Strategies[a]

Ineffective	Effective
Rereading learning material or re-watching videos[b]	Creating new mental connections to existing knowledge
Highlighting or underlining	Organizing thoughts and creation of own tables, chart, flash cards
Listening to didactics	Teaching, elaboration, self-explanation
Ending a lecture cold or with a couple of general summary statements	Ending a lecture with an unknown question or two that requires information application

(Continued)

Table 3.2 Comparison of Ineffective and Effective Learning Strategies[a] (Continued)

Ineffective	Effective
Rote memorizing	Applying material to new problems
Recognizing previously learned material	Actively retrieving information
Problem-solving after a solution has been taught	Taking practice tests and problem-solving without looking at an answer key first
Cramming	Leveraging spaced repetition
Learning one topic at a time	Interleaving[c]
Relying on low-effort recognition exercises	Practicing high-effort retrieval techniques once information has been partially "forgotten"
Depending on classroom learning[d]	Caring for patients
Never revisiting prior experiences	Reflecting
Emphasizing mnemonics	Understanding how something works
Consuming factual nuggets on social media	Creating high-quality content for social media

Note:
[a] Concepts are adapted and modified from multiple resources including making it stick, Dunlosky, Bjork, D'Souza [44, 50, 58, 91]
[b] Applies to rereading for review. Reading a topic that is difficult to understand twice to gain a basic grasp of concepts. There is more direct data on rereading than on re-watching videos.
[c] Interleaving refers to alternating the subjects of study.
[d] Classroom learning, when well done, has its place, but ultimately direct clinical practice is needed.

teaching-testing philosophy can be a disservice to learners, by making the column one-style learning the path of least resistance.

There are additional strategies you might find useful. For example, you might be better off varying your study location to practice retrieval in different contexts and environments despite the common advice to maintain a consistent study location.[70] As another example, if you are a note-taker in class, consider taking some or all notes just after class instead to engage active recall.[70] Additional learning concepts can be found in the excellent references for this chapter.

Online Learning, Videos, and Flashcards

Online Learning and Videos

Online learning resources are a mixed blessing. On one hand, these are often free, image-rich, animation-compatible, and readily accessible. There is also potential peer interaction and community building. On the other hand, these resources are inconsistently peer-reviewed, have variable quality, and can exacerbate the illusion of learning. There are also too many options to sort through, making it difficult for learners to identify the well-vetted premier resources. Trainees sometimes replace traditional staples like textbooks with an assortment of online options outright, but swapping out a coherent approach for the online wilderness can leave large knowledge gaps.

17

Online videos are a popular learning medium these days. Evidence on learning from videos is mixed, but videos can be effective pedagogical tools when done well.[72] They engage both visual and auditory working memory streams but must be clear, level-appropriate, appropriately paced, and promote active thinking. Effective videos are often short, since viewership is known to wane exponentially after just six minutes.[72]

Videos are particularly useful for learning processes that have dynamic spatial considerations, like learning MRI physics, physiology, or procedural skills.[73] Major sources like the *New England Journal of Medicine* (*NEJM*), reputable societies, or experts produce high-quality videos that are useful to view.

There are some major caveats to learning with videos, however. Compared to static images, animations are often *less* effective due to the fleeting format and clog our working memory with extraneous distractions.[74] Video viewing also easily slips into passivity—one study found that students who prepared for the United States Medical Licensing Examination (USMLE) Step 1 examination answering question banks outperformed those viewing passive videos.[75]

Another study evaluating 74 YouTube videos found that 68% were of inadequate quality and that those submitted by nonmedical sources were more popular than those submitted by medical professionals.[76] Online videos can also be posted by anyone and are ripe for misinformation. Perhaps most importantly, it is difficult to create (and thus find) short, high-quality videos for every learning level, and there is little incentive to do so.

Flashcards

Flashcards are also a mixed bag. As with videos, how flashcards are used and their quality matter a lot. In the favorable column, flashcards are amenable to spaced repetition, are portable, and can fill small gaps of downtime—especially portable electronic versions like Anki flashcards. If you create your own flashcards (or simple notecards), it is far better to use your own words (instead of verbatim copying text) draw connections, find your own meaning and patterns among topics, or perform elaboration and self-explanation, than simply restate information.[77] When reviewed as unknowns, they promote retrieval. Anki flashcards also allow for spaced repetition, keeping track of errors, and borrowing premade cards (to be used cautiously).

However, many trainees rely too heavily on Anki-type flashcards these days, sometimes viewing them as a panacea to learning challenges. What's not to like? Well, these take substantial time to create, manage, and work through.[1] The content is stuck in a narrow *carbon-copied context* where you can end up memorizing the cue. It would be like taking a basketball shot from the same location on the court, with the same foot position, on perfect balance repeatedly—no crowd, no teammates, no opponents, no surprises—and then being put in a real game.

That is, the context of retrieval is static, and you might have difficulty retrieving the same information in other settings like test questions or patient care settings. Flashcard fluency can promote the illusion of knowing, while substantial gaps in understanding may remain.

Further, you can get lost in the details without grasping the overarching concepts like learning to dribble a basketball without knowing that the goal is to score more points than the other team. It is also hard to actively apply flashcard concepts and—using our basketball analogy—may be akin to ignoring gameday strategy. Flash card information too often provides unconnected snippets of knowledge, like not learning how a basketball shot relates to passing and dribbling. Most flash cards promote *lower order understanding*, like memorizing multiplication tables instead of applied word problems. That is, flash cards do not easily capture the complexity of medicine.

Many students borrow premade Anki cards, which save time for them. However, the value is diminished, because creating the flashcards produces much of their value, and the flashcards may not be tailored to their needs. Converting a textbook largely amounts to indiscriminate reshuffling of information and provides an illusion of productivity. This method also disrupts the organization and cohesion of the textbook information, stripping knowledge away from the underlying story.

By analogy, consider your favorite full-length story, either a movie or a book will do. Imagine dividing each scene into several fact-based question cards, randomly removing a few of them—especially those about the backstory and shuffling them around. Now, if you only had the cards, you could memorize the answers and *still* have little idea of the premise and plot, tone, character development, or take-home message.

Types of Memory

Working Memory

To further understand how we learn, let's explore the different types of memory involved. We can break down memory in terms of duration and type. Working memory is fleeting, and the capacity is easily overwhelmed. It can process either new information or information drawn from long-term memory. Over-reliance on working memory of new information is a potential drawback of using problem-based and experiential learning too early in training, discussed further in Chapter 6.[78]

Long-Term Memory

Long-term memory capacity, on the other hand, is well-ingrained and has nearly boundless limits. Some things in long-term memory are recalled more readily than others though, and we'll explore why this concept matters for learning medicine in Chapter 35. Long-term memory consists of *declarative (explicit) memory* and *non-declarative (implicit) memory*. Declarative memory can be retrieved consciously and consists of both semantic memory for facts and episodic memory for experiences (episodes). Memorization of medical facts such as those typically taught in the formal curriculum falls in the declarative memory category.

Beyond declarative memory is non-declarative memory, which plays a significant role in skill acquisition and habit formation. Non-declarative memory lies in the subconscious and includes associative and procedural memory. *Associative memory* consists of *classical conditioning* and *operant conditioning*. Classical conditioning involves learned associations between involuntary stimuli and an outcome. For example, through rewards, trainees are conditioned to display traits such as clinical efficiency, confidence, proactivity, and a positive attitude.[42,79] In contrast, operant conditioning involves learned associations between voluntary actions and outcome. Associative memories like odors, places, and the effects of actions influence many experiences in medical school.

Procedural Memory

For procedure-oriented trainees, the opportunity to think *and* work with your hands is an appealing part of medicine. Specific considerations for learning procedures are explored in Chapter 41. The term *procedural memory*, as used here to apply to medical interventions, should not be confused with the term procedural knowledge.

Habituation

Habituation is a form of non-associative learning that decreases a behavioral response after repeated exposure to a stimulus (without a punishment or reward and without sensory adaptation or motor fatigue).[80] Simply stated, we get used to something. More generally, habituation is believed to facilitate learning by filtering out routine stimuli, allowing focus to be on novel stimuli.[80]

Habituation occurs on multiple levels in medicine with both positive and negative effects.[81] Beneficial examples include increased ability to remain focused and unperturbed in the face of exposures that would be dreadful in other settings, such as those surrounding trauma, surgery, or cadavers. More dubious examples can sneak up on us through a gradual slippery slope onset. Examples include becoming used to lying, injustices, paternalism within medicine, and unquestioned obedience to authority.[81,82] So, there are some types of habituation you should resist.

Social Learning

In addition to individual learning strategies, social learning significantly impacts our professional development. Specifically, observation and interpersonal interactions play a large role in the development of a trainee's professional persona, identity, and skillset.[83] It is useful to understand the myriad factors that influence this process including conformity, display rules, in-group effects, medical culture, role modeling, rites of passage, and storytelling.[84] For these reasons, the effects of social learning make many appearances in this book.

For now, let's see how social learning transpires. In large part, we acquire professional behaviors by association, observation, and habituation. We also hold pre-existing internal concepts of social situations called schemas.[85] Once solidified, schemas are hard to crack. If we encounter new information that contradicts pre-held notions, we tend to *assimilate* into the existing schema as a slight modification instead of changing the schema outright.[86,87]

For example, imagine you believe that surgeons are *black-and-white thinkers*. You may interpret an instance of gray-area thinking of a surgeon you meet as an exception rather than considering that many surgeons might not be black-and-white thinkers. It is therefore useful to be aware of your established beliefs and make efforts to think flexibly when a situation calls for it.

Everyday interactions with medical professionals around you cast a vision of how a doctor should present himself and what emotional displays are acceptable, a phenomenon known as *display rules*.[88] The tone taken with nurses or administrative assistants, interactions with other colleagues on consulting services, clinical communication style, sentiments of cynicism versus optimism, and much more fall into this category.

For example, if your attending shows subtle stigma and judgment when evaluating an overweight patient, the message to you is that this is an appropriate way to view and treat patients.[89] So, be aware of the typical display rules and try to selectively adopt the most positive and effective ones.

Memory Aids

Memory aids are another commonly used method to learn medical school material. *Memory athletes* memorize mountains of data with specialized techniques like *mnemonics* and visual associations. Even though mnemonics are a mainstay for many medical trainees and improve memory in the short run, the long-term retention is low.[58] In fact, overusing them may result in "accelerated forgetting" as it is an indirect two-step process with need to decode a key word.[58]

Table 3.3 HACEK Group of Bacteria

Letter	Bacteria
H	*Haemophilus* species
A	*Aggregatibacter actinomycetemcomitans*
C	*Cardiobacterium hominis*
E	*Eikenella corrodens*
K	*Kingella kingae*

You must also either find or create memorable mnemonics. If you do use them, these may be best for topics that comprise a tangible list (e.g., differential diagnoses for various clinical scenarios) and less effective for abstract concepts. For these reasons, mnemonics are generally considered low-effective learning strategies.[50,58]

Managing a real-life situation usually requires more in-depth understanding anyways, such as differentiating features of diseases. For example, residents use the mnemonic MAGICAL DR to recall the top ten or so causes of rim-enhancing masses on brain MRIs. However, never are all categories serious considerations, and sometimes the MRI appearance is even pathognomonic for one diagnosis (called an "Aunt Minnie" in radiology, because identification of those entities is akin to recognizing the face of a beloved family member). Therefore, mnemonics like this have limited use.

That said, a few key mnemonics may be useful for select topics like recalling the relationship of artery or nerve branches or remembering members of a group like HACEK oropharyngeal gram-negative bacteria that cause infective endocarditis (Table 3.3). Overall, mnemonics are useful for select situations, but do not become overreliant on them.

Impact of Sleep and Alcohol on Learning

Beyond the effective learning methods discussed, factors like sleep and alcohol consumption significantly impact our ability to learn. Studies show a profound relationship between the quality of sleep and learning and that sleep disruption from even a small amount of alcohol before bed degrades memory formation.[90] We explore these topics further in Chapter 17.

Key Takeaways

There are many considerations for learning medicine, including use of effective learning techniques, types of memory, social learning, and other topics in well-being and productivity that will be discussed later. We'll build on these topics in Part IV with several specific strategies for learning during clinical rotations and managing information overload. Next, we'll turn to a specific, but critical, topic for learning medicine: learning and mastering medical vocabulary.

Note

1   The time commitment to create flashcards can be ameliorated using AI technology, but the general critique still holds.

4

Medical Vocabulary

Vance T. Lehman

Medical Terminology

Mastering medical vocabulary is a critical task that medical trainees face, yet it is a major challenge due to the sheer number and complexity of medical words.[92] As with other learning topics, the formal curriculum excels at delivering information (words) but falls short in teaching us how to understand them. Although we are in the age of medical English, medical words are primarily derived from Latin and Greek origins. The precise etymology is less important than the meaning, though clinical terms tend to come from Greek (as modern medicine began in Greece) and anatomic terms tend to come from Latin (as anatomic knowledge increased during the era of medical Latin).[93]

While these terms can seem overwhelming, learning bases, prefixes, and suffixes can become a shortcut to recognizing words or deducing the meaning of unfamiliar words since they can be recombined in many ways. For example,

OSTE + oma = osteoma, a benign tumor of bone translates to "bone" + "tumor arising from or composed of."

In addition, the base *OSTE* and the suffix *oma* are each found in many medical words related to bone and tumors of a specific type, respectively.

You already know many of these like *corpus* (body), which is related to the words corporal or corpse. After a basic anatomy course, you will know that the corpus callosum connects the cerebral hemispheres. Others are more obscure like the Latin word *limbus* (border or edge), which is related to the common word *limbo*. In medicine, we apply it to the term limbic system (border between the cerebral hemispheres and brainstem) or to limbus vertebrae where a portion of the ring-like edge of the bone remains unfused.

Some medical terminology is borrowed from other languages, like *cri du chat* (*cry of the cat* in French) which is a 5p deletion syndrome, *mittelschmerz* (*middle pain* in German) describing menstrual pain, or moyamoya disease (cited as *puff of smoke* in Japanese[1]) characterized by idiopathic occlusion of arteries supplying the brain and proliferation of collaterals.

Finally, while the number of base words and word parts from other languages is overwhelming and simple rote memorization is an inefficient use of time, I think it is useful to visualize the words (a border for "limbus" and so on) and consider how the form applies to the medical term.

DOI: 10.1201/9781003633389-5

Defining Health

When we think of medical vocabulary, we usually think of formal words (jargon) like the words just mentioned, but learning the nuanced connotations of common vocabulary when applied in the medical setting is just as important and less often discussed. Words have power and we must be sure we use them correctly and understand the full breadth of the meanings they engender. Unfortunately, the definitions of many words are simply assumed as givens in medical education without examining what they really mean. It took me a long time in medical practice to discover the importance of the specific meaning and nuance of many words I had mistakenly taken for granted.

For example, the first medical school lesson could center on the importance of vocabulary, starting with the meaning of the word *health*. How would you define *health* for a patient? If one of the central goals of *health* care is helping people achieve and maintain optimal health, shouldn't we share an understanding of what the word means? How else would we set our primary aims and strategies for all care and advice we deliver?

It turns out the word *health* means different things to different people.[94,95] We can view it as the *absence* of organic disease or also with the *presence* of features like a psychological state, being physically fit, well-rested, in a state of equilibrium with our surroundings, the ability to cope with daily life demands, and more. The same person may be healthy by some definitions yet unhealthy by others. Your patients and even your attendings may have various opinions on what it means to be healthy, and it is often useful to find a mutual understanding.

The World Health Organization (WHO) defines health as a state of complete physical, mental and social well-being and not merely the absence of disease or infirmity in the preamble of its constitution.[94] This definition is lauded for being "holistic" but critiqued for being "utopian."[96] It also lacks operational value for research and is irrelevant to physicians focused narrowly on diseases.[94] Such a broad definition of health encompasses multiple domains including physical, subjective, behavioral, functional, psychosocial, social, and cultural.[97] So, a person could be healthy in certain domains but not others.[97]

Who determines what defines a healthy state for a given patient? Is it the patient, the physician, or both? Certainly, we can agree there are things about health the patient might not fully understand or acknowledge (like the short- and long-term health risks posed by consuming too many daily servings of alcohol), but there are also perspectives only the patient can provide like his philosophy, priorities, and goals. Evaluating a person's life goals (realistic or aspirational) is a key component of treatment decision-making, which should start with mutual understanding of the patient's level of health.

The meaning of health also depends on age. For example, you will never see a radiologic imaging study of the spine in a patient over 50 years old that looks "normal." While certain findings are pathologic and symptomatic, most are not. Family and friends of radiologists often ask them, "Should I be concerned with all this arthritis and degenerative change the MRI found in my spine?" in reference to incidental age-related findings. In fact, differentiating normal aging from pathology is one of the basic, but often challenging, tasks of medicine.

Defining Disease

Just as the definition of health is complex, so, too, is the definition of disease. It is essential for you to understand what a disease is, but it turns out that there is no single accepted definition. We could define disease as any deviation from health, but this is problematic given the many definitions of health. Everyone might be in a state of disease if we define it as any deviation from the all-encompassing WHO definition. Several definitions of disease have been proposed but there is no consensus.[96,98–100] In fact, the National Cancer Institute, U.S. Food and Drug Administration (FDA), American Medical Association (AMA), and numerous authors have all defined disease differently.[101,102]

What's more, there are points of controversy and complexity about disease category designations. Diseases are added, subtracted, and modified over time. They evolve with diagnostic capabilities and medical knowledge. Disease states can depend on sociocultural values. Genetic predisposition to diseases can be detected in patients who have not developed that condition.

A diagnosis also has a psychological impact on patients, for example by providing clarity of their situation or medicalizing normal states.[96] Patients, health professionals, insurance payors, Big Pharma, and legislators, for example, have different viewpoints on what should be considered a disease.[100]

Consider that homosexuality was long considered a disease and went through several iterations of disease classification and treatments that would be unthinkable today, including electroshock therapy and hormone injections before the disease label was removed from the *Diagnostic and Statistical Manual of Mental Disorders, Fourth Edition* (*DSM-IV*) in 1974.[96] Osteoporosis was written off as an unavoidable part of aging in some individuals until it was recognized as a disease by the WHO in 1994.[96]

Some recent disease designations have even stirred controversy. For example, there has been substantial debate over the disease designation of obesity with consideration of numerous pros and cons to the designation.[102,103] Even nonmedical reasons can enter the calculus, such as the implication of health policy and access to research funding for obesity.[103]

A final point of controversy in disease designations and diagnoses is the opinion that industry is often too influential.[104–106] It turns out that industry can influence disease definitions and frequency of diagnosis through multiple mechanisms.[106] This transpires directly through lobbying and industry involvement at medical conferences, for example.

Industry-driven approval of a medication could also influence diagnostic frequency through various mechanisms because a cure implies that a diagnosis is possible. Direct-to-consumer advertising could imply that diseases are more common than they are or promote treatments for conditions that could be viewed as normal parts of aging. So, as you progress through medical training, it is useful to keep the dynamic, nuanced, and potentially problematic origins and viewpoints of disease designations in mind.

Other Medical and Common Words with Hidden Meaning

It is also critically important to carefully consider the nuanced definitions and connotations for many other medical words (jargon) and common words that are relevant to patient care.

First, you should be aware of how medical terms can be (mis)interpreted by, or influence, patients in ways you medical professionals might not predict. For example, some patients find the term *incompetent cervix* referring to a weak cervix at risk for premature delivery to be a stigmatizing term, in part because the term "incompetent" can be interpreted in a different way.[107]

In addition, the words used to describe a medical diagnosis influences the aggressiveness of patients' preferred treatment.[108] For example, patients with ductal carcinoma in situ (DCIS) who are told they have *preinvasive cancer cells* more often opt for treatment (instead of watchful waiting) and have a greater level of concern compared to those who are told they have *abnormal cells*.[108] While it is impossible to predict every possible way patients will construe every word, it is worth staying cognizant of how laypersons may interpret commonly used medical terms.

Second, a variety of unofficial terms have been used in the medical profession to describe patients, patient situations, or patient actions that may be considered pejorative.[109] For example, stating that a patient "complains of something" or "denies doing or experiencing something" subtly implies judgment. The term *patient compliance* entails judgment and could be considered paternalistic. A variety of other terms such as *bounce back*, which is used to describe a patient who is readmitted shortly after leaving the hospital may strip patients of their humanity, imply judgment, and/or imply a failing on the part of the patient.

It is easy to normalize and adopt these statements if you do not consciously recognize the potential underlying meaning. You should try to minimize the use of these terms and phrases given implied connotations can impact how a situation is perceived. In addition, some of your peers and attendings will be attuned to it and will overtly or covertly disapprove.

Third, many common words have more layers and depth to their meaning in ways that matter. Consider that for international treaties, a security *assurance* offers only a promise of protection, which can be easily sidestepped once a country is threatened, while a security *guarantee* is a stronger legally binding agreement that is difficult to dodge. As with legalese, the nuanced definitions of words in medicine matter a lot.

Some of these words that we'll explore in this book include compassion, culture, disease, emotion, empathy, failure, fatigue, happiness, motivation, probability, religion, reward, science, spirituality, stress, and well-being. Learning these definitions is more than an academic exercise; it is a pathway to a deeper understanding of medicine. The take home point is that for many common words, it is useful to take time to learn the depth of their meaning and what significance they have for you, your colleagues, and your patients.

Finally, building a strong base of medical knowledge, including vocabulary, is just the beginning. The practice of medicine entails the art of applying this knowledge to real-life scenarios and medical decision-making, which is discussed next.

Note

1   This meaning is popularized in the English literature to represent a proliferation of abnormal blood vessels, but primary Japanese sources often give a more abstract and nuanced definition such as *hazy* or *murky*.

5

Medical Decision-Making

Vance T. Lehman

A Challenging Scenario

At first, it seemed like just another routine examination—an MRI of the brain to follow-up a benign tangle of channels of slowly flowing blood called a cavernous malformation.[1] Although the patient was new to our practice, seeking a second opinion, modern integrated health system records showed that they had undergone several MRI exams elsewhere over the past couple of years. Each radiology report described a round lesion composed of blood that was felt to be most consistent with a cavernous malformation. Importantly, there was no evidence of a soft tissue component, as one would expect if it were a tumor, but because the patient reported some neurologic symptoms, the medical team was keeping a close eye on it.

The indication for the new MRI said, "Follow-up cavernous malformation" in bold letters. Sure enough, the lesion was stable in size and appearance compared to an MRI performed several months earlier. I had seen countless cavernous malformations before; this lesion seemed to fit the bill, and it was easy to stay in automatic mode based on intuition and experience.

I clicked the "sign" button on my report, but as the case disappeared from the screen, an unconscious alarm went off in my head. I had a gut instinct that I should take one more look. Perhaps it came from a few atypical features (the presence of edema, the absence of "popcorn" appearance of internal blood locules, a classic but not essential finding in hemorrhage), an inner voice advising that more clinical information is needed, or something else—impossible to know for sure. Fortunately, we are given a grace period of a few seconds to undo a signed report and call it back before it is released to the clinicians and the patient. That is what I did.

It was time to switch into an active problem-solving mode. First, I laid out all the available comparison examinations side by side to closely examine subtle incremental changes from one time point to the next. I also fused the images from the initial study to the current one, so the corresponding anatomy was perfectly transposed.

What I found was alarming. Even though there was little detectable difference at all between any one scan and the immediate one before, when careful measurements were placed in exact locations on serial examinations, very subtle growth of the lesion over time was evident. On any single comparison to only the immediate prior MRI, this could easily be chalked up to measurement error, but taken together, the evolution over a longer time scale was undeniable.

Sure enough, the edema, or fluid surrounding the lesion, had subtly increased as well. All these findings were atypical for a benign cavernous malformation. This was enough to raise serious doubt about the presumptive diagnosis. It was time to tackle the arduous task of sifting through outside clinical notes. Even though the indication for the examination had been "follow-up cavernous malformation," the outside records revealed a critical clue: the patient had a history of renal cell carcinoma, a highly vascular tumor of the kidney.

DOI: 10.1201/9781003633389-6

Since the kidney tumor had been removed and the patient had no known metastases elsewhere, and since the features were more typical of a vascular mass rather than of a typical metastasis, no one stopped to think that the brain mass might not be a cavernous malformation after all. As a result of carefully chosen verbiage in my report and discussion with the team, the mass was surgically resected and proven to be a metastasis in need of treatment instead of a cavernous malformation only requiring surveillance.

This anecdote demonstrates the differences between System 1 and System 2 problem-solving, the influence of biases, the virtue of an unhurried examination, and the importance of using problem-solving tools for atypical and complex scenarios. Let's break this down in the context of our scenario, first with a little background information.

System 1 and System 2 Thinking

Formal medical training often focuses too much on fact memorization and too little on medical decision-making. Often, decision-making is learned tacitly by observation and experience, but a lack of formalization risks leaving gaps in trainees' abilities.

There is an entire body of literature describing how humans make decisions, including the concepts described by Daniel Kahneman and Amos Tversky.[110] They proposed two general systems of decision-making: System 1 (thinking fast), which entails fast, intuitive, emotional, pattern recognition otherwise known as heuristics, and System 2 (thinking slow), which entails slower, in-depth deliberation (thinking fast and slow). This concept is now well known in a broad sense, but it is worth exploring how this specifically applies to medicine. To start, both System 1 and System 2 decision-making processes have roles in medicine, but overreliance on one without the other is rife with pitfalls.

In the case example, I was using System 1 decision-making by fitting the brain lesion to a cavernous malformation by pattern recognition, even if it wasn't a perfect match. System 1 is useful for common scenarios and classic presentations, and allows you to use heuristics, or mental shortcuts, for making diagnostic and treatment decisions in patients with classic manifestations of disease.

Other common examples of System 1 decision-making in medicine include assigning a diagnosis of acute otitis media in a child with the classic presentation of earache, fever, and bulging tympanic membrane. But we can see in our case example that using System 1 introduces liabilities when scenarios veer too far away from classic presentations, rendering us susceptible to biases, logical fallacies, and mistakes such as overfitting a diagnosis to the most similar classic one.

In this case, unchecked System 1 thinking initially made me susceptible to several cognitive biases. First, I could not help but be influenced by the opinions of the prior radiology reports and the stated indication of the exam, both pointing to a presumed (but incorrect) diagnosis of a cavernous malformation. This is called *prior report bias*. This bias is related to *confirmation bias* since I started out with a diagnosis in mind and then gave most weight to imaging findings that supported the initial possibility. For this reason, radiologists (and pathologists) will sometimes try to interpret a study first without clinical information and, only after she has rendered an opinion, factor in the clinical information. However, this approach is often impractical since the indication is usually known ahead of time.

Second, I initially perpetuated the original diagnosis, a phenomenon known as *anchor bias*. I overcame this bias, but only after switching to System 2 thinking. Third, some key clinical information was buried, and so I relied too heavily on the information readily available to me and the examples of lesions I already had in mind from past experience, which is called *availability bias*. Fourth, one could make the case that I initially showed *overconfidence bias*, as I was ready to outright call the lesion something it was not. Cognitive biases are further discussed in Chapter 29.

Fortunately, I activated System 2 just in time. The trigger for this was based on experience and intuition, but the decision was deliberate. I could have chosen to ignore the gut feeling and just moved on. The identification of clues that should prompt System 2 thinking is one of the core skills physicians learn through experience. But this is harder than you might think. Overreliance on System 2 thinking can lead to over-deliberation, unnecessary energy expenditure, lost time, and potentially worse clinical decisions. If we spend too much time questioning everything that is not textbook perfect, we will be paralyzed or led astray by over analysis.

It is not possible to learn how to know when to switch to System 2 thinking from book-learning alone. While most medical trainees will naturally use both systems, you should self-monitor to avoid overusing heuristics when you need more in-depth thought or conversely avoid spending too much time and mental energy on routine tasks. However, it takes time to develop enough experience to safely use System 1 in many settings. So, it is usually best for new trainees to favor System 2 in many, if not most, circumstances since they do not yet have the experience to rely on pattern recognition.

Street Smarts

In his book *How Doctors Think*, Dr. Jerome Groopman sums up the value of an experience-based approach to medicine as "flesh and blood decision-making."[111] [2] Similarly, our case illustrates the importance of experience-based *street smarts* (or having good situational awareness and common sense) in medicine. I've observed that physicians who start off favoring the virtues of book knowledge and discounting street smarts—potentially conditioned this way by two decades of classroom learning—often reverse their opinion after observing great physicians from the generation before. That is, most physician skills are learned outside of formal reading materials. There are many reasons why this is true.

Medical Decisions Are Often Complex

First, real-life medical decision-making is often complex. Clinicians usually cannot assign probabilities to every decision-making factor, and there is no comprehensive list of guidelines for every conceivable decision point, so intuition often plays a role. So, each situation is unique and may not fit perfectly into an algorithm or *evidence-based* guidance from expert consensus or meta-analyses.

Additionally, although physicians should usually adhere to standard practices, at times they must carefully sidestep simple algorithms and black-and-white thinking. They must be cognizant of decision-making principles but also be facilitators of shared decision-making and synthesizers of multiple types of information—published guidelines, effects of comorbidities, patient goals and motivators, ethical considerations, insurance ramifications and more.

Further, clinical decision-making often involves complex calculus of balancing benefit versus risk, as well as likelihood and degree of effect thereof. For example, a risk could be likely but inconsequential, unlikely but devastating, or other combinations. Similarly, a benefit could be probable but mild, unlikely but dramatic, or other combinations.

Medical Decisions Often Depend on Procedures and Perceptions

Second, many clinical decisions depend on knowing a procedural approach or having certain perceptive skills, both things that are difficult, or just too mundane, to convey in books and guidelines. Consider just one example in radiology: one of the most important things I do every day is simply labeling the vertebral bodies in a spine examination and commenting on whether there is a conventional or variant number of them in the report. It's a relatively trivial task (for an experienced radiologist) that ends up mattering a lot. I've never seen this emphasized in a book (though perhaps it is somewhere); it is just something you do. When this step is skipped, wrong level spine interventions in patients with variant anatomy, such as an extra vertebral body, may occur.

There are analogous examples throughout medicine, like knowing when to get a second opinion on a critical diagnosis in pathology, double-checking 3D coordinate parameters on a headframe for an invasive stereotactic head procedure in neurosurgery, reviewing patient anatomy prior to a procedure, and so on.

Further, as mentioned in Chapter 3, much of medicine relies on visual (or other sensory) perception including the physical examination, interpreting tests like EKGs, and interpreting pathology slides or radiology images. Each task is unique, but what each has in common is that the abnormalities may look no different than the normal background to a layperson. To the trained eye, however, pathological or other relevant features stand out against the background; the mind learns to zero in on the important things and to ignore others.

The Content of Books and Tests Often Do Not Reflect Real Practice

Third, the distribution of problems you will encounter in your future clinical practice more closely matches the distribution of problems you have encountered during clinical practice training than the distribution of those contained in formal learning materials (and tests). It is often more useful to understand the rich array of variations of common problems that arise in real practice than knowing classic facts about uncommon problems.

For example, in real-life radiology, I see dozens of cases of run-of-the-mill lumbar spinal canal stenosis for every oddball case of a spinal cord tumor or unusual inflammatory condition. Further, spinal canal stenosis can arise from many different combinations of degenerative cysts, other fluid pockets, bone overgrowth, intervertebral disc bulges and herniations, slipping vertebral bodies, overabundant epidural fat, and/or a congenitally narrow spinal canal. What's more, an area of stenosis might only be evident when a patient is standing and mostly occult when he is lying down during the MRI exam; such positional stenosis is easily missed if the radiologist does not know the subtle clues.

The most useful resources would teach us mostly how to characterize the full spectrum of such common, but potentially tricky, combinations. The other uncommon conditions are important too but should not dominate our learning materials. Nonetheless, too many formal resources will spend a fraction of the space on what is commonly needed for practice and too much space on arcane things that are not encountered during most working days.

Above All Medical Decisions Require Focused Attention

Fourth, but perhaps most important, the most basic requirement for excellent decision-making is simply being unhurried, attentive, and focused. Maintaining professional poise in the face of time pressure and finding the right speed for a given situation takes experience, though. If in doubt, it is usually best to err on the side of slowing down, especially early on. Remember, a high IQ and a deep fund of knowledge do little good if you rush too much to apply them well. For challenging clinical situations, taking ample time to think things through, and learning from experience trump relying on book knowledge

The takeaway, though, is that, in real life, physicians often start with experience-based heuristics but remain aware of the need to modify their instincts in certain circumstances by using a variety of formal decision-making processes and tools. So, although experience is paramount, it is essential to couple it with in-depth reading, an understanding of evidence-based medicine (EBM), and awareness of cognitive processes. In practical terms, this means you ought to be reasonably proactive in seeking out real-life experiences while on duty and then study reasonably intensely when at home.

Formal Reasoning

We'll finish up Part I with a brief introduction to formal reasoning. Although most physicians do not actively consider the type of formal reasoning they are using in the moment in clinical practice, the concept is useful to help understand clinical decision-making, establish the role of base rate determination in Bayesian reasoning and statistical analysis (Chapter 27), and clarify the scientific method (Chapter 26).

A medical diagnosis (and research) can be based on different forms of reasoning—deductive or inductive.[3] Strictly defined, *deductive reasoning* draws a specific conclusion from general premises. For example, say a patient has a Huntington disease gene mutation. This Huntington disease gene mutation is 100% correlated with the development of Huntington disease with time. Therefore, this patient will develop Huntington disease if he lives long enough. Thus, physicians can offer patients a high degree of certainty for deductive conclusions.

Strictly defined, *inductive reasoning* draws general conclusions from specific premises. In practice, this usually refers to a Bayesian process of updating initial probabilities (such as base rate of a disease, likelihood ratio of a positive test, or likelihood of having a condition based on past clinical experience) to update the probability of a diagnosis. Inductive reasoning is probably more common in everyday practice. This takes advantage of similarity of situations to those encountered in the past, which can be a useful shortcut but also leaves us susceptible to overgeneralization, stereotyping, and reaching invalid conclusions since incomplete information is usually available including exact baseline probabilities.[112]

This concludes Part I, where we have learned the basic types of curricula and an overview of the origins and definitions of the hidden curriculum. We have focused on the blurry boundaries between the hidden curriculum and the null and formal curricula, especially how the need to learn and apply a vast amount of information can create challenges if not managed well. We'll now turn to Part II, where we'll delve into the 12 themes at the heart of the hidden curriculum.

Notes

1 All real-life scenarios in this book are composite and anonymized using analogous substitution of details but maintain the primary educational message.
2 The term "flesh and blood decision-making" dates back to the 1990 book *Human Error* by James Reason.
3 Another type of reasoning, abductive reasoning, which uses a component of intuition to arrive at a best guess is closely related to inductive reasoning, but the distinction is not highly important for clinical decision-making and not further discussed here.

Part II

Themes

Part II will explore the themes, or common threads in the hidden curriculum, beginning with those that provide essential background for the rest of the book related to human history, culture, and hierarchy.

DOI: 10.1201/9781003633389-7

6

History

Vance T. Lehman

Relevance of Natural History

To start, it is essential to reach beyond the formal curriculum and learn more about the history of human nature as it relates to human evolution, the transition from hunter-gatherer to modern-day cosmopolitan, and the development of modern medical education norms. For this, we'll first discuss the importance of evolution in medicine and the multifaceted impact of evolutionary forces on many areas of the hidden curriculum, including how we learn, thrive, and interact with others.

The Theory of Evolution was emphasized in medical training during the first half of the 20th century, paralleling great scientific strides during this time. But medical educators sidelined this topic in the mid-20th century, partly in reaction to the eugenics movement.[113] In more recent years, medical training has revived this topic under the term *evolutionary medicine* with application of knowledge of the human genome and epigenetics.

Still, evolution remains undertaught in medical school largely due to time limitations and concern over topic controversy.[114,115] This trend is surprising since the practice of medicine is solidly rooted in the biological sciences, which depend heavily on the central tenet of evolution. This is a clear example where politics and reaction to a historic catastrophe will influence your medical educational experience.

In response, you should consider investing time to view major topics in your curriculum through an evolutionary lens. This can enhance your understanding of many topics like antibiotic resistance, oncologic principles, women's health topics (as reproduction is heavily affected by evolutionary selection pressures), human nutrition, and population disease susceptibility.[114,115] An evolutionary perspective can also help you answer the *why* questions that students and patients might have for disease and human biology.[116] In the years after training, I have found that additional study of evolutionary concepts is enormously helpful for understanding both medicine and the medical training environment, especially the ways in which our evolutionary driven ancestral traits help explain many of our modern-day challenges.

Misplaced Cavepersons

To fully understand our modern educational and workplace experiences, we must travel back in time to the era of our caveperson counterparts and see how they survived through learning, socializing, and working together. Evolutionary concepts introduced in this chapter will help explain many facets of the hidden curriculum that we'll consider in this book (Table 6.1).

DOI: 10.1201/9781003633389-8

Table 6.1 Relevance of Human Evolution to Medical Training[a]

Social learning
Culture
Language, gossip, and storytelling
Supranormal stimuli
In-group and out-group effects
Goodness paradox
Hierarchy and egalitarianism
Shared beliefs (social collectives, oaths, fiction)
Teamwork, collegiality
Leadership
Empathy level
Personality types and behaviors
Stress response
Cognitive biases
Mindfulness, attention, and well-being
Genetic susceptibility to disease

[a] These points are elaborated on throughout the book.

Consider that for over two million years, members of the Homo genus have taught each other to use stone tools, not with written words but through demonstration of procedural knowledge and mentorship.[117] Prior to written language, storytelling was probably a key mode of learning.[118] Hunter-gatherers learned from stories and observing others since they were not born with the ability to survive in the wild on their own.

Further, stories seem to have deeply rooted social educational purposes, such as teaching egalitarianism within a tribe or cautionary lessons.[118] The development of key aspects of language—storytelling, gossip, and ability to describe abstract concepts—were instrumental to human evolution and domination over all other species.[119]

In fact, some experts argue that social learning and large-scale cooperation, aided by language, are major features that distinguished Homo sapiens from other species.[120,121] With these skills, humans collectively dominate the earth. Human toolmaking and weaponry genius eventually became too complex to encode entirely in our DNA.

Instead, we mostly learn these and other basic survival skills through direct experiential learning that is propagated through generations via a culture. The broader implication is that the primary way we learn the practice of medicine is the same way humans have learned life skills for millennia—through stories, experiences, teamwork, and teaching rather than in a classroom or (too much time) studying at a desk.

Beyond learning, atavistic tendencies have a great influence on how we think and feel, and in turn, our well-being. Shifting attention helped keep cavepeople alert and alive, but today can lead to mind-wandering and rumination.[122] An overconfident caveperson could save the tribe from predators but today could be dangerous. Common threats were true threats to life, but now these are more often threats to ego.

The need for cooperation for learning and survival has also endowed us with natural empathy and compassion for our fellow humans.[122,123] This preview of things we'll discuss in more detail tells us that thinking like a caveperson can create problems for us today, but showing compassion like a caveperson can be beneficial.

Now, for around the last 70,000 years, humans have been the dominant species on our planet and are thought to have become genetically akin to modern humans around 40,000–50,000 years ago. Accordingly, we are still genetically hardwired to be hunters and gatherers even though we have since developed a socially alien industrialized world. Over time, hunter-gatherers developed a tendency for peaceful egalitarian cooperation when working in small groups. We'll come back to how in-group cooperation and related factors underlie evolutionarily driven in-group effects, tensions between hierarchy and egalitarianism, and perceptions of fairness in the modern workplace.

But even for the cavepeople, not everyone fit into the tribal mold. There were outliers like psychopaths who sometimes were able to remain under the radar and benefit from the collective generosity of the rest of the tribe, but other times they were outed. Evidence suggests that capital punishment was employed as a mechanism to deal with some sinisterly dictatorial or psychopathic tribe members.[121,124]

Still, many psychopathic individuals found an evolutionary loophole letting them evade cooperation and today can infiltrate any modern workplace type, including in medicine. We'll also see in Chapter 29 how this aspect of the story relates to a concept that helps explain human behavior called the goodness paradox.

Also, notice what did not mold human evolution—soda, candy bars, smart phones, shiny sequins, and airbrushed models on magazine covers. These can be considered *supranormal stimuli* that are more enticing than things found in nature because they exceed our evolutionary thermostat setting for stimulation. These can hijack our attention and may contribute to over-indulgence in a variety of modern-day vices such as substance or gambling addictions, unhealthy food, and excessive screentime.[125] By this view, supranormal stimuli present health and well-being challenges for medical trainees and their patients.

Post-Agricultural Revolution Changes

Human dominance on Earth surged into overdrive 12,000 years ago as the recession of the glaciers ushered in the Agricultural Revolution.[119] And it turns out that we can draw a straight line from this revolution to modern-day psychological and social norms.

Along with the Agricultural Revolution, humans acquired possessions and landownership rights, and with this change came increased trade, the need for law and order, and an increasingly stratified social hierarchy. Diet diversity diminished and patterns of infectious disease shifted. Religions that placed humankind and God above animals and nature replaced the animistic beliefs of hunter-gatherers.[119,126] [1] Several changes in social structure and culture set the stage for a deeply entrenched patriarchy.[127]

It turns out that all these post-Agricultural Revolution trends including social hierarchy structures, diet, disease patterns, religious practices, and male-centered leadership directly impact medical practice and training in ways seldom discussed. One effect is that these trends have stamped deeply embedded assumptions in our societal and workplace culture that are often at odds with our real-life experiences that we'll consider in the upcoming chapters.

Recent Human Evolution and Technology

Finally, there are several other intriguing viewpoints on recent and continued human evolution that are detailed elsewhere, including the intricate interplay between technology, genetics, and behavior.[120,128–130] In brief, humans have evolved under the heavy influence of technology since we started using simple tools. Additionally, one viewpoint holds that human evolution in certain respects has accelerated in recent millennia due to the rapid expansion of the population.[121] From these perspectives, how we learn, how we socialize, and who we fundamentally are as a species may be rapidly evolving in this era of technological leaps. Technology, to some extent then, may already be interwoven into the human condition as a counterforce to the caveperson-modern life mismatch.[2]

Major Events Impacting Modern Medical Education

Now, let's turn our attention to major events important for medical education. The evolution of modern medical education is profoundly shaped by key historical events and figures, medical culture, and ongoing shifts in medical practice.

William Halsted's Influence

A pivotal figure in this evolution was Dr. William Halsted, whose pioneering work at Johns Hopkins established the American surgical residency paradigm around the turn of the 20th century. He was one of Hopkin's *Big Four* founding physicians and educators (Figure 6.1). Halsted, a transformational surgeon vaunted for superb technical skills, although sometimes hindered by substance use, initiated the first American surgical residency program. He developed a progressive mentorship program where residents gradually assumed responsibility and status in the medical hierarchy.

In Halsted's program, residents learned the basic science of medicine, taught their juniors, and ran the clinical practice. For years, they lived in the hospital with little time off (hence the term *residency*), usually remained unmarried, and had no guarantee of finishing the program.

The culture of Halsted's residency spoke to complete dedication, extreme focus, and continual availability to patients. The program formalized the training structure and ensured

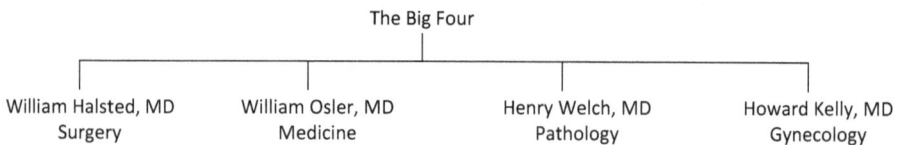

The Big Four

William Halsted, MD	William Osler, MD	Henry Welch, MD	Howard Kelly, MD
Surgery	Medicine	Pathology	Gynecology

Figure 6.1 The *Big Four* are the original physicians of Johns Hopkins University. William Halsted started the first modern U.S. surgical residency program. The others started residency programs as well, although these were generally more personal and less regimented. Although there has been substantial modernization in recent decades, the continued influence on the structure and culture of modern residency programs is undeniable.

generational propagation of skill and knowledge. Persisting throughout subsequent generations of medical trainees, this total immersion model has now trained generations of physicians and continues in a modified form today.

However, the seemingly unwavering dedication demanded by Halsted's program concealed a darker side consisting of a complex interplay between innovation, addiction, and trainee exploitation. Inspired by Sigmund Freud's insights relating to the potential medical uses of cocaine, Halsted ingeniously spearheaded the use of cocaine-based local anesthetic.[131]

While he mostly tested this innovation on his medical student *volunteers*, he also engaged in self-experimentation and became hopelessly addicted.[131] In effect, the residency program provided cover for Halsted's addiction by allowing teaching and clinical care responsibilities to be delegated to continuously available senior residents.

We could debate the merits and appropriateness of the extreme residency conditions on their own terms, but hidden motives and apparent hypocrisy certainly taint the setup. Although Halsted worked long hours at times, potentially facilitated by cocaine use, he also indulged in regular prolonged sabbaticals to his summer home and Europe. He was married (unlike his residents),[3] had no children, smoked tobacco (as was common in the day), had time to socialize and pursue hobbies, and enjoyed many luxuries.

Today, the demographic, technological, medico-legal, and well-being realities bear little resemblance to Halsted's era. For example, Halsted only trained men, who had no need to balance pregnancy or dual-working households. Completing a residency was optional back then, while physicians today must participate in a residency program if they intend to receive state medical licenses and to be recognized by national medical boards.

Despite substantial modernization of training programs in recent decades, they are still heavily influenced by the Halstedian model. While Halsted's legacy continues to influence residency training, other significant events have also shaped the trajectory of medical education.

The *Flexner Report*

The 1910 *Flexner Report*[4] dramatically altered the landscape of American medical education, standardizing curricula and emphasizing the biomedical model but also introducing unintended consequences.[132,133] At the turn of the 20th century, numerous low-quality, for-profit American medical schools lacked standardization.[132] The *Flexner Report* shuttered many of these and prescribed many standards including two years of basic science before clinical training.[133]

While fortifying science education before medical school has clear advantages, critics of the *Flexner Report* point to its limiting secondary effects, as summarized in Table 6.2.[134,135] Today, all these secondary effects impact the hidden curriculum. Thus, the legacy of the Flexner Report, along with subsequent developments, continues to shape the challenges and opportunities faced by today's medical students and residents.

Modern Curriculum Refinement and Challenges

The modern medical curriculum, while constantly evolving, presents both advantages and limitations, as illustrated by my experience with a smoking cessation mini course. As part of a well-intended effort to introduce some practical clinical skills to new medical students who were otherwise focused mostly on basic science, I was given a mini crash course in how to motivate patients to quit smoking.

For this exercise, we were taught how to move patients from the precontemplative stage to the contemplative stage, and from the contemplative stage to the action stage. To do so required

Table 6.2 Major Secondary Effects of the *Flexner Report*

De-emphasis of Psychology in Medicine
De-emphasis of Spirituality and Religion in Medicine[a]
Divide Between Science and Clinical Based Philosophies of Medical Education
Enhanced Selection of Privileged Medical Students
Increased Physician Authority and Dominance
Promoted a Medical Spirituality of Immanence[a]
Closure of Most Black Medical Schools
Barriers for Female Medical Trainees

[a] A spirituality of immanence entails healing focused on bodily and physical health without focus on spiritual health, further discussed in Chapter 22.

probing for barriers to change, and helping patients arrive at their own conclusion that they should quit smoking.

This exercise helped convey principles of motivational interviewing, but I lacked knowledge of available pharmacologic interventions, the underlying evidence or success rates of the intervention techniques, or real details of the medical risks of smoking. I felt like an outright impostor—we'll see in a moment why this result matters.

Your medical curriculum will likely be the only one you have ever known, so it will probably seem well vetted and stable on the surface. But the truth is that it is fluid and your curriculum will be a snapshot in an ever-evolving experiment. Sometimes the curriculum changes for the better and sometimes for the worse. What's more, the changes in recent decades have accelerated—spurred by changes in teaching philosophy, an increasing body of knowledge, heightened focus on trainee well-being, and enhanced trainee/patient protections.

These changes mean you will face limitations of the formal curriculum that you are unlikely to recognize without understanding a little history. The trick is to leverage as many advantages of the current curriculum and of the older, partially forgotten, ways as possible while minimizing the disadvantages. So, what are some of the key recent changes, and how can you leverage both the historical and modern advantages?

To understand this, it is useful to imagine what training was like in the post-Flexner era until recent years. Medical school typically involved two years of basic science coursework, including subject-based classes, traditional tests, and grades. These grades brought both incentives and stress.

While there was always some heterogeneity and changes in content over time, modern times have brought marked changes in medical education, including the full-fledged emergence of integrated curricula (teaching basic and clinical sciences across subject matters together throughout medical school), problem-based learning, P/F grading, and increased emphasis on social aspects of health and the humanities.[4] Other changes often include widespread introduction of remote learning or recorded lecture options, increased numbers of days off (e.g., wellness or study days), and less time in the anatomy lab, for example.

Residency training commonly prescribed 100-hour or longer work weeks with regular 36-hour marathon shifts.[5] Medical teams (attending, resident, intern, and medical student) often worked closely together for more extended periods of time compared to today (e.g., over weeks). Inpatient practice involved fewer shifts and handoffs, and uninterrupted patient care was easier. Being in-house, residents were available to benefit from spontaneous experiences, especially medical or surgical emergencies or new hospital admissions. The work hours were seen as necessary to garner sufficient experience.

Overall, I think we must acknowledge that this system offered many educational benefits. The system recognized that residents are relatively inefficient early on, in-patient care is complex and requires constant attention, experiences arise spontaneously at all hours, longitudinal teamwork is beneficial, and experiential learning is paramount.

On the other hand, some trainees experienced being in a chronic zombie-level state, not quite functioning in high gear. Trainee well-being, personal relationships, and possibly even patient safety sometimes suffered; the demands could grow to be excessive, and cynicism could take hold.[136] Some patient care activities were perceived as *scut work*, and trainee treatment was sometimes perceived as abusive. Attendings were sometimes absent, leaving the teaching and ultimate responsibilities to the senior residents.[136] There was often less time for formal studying.

Then, the 2003 ACGME reforms limited the average work week to 80 hours, with guidelines for shift length and days off.[137] In 2009, the Institute of Medicine published a detailed report on the effects of prolonged work, sleep-deprivation, program adherence, focusing on well-being, and avoidance of errors. Further modifications in 2011 included restricting interns to work no more than 16 consecutive hours and to encourage residents to assume greater personal responsibility regarding alertness.[138]

How to Navigate the Changing Curriculum Landscape

Integrated Curricula

Understanding the historical context of these changes is crucial for navigating the complexities of the modern medical curriculum and maximizing its benefits. First, you should recognize that educators debate whether the traditional approach of science-based curricula preceding clinical training is a time-tested blueprint for success or a flawed obsolescence.[139]

The integrated curriculum, while offering potential advantages, also presents challenges. Potential benefits include incorporate active learning, repetition of ideas in various contexts, emphasis on relevant topics, and training on delivering clinically focused presentations for example. It can also help introduce principal concepts like communication skills and *shared decision-making* earlier in a medical student's experience.

However, some also believe that a basic science foundation should come first, so it can later be applied to learning the practice medicine.[139] Problem-based learning taxes our working memory, which has potential for high cognitive load that could even hinder long-term memory encoding, especially when working memory draws from new information instead of long-term memory.[78]

While an integrative approach makes valuable connections across subjects, it is difficult to have a strong knowledge base in all these areas at the start; I believe this is one reason that the smoking cessation mini course did not work well for me. In addition, integrated curricula can shortchange important topics ranging from nutrition to various fundamental science concepts.[140] Finally, an integrative curriculum risks instilling a false sense of burgeoning clinical knowledge before trainees have truly mastered it and before they even have the foundational knowledge necessary for context.

The integrative medical school curriculum of today has even been called "organized anarchy," a term reflecting the flexible (but inconsistent) topics, insufficient hours of planning available to physician-teachers, and physician-teacher overconfidence; all of these facets can cumulatively create a smokescreen to obscure curricular inadequacies.[141] While I do not entirely agree with this characterization, it does suggest the need to introduce some structure and context to our own education.

For all these reasons, trainees must be more proactive than ever in preparatory studying and subject review and reflection to reap maximum benefits. Since learning basic science within confined contexts may make it more difficult to generalize the knowledge later, it may be useful to consider how your learning material applies to clinical areas. In addition, you may need to identify the major gaps in your curriculum and supplement your own learning for both breadth and depth.

Pass/Fail Grading

P/F grading systems, while intended to reduce stress, have unintended consequences that require careful consideration. Pure P/F schemes award the same evaluation to the top student as one who barely passed, which is a lost chance to differentiate yourself. Therefore, attempts to curtail competition can paradoxically increase stress for high-achieving students. This system may also lower the incentive to study material in its greatest depth.

However, many medical schools have multiple tiers like *high pass*, which then become essentially code for traditional letter grades. Since it is difficult to differentiate among so many students, understanding the hidden curriculum is a key method to elevate your grade to a high pass.

Thus, be aware that you will still probably be ranked by quartile (or something similar) on Medical School Performance Evaluations (MSPEs—formerly known as Dean's Letters), suggesting that the lack of official grades offers only the illusion of rank-free reporting. Therefore, you should not view P/F grading systems as a free pass to coast. Finally, P/F grading systems may confer advantages to students from prestigious schools over others.

That said, there are numerous purported benefits to P/F grading systems, such as possibly decreasing learner stress and encouraging collegiality over competition, without compromising learning.[142] The best approach is to leverage these benefits while staying aware of the real reporting system (not just the illusion), and to commit to your own learning. Finally, P/F testing increases the impact of doing curriculum vitae (CV)–building side endeavors and may increase free time for leisure pursuits.

In this P/F era, you should consider finding opportunities beyond the classroom to help differentiate yourself from your competition. Consider doing the extra activities largely in the offseason, though, so you do not shortchange your formal (and informal) medical education.

Modern Residency Training

Modern residency training, while offering improved work-life balance, demands efficient time management and proactive engagement. In residency, you can benefit from better rest, less fatigue, and more potential study time than in years past. The work may be compressed, however, requiring you to find efficiencies, and proactively seek out experiences, look for ways to learn secondhand from missed (off-hours) opportunities (like sharing stories with colleagues), and polish hand-off skills.

Additionally, since you may work with attendings for one shift each day for a limited time they are on service, it is more important than ever to make efforts to interact with them effectively so that they are fully invested in your success. Finally, time away from work is for rest and recovery, but the truth is that if you want to be at the top of your game, there will be work to do then too (e.g., studying, research).

Key Takeaways

Understanding the history of medicine and medical education is crucial for navigating the hidden curriculum. By recognizing the influences of evolution, cultural shifts, and landmark events, medical trainees can better understand the human tendencies, culture, and expectations that shape their training experiences. Thus, this chapter sets the stage for much of the rest of this book, including the central theme of culture as a dominant force shaping how we live and learn, which we'll explore in the next chapter.

Notes

1 Animistic beliefs generally hold that all natural things are animated by souls (and may also recognize spirits). These are related to integration of all living things on earth and generally consider humans to be one of the animals.

2 In fact, some refer to this transformation as *Homo technologicus* and philosopher Yuval Noah Harari argues we may become a technological-human super hybrid called *Homo deus.*

3 Some sources suspect this was a marriage of convenience.

4 The author, Abraham Flexner, also had close connections with, and was influenced by, the Hopkins Big Four (Duffy).[133]

5 Substantial changes in medical education began in the later part of the 20th century after the *Libby Zion case* catalyzed a series of resident duty hour reforms. In 1984, Libby Zion, an eighteen-year-old admitted to a New York hospital with a fever, received meperidine (trade name: Demerol) prescribed by an intern, resulting in a tragically fatal serotonin syndrome. This judgement culminated in recommendations made by the *Bell Commission* and subsequent national reforms.

7

Culture

Vance T. Lehman

Consequences of Culture

During training, I would have dismissed discussion of workplace culture as academic drivel. I now know better. Culture serves as a command-and-control center, a force that sets the tone for *everything* else in an organization. Culture drives safety, decision-making, behavior, satisfaction and retention, financial performance, and more. When culture falters, governments fail, space shuttles explode, and businesses suffer. There are intelligent and capable people in any medical institution around the globe. Yet, a key to the success of any organization is workplace culture because it can bring out the best (or worst) in people.

As a trainee, it is challenging to understand how much culture drives your workplace behavior. This is likely because we live, learn, and survive within social groups. The glue that holds these social groups together and provides longitudinal stability is culture. It follows that the hidden curriculum is largely embedded within medical culture. In fact, many articles define the hidden curriculum as a sociocultural concept of transmitted values, beliefs, culture, and behaviors.[5,143] In this chapter, we'll explore the origins and unpack the concept of culture.

Conveniently for the purposes of this discussion, it turns out that several types of culture—that of the workplace, a community, or a major world religion, for example—share some basic traits. Before we define these traits, recall that the concept of culture has been a vehicle to pass on traditions, knowledge, and the purpose of our existence for millennia.[144,145]

All in all, workplace culture will probably have a far deeper impact on your training and career than you would have thought. Culture helps define who we are as physicians and our likelihood of professional success. During training, you must quickly adapt to the cultures of different services. Otherwise, carrying over the cultural assumptions from one service to the next can be an impactful mistake. The culture of an institution should be a prime consideration when creating a residency rank list order or, after training, searching for a job.

Layers and Levels of Culture

To understand workplace culture though, we need to turn to insights from business experts. Management guru Peter Drucker allegedly said, "[C]ulture eats strategy for breakfast."[146] In other words, an organizational culture cultivates workers' beliefs, values, and identities, which in turn spurs motivation and productivity; the impact of these factors outweighs any from strategy alone. That is, your workplace culture will probably have a major impact on your professional development.

DOI: 10.1201/9781003633389-9

Table 7.1 The Three Levels of Culture

Artifacts	Visible, realized features of culture or what is done. Typically reflect the basic shared assumptions.
Espoused Values	Overt statements or gestures representing what the organization officially says it values or aims to do.
Shared Basic Assumptions	The true core organizational values, which drive artifacts but may or may not be reflected in the official espoused values.

Cultures of any kind are more complex than they appear on the surface. In society, for example, there are many *layers of culture*, including national, organizational, ethnic, and familial. Regardless of the category (or layer) of culture (society, work, etc.), culture manifests itself on three basic levels: artifacts, espoused values, and shared basic (implicit) assumptions (Table 7.1).[147] *Artifacts*—actions and items in plain sight—are important visual culture indicators.[147] In the workplace, artifacts consist of a wide variety of visible features, such as awards, bonuses, accolades or praise, behaviors, attitudes, actions, or an interior lobby design.

Espoused values, overtly stated cultural values, form the second layer of culture. Salient examples in medical organizations include a practice mission statement or a committee charter. Espoused values are a culture's veneer, which may or may not reflect the artifacts or the third and deepest level, the *shared basic assumptions*.

Shared basic assumptions are the core values of an organization. These are signaled by actions but also transmitted by subtle means such as observing and modeling behaviors. Shared basic assumptions, rather than the stated espoused values, drive artifacts. Shared basic assumptions may be broader values, such as revenue optimization, whereas artifacts are specific observable examples, such as raising prices on a certain product.

The good news is that there is no need to memorize the names of these levels. The important things to remember are that organizational culture matters a lot, is learned through a socialization process, and partially resides below the surface of the formally stated institutional mission.

Origins of Medical Culture

We have seen how culture manifests, but where does it come from, and why do we need to consider its impact on business and medical practice? For one thing, we can usually draw a straight line between the values of an organization's founders and the culture of an organization.[147] In fact, founders are said to establish an organization's DNA; while the DNA can mutate and evolve, the original imprint usually remains paramount.

So, when evaluating potential training programs or jobs, it helps to consider an institution's founding principles, even if these are old. Through concerted efforts, though, organizational culture can be modified substantially.[147,148] Such efforts have demonstrated remarkable results in medicine[148] and are a sign of well-adjusted practice priorities.

Looking deeper, other sources of culture in medicine are more fundamental than the founders of any given healthcare organization. Reflecting the small size and function of tribes during hunter-gatherer times, it turns out that human leaders only function effectively through first-hand interactions in groups of up to around 150 people.[119] Any larger group requires a uniting narrative (or indoctrination) of shared values, assumptions, or goals to maintain group cohesion called a *social collective*.[119]

In medicine, this shared narrative arises in part from the broader sense of professional identity and commitment to universal oaths. In addition to medical training oaths, the shared basic assumptions (reflected in a social collective) of modern training remain heavily influenced by post-Agricultural Revolution societal norms such as patriarchy, and more proximally, the philosophy of the *Big Four*.

These assumptions were further engrained by the effects of the *Flexner Report* and the relationship between medicine, religion, and spirituality (Chapter 22). Yet, despite the deep and central role of culture in medicine, culture is maintained by everyone in the collective and is the sum of countless micro actions. So, whether we realize it or not, during medical training, we are incorporated into a group identity formed by shared beliefs and influences.

Culture and Conflict

Now, let's consider how culture can create conflict when the three layers are out of sync (Figure 7.1), first with a deep, pervasive example and then with some everyday examples. The deep conflict of medical training culture is critical to understand because it lies at the heart of many of the challenges we face today.

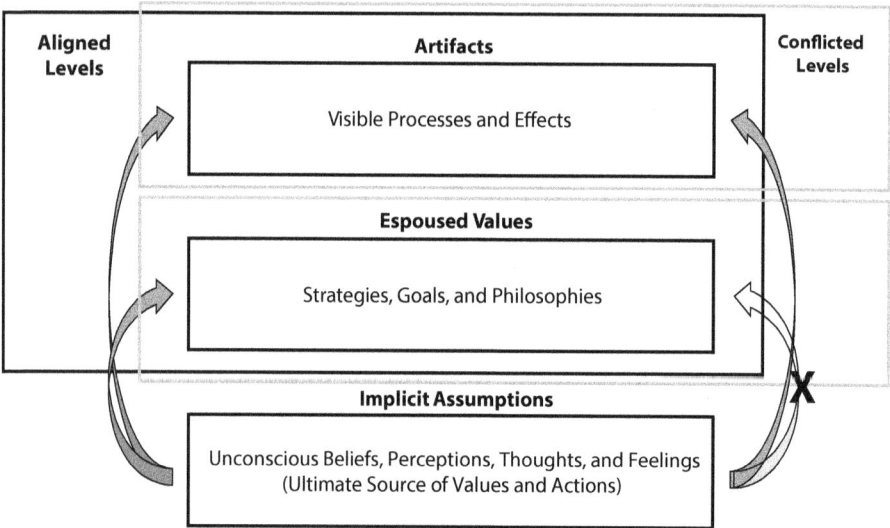

Figure 7.1 The levels of culture. The three levels of culture are artifact, espoused values, and implicit assumptions. Implicit assumptions are the deepest and least visible aspect of culture. When artifacts and espoused values reflect implicit assumptions, all three layers of culture are aligned (lefthand column). Conflict arises when artifacts or espoused values contradict implicit assumptions (righthand column). For example, espoused values can differ from both artifacts and implicit assumptions. For example, an organization may formally declare that it values teamwork above individual efforts and accolades (espoused values) but recognizes individuals instead of groups (artifacts), through initiatives like "employee of the month," "teacher of the year," or individual promotions. This reflects implicit assumptions of individualism, conflicting with the espoused values. Generally, artifacts reflect implicit assumptions (as seen in both the lefthand and righthand columns) unless external forces, such as regulations (e.g., resident duty hour limits), influence the artifacts.

46

Consider that, for decades following the Halsted era, the shared basic assumptions, espoused values, and artifacts were mostly aligned, reflecting an all-encompassing work culture. People may have worked exceedingly long hours and even experienced exhaustion, but most everyone had some internal peace because the values and mission were congruent.

Then, a variety of factors led to the development of work-hour restrictions and other reforms. While these changes are positive overall, they have cast us into a transitional period of cultural conflict. We are told that the system values reasonable work-life integration and trainee wellness (the espoused values), and, thanks to rules and oversight, this is largely what plays out (the artifacts), but all this grates against the persistent older deeply rooted shared basic assumptions, creating an unspoken tension.

This is not to say that there was no work culture conflict in the past era. Indeed, conflicts between espoused values and reality are captured in articles and depicted in *House of God*. Interns have felt "abused and neglected" during a year described as "traumatic" and a "baptism by fire."[136] Our current conflict, however, puts the deepest professional assumptions and values at odds with reality. For these reasons, the current environment is, in some respects, more challenging and disharmonious than that of the past.

There are many specific examples of conflict between the different layers of the medical culture that can result in internal conflict for trainees. Common examples include the following:

- Patient care is the top-stated institutional priority (espoused value), yet policies put profits over patients (artifacts that reflect shared basic assumptions)
- Teamwork is formally valued over individual effort (espoused value), yet "Teacher of the Year" awards recognize individuals instead of teams (artifact that reflect a shared basic assumption)
- Preventive care and well-being are formally prioritized (espoused value), yet there is an absence of an on-site exercise facility or healthful meal options in the hospital cafeteria for staff and time constraints make it difficult for physicians to devote time to exercise, cooking, or scheduling their own preventative health exams (artifact that reflects a shared basic assumption)

Workplace culture conflicts can directly affect trainees in subtle and paradoxical ways. For example, the introduction of well-intentioned trainee wellness and resilience initiatives may seem like a mixed message in a work culture that otherwise rewards self-sacrifice and frames burnout management as a personal rather than organizational responsibility.[119] While there is sometimes little you can change in a system, it is helpful to understand these forces since this can provide clarity to mixed messages, can be at the heart of trainee-attending tension, and can optimize your ability to manage culture conflict when it arises.

Key Takeaways

Understanding workplace culture is essential for medical trainees. Trainees can navigate the hidden curriculum more effectively by considering the layers and levels of culture, the origins of medical culture, and the related potential for conflict. In the next chapter, we'll discuss one indelible aspect of the medical culture—the theme of hierarchy.

8

Hierarchy

Vance T. Lehman

Why Medical Hierarchy Matters

Hierarchical forces are deeply ingrained in the medical culture and will have profound implications for your professional development, evaluations/grades, and patient care. What challenges do hierarchies bring and why is it so important to understand this topic? To answer these questions, we need to briefly revisit our evolutionary-driven nature.

In the wild, mammal species that live and hunt in groups have well-established hierarchies, with alpha males and alpha females.[112] Thus, a tendency for hierarchy seems to be encoded in our primal DNA. But it is not so simple for humans because as we evolved, several forces put the brakes on this tendency, promoting a desire for relative egalitarianism within a tribe. Thus, it is useful to consider the factors that push us to be egalitarian on one hand and hierarchical on the other since it is a setup that can create tension in the training environment.

Major reasons that humans gained egalitarian tendencies center around the need to cooperate for strategic hunting, social learning such as toolmaking, and raising high-demand children.[150] Storytelling skills were used to teach cooperation and egalitarianism.[118] The nomadic lifestyle limited the number of possessions, curtailing wealth inequity.[145] Advancements in communication and cooperation helped a tribe band together to overthrow members who were too dictatorial.[121,150] The net result is that humans are believed to have self-domesticated, showing little in-group violence, and having a relatively loose hierarchical structure.[150]

Workplace Hierarchy Is a Permanent Fixture

However, as hunter-gatherers formed larger groups and the ability to develop shared perspectives leading up to the agricultural revolution, broader hierarchical frameworks were probably required to maintain social order.[119,151] Modern societal and corporate structure have gone much farther and have introduced large and complex hierarchies that we did not evolve to manage. This creates a conflict between our intrinsic preference for relative fairness and egalitarianism versus the desires of those maintaining hierarchical systems. Although many have called for flattening of the corporate hierarchies, organizational psychologist Harold Leavitt dashes any hope, contending that they are—despite major drawbacks—permanent fixtures since we have found no better alternative.[152]

Likewise, the medical hierarchy is a permanent fixture. So, we may be better off taking Leavitt's advice to learn how to manage hierarchy and thrive within it.[152] But this is a major challenge. I think it is normal for you to dislike, even disdain, the medical hierarchy at times because it grates against the innate part of us that demands egalitarianism. In medicine though, like the military, if the hierarchy breaks down, the entire system could fail, and people could suffer or die.

 DOI: 10.1201/9781003633389-10

Table 8.1 Potential Effects of the Hierarchy on Physicians in Training

Positive	Negative
Can instill social order	Can make trainees reluctant to reveal ignorance/close gaps in understanding
Can enhance patient safety in some settings	Can discourage individuals from speaking up against safety concerns
Can reduce trainee anxiety	Can increase trainee anxiety
Can promote professionalism	Can perpetuate old-fashioned, disrespectful, or otherwise maladaptive methods of interpersonal communication
Can encourage positive action via praise and reward	Can discourage disclosure of medical errors via punishment

Virtues and Perils of the Medical Hierarchy

Is the medical hierarchy a good or bad thing? Consider that hierarchies can be functional, oppressive, or some combination of the two. Showing how murky the topic can be, the Code of Hammurabi defined three classes of people—superiors, commoners, and slaves. This is relevant because it illustrates how hierarchies, while providing social structure, can also be inherently unjust and discriminatory. The hierarchy in medicine is also best considered as a mixed example (Table 8.1).

On balance though, the modern medical hierarchy, when benevolent, is beneficial for you because it establishes a clear-cut system for decisions, training, safeguards, and accountability. Important decisions or tasks are routed to the most knowledgeable or capable individuals and delegated efficiently. It promotes cooperation, decreases conflict, and can protect you from getting in over your head. Thus, you should embrace the positive aspects of hierarchy. Of course, there certainly is potential for negative effects as well, though these have been partly offset by protections.

Because of these reasons, it is in your best interest to honor the hierarchy unless there is a serious safety or ethical issue. In fact, infringements on hierarchical norms often prompt negative evaluations. Things to avoid include being overly questioning or skeptical about an attending's opinion; ignoring feedback, which can give the impression a trainee knows better than the attending; overcorrecting of staff over minor things; expecting staff to accommodate trainee schedules for meetings (instead of vice versa).

In sum, it is useful to develop a sense of why hierarchical norms are important to those you answer to and why breaches could be perceived as a personal slight and a violation of professional culture and norms.[153,154]

Nuances of the Medical Hierarchy

Medical hierarchies weave a complex web within and between physicians, trainees, nurses, technologists, and other medical staff. Power and the ability to influence others may work down, laterally, or upward within the hierarchy.[155,156] For example, shrewd trainees who surmise what their attendings want and then make a positive impression are influencing those above them.

Some hierarchies are fluid, as with a trainee climbing the ranks, whereas others are calcified.[156] In medicine, we must constantly pivot and adapt to new positions, which means you should carefully calibrate your actions to your current position. Additionally, the effects depend heavily on how hierarchy is implemented. For example, subordinate anxiety heightens if there is constant fear of negative responses if asking for help is considered a weakness, but anxiety reduces if asking for appropriate help is welcomed.

Exceptions to Medical Hierarchy

There is a key exception when hierarchy should be challenged—when needed to protect patient (or own) safety. For example, trainees should always speak up if they believe a mistake will negatively impact patient care. In addition, individuals higher up in the hierarchy have a duty to create and maintain a Culture of Safety in which team members feel comfortable speaking up. Still, if you must call attention to a potential safety problem, remain respectful and tactful.

It also turns out that physicians benefit from relaxing hierarchical stratification in certain settings. For example, when working together in small groups or committees with physicians at various stages and nonphysicians, hierarchy can stifle creativity and psychological safety.[157]

Authority and Conformity

Although the medical hierarchy can be functional, we'll now turn to a few examples that help us understand what can happen when a strict hierarchy with strong authority figures goes awry. As medical trainees, you should be familiar with two famous experiments that investigated this setup: the Stanford Prison Experiment and the Milgram Shock Experiment.

The Stanford Prison Experiment

During the 1971 Stanford Prison Experiment, a group of study participants assumed a toxic authoritarian stance, now called the *Lucifer Effect*.[158] Specifically, college students randomly assigned to be "guards" showed extreme abuse to the randomly assigned "inmates" and has been called "one of the most notorious and controversial psychology studies ever devised."[159] The effects of this experiment occurred within days, so the potential effects in long-term systems like medicine are sobering.

The Milgram Shock Experiment

Stanley Milgram performed another famous experiment in this realm that you should know. Here is the set up: Two unsuspecting study recruits were summoned to a room. It was a sterile setup with a strange switchboard with some controls, a monitor, and a scientist wearing a gray lab coat. The recruits were briefly introduced, and one, a pleasant plain-clothed gentleman, was selected by a rigged paper draw to be ushered to the next room over. The scientist then reiterated the study's purpose to the first recruit, a test of punishment's impact on learning. This recruit would be the *teacher* while the other would be the *learner*. The scientist administered a low-level shock to the *teacher* to give him a reference of the shock voltage effect and to instill credence.

The learner and teacher were separated by a wall but could hear each other. The teacher recited a list of word pairs and then quizzed the learner. Every time the learner made an error, the teacher was instructed to administer an electric shock. With each shock, the scientist instructed him calmly but firmly with a predetermined script to increase the voltage. With increasing voltage, the learner appeared to give verbal protest or bang a table in agony, but everything was a show. The learner paused and questioned if he should stop but ultimately continued to the highest voltage which was labeled "Danger, Severe Shock."

This experiment was repeated many times under different circumstances; the bottom line is that around two-thirds of *teachers* continued administering electric shocks to the highest possible voltage. One interpretation is that we are far more susceptible to the commands of authority when those commands violate our conscience than most would predict. In this case, the authority was even a stranger, not an attending with influence over your future career.

The electric shock studies by Milgram have been heavily critiqued, both on ethical grounds and interpretations of results. Practically speaking, training in medicine is different in that we are indoctrinated over time and subject to behavior *normalization*, depend on the system for our livelihood, and act in more subtle ways than administering shocks. The results then may not translate perfectly to medical training, but the experiment remains one of the most compelling explorations of human nature in a hierarchical setting that bears certain resemblances.

It is also interesting that the subjects complied even without invoking *dehumanizing* language toward the people *receiving* the shocks, though they were behind a wall and could only be heard, not seen. Instead, only basic *justification* was needed—use of shocks in the name of science. This shows the powerful influence that an authority has over human actions, which has been shown many times over, including the strong influence that physicians exert.[160] Why would this be? It seems that obedience to authority is instilled in us from an early age and usually functions as a useful heuristic since experts typically point us in the right direction.[160]

Other Extreme Examples of Authority and Conformity

In *Man's Search for Meaning*, Viktor Frankl chronicles his experiences as a prisoner (and physician) in WWII concentration camps, exploring themes of conformity, good, and evil.[161] He recalls that few guards covertly helped the prisoners while a subset of the prisoners who were given elevated status over the others became more monstrous than some guards.

So, while many people conform to their environment, even when it is infected with evil influences, responses vary. The desire to understand the human potential for situational human brutality was a key impetus behind both the Stanford Prison Experiment and the Milgram Experiment.

Fortunately, the extreme brutality tested in the Stanford Prison Experiment and the Milgram Experiment does not reflect the typical training experience in medicine. These are also artificial situations and more recent evidence suggests that the results of the Stanford Prison Experiment do not always replicate in other circumstances.[162] Still, some concerning parallels on a smaller scale must be considered. Specifically, it is important to understand that the influence of authority upon us, or by us on others, can drive otherwise unthinkable behavior if we do not keep the influence in check.

Other Insights from Psychology and Social Psychology

Beyond these extreme examples, a large body of literature shows a strong general human tendency to conform to their environments, including in medicine. For example, studies by psychologist Solomon Asch found that many people provide absurdly wrong answers to quiz questions when everyone around them does too and will join the group in facing the wrong way in an elevator.[163]

The medical training environment may be a particularly strong setup for this natural tendency, in part because conformity can help trainees navigate a new, uncertain environment.[160] While conformity can have a positive effect when it teaches good medical practice, it can also lead to incorrect procedural approaches, incorrect diagnosis, inappropriate treatments, or undesirable behaviors.[164,165] Unchecked conformity can also normalize counterproductive activities such as working past the point of exhaustion at the expense of personal well-being.

There are also many insights from the social psychology literature.[160] In brief, many of the rites, ceremonies, and practices of medicine are aligned with practices that are known to influence human behavior. These include public commitments (such as oaths), social proof (exposure to like-minded individuals), and self-sacrifice. These factors can alter a self-image and encourage behaviors that maintain the new image. In fact, medical training has been said to create a new professional identity and, to maintain this self-image, trainees will naturally act in ways to preserve it.

Additionally, consider that initiation events, often difficult, embarrassing, or painful, are performed across cultures, situations and time. Such barriers to access and sacrifices have been shown to increase members' commitment and affiliation to a group and the attractiveness of a group because things that are difficult to obtain are valued.[160] Though this is not the consciously intended, nor the only, reason for difficult training, an intriguing parallel can be seen in the physician training journey.

Countermeasures

There are clearly some situations and influences at play that we cannot change, at least in the short term. For these examples, I believe it is still useful to understand the forces behind your own experiences. It offers some sense of agency and enlightenment.

For other situations, with appropriate awareness, you can make informed decisions and, when an approach is in doubt, seek out additional information. Additionally, as you gain rank, it is useful to encourage open discussion and welcome questions during informal teaching sessions/rounds.[165] Otherwise, unquestioned deference to your orders by physicians and other staff lower on the pecking order can lead to medical errors since even egregiously inappropriate requests are sometimes followed by those who intellectually should know better.[160]

Key Takeaways

It is critical to understand the opposing forces for hierarchy and egalitarianism, but corporate hierarchy, for better or worse, is an indelible feature of medical training. As a trainee, you must maintain appropriate respect for those higher on the hierarchy ladder and resist forces that might tempt you to mistreat those on lower levels. In addition, social forces underlying authority and conformity have potential to exert a greater influence on you than may be apparent, especially if the underlying forces are not recognized.

Next, we explore conflict, a theme that must be managed well to avert problems in training and beyond.

9

Conflict

Vance T. Lehman

Introduction

My initial exploration of conflict's role in the hidden curriculum led to a surprisingly extensive list of ways it affects trainees. When my list ballooned past 50, I had to stop. Two things were clear: (1) conflict is pervasive in medical training, and (2) a comprehensive list of its sources would be unwieldy and unproductive. Instead, I've included a few examples that demonstrate major types of conflict.

In fact, we have already seen conflicts that arise from the mismatches between our caveperson instincts and modern reality, as well as from misaligned levels of medical culture. Additional types we'll consider here include careerism, conflicts of interest, mixed messaging, conflicts of time and priorities, internal conflicts, and interpersonal conflicts. These conflicts are relevant because some are hidden, making them particularly challenging to manage. Addressing them requires navigating stress, moral dilemmas, interpersonal tension, and confusion.

Conflicts and Careerism

Let's take an example. Say you are listening to a lecture given by a visiting professor, Dr. Special, a world-famous researcher on the treatment of Tumor X. Dr. Special proudly presents a series of studies performed in his lab, showing the bench-to-bedside way his team developed a new treatment for Tumor X, a drug called Silver Bullet. He has, in fact, been so laser-focused on developing Silver Bullet that this has become the primary focus of his career. The compelling data he presented clearly demonstrated this. Silver Bullet is clearly a game changer in the treatment of Tumor X, you think.

Just then, one of your professors, Dr. Pragmatic, diplomatically points out a few apparent flaws in Dr. Special's results. First, she noted the highly selective patient population, questioning the generalizability of the results. What's more, the handpicked case studies used in the presentation, including patient images and testimonials, seem to show the outliers with the best results. In turn, Dr. Special subtly implied Dr. Pragmatic's adherence to the conventional treatment stemmed from her involvement in its development

While visiting professors are usually given red-carpet treatment, and their work and statements may go unchallenged, this scenario is otherwise not so out of the ordinary. What types of conflict are illustrated here, and why should you care? Well, around the time I learned about the replication crisis (Chapter 28), I saw a physician promoting his research on national TV. The message, at best, presented premature optimism, particularly for the public. Immediately, it dawned on me that even while in medical training, I, too, had been in that

DOI: 10.1201/9781003633389-11

target audience and taken for a ride. I had been swayed by careerism-driven messaging. This had put me at risk of making decisions based on claims that were not as well-established as some of the experts had implied.

Careerism

Careerism is a common type of conflict of interest (COI) that is basically defined as a primary focus on advancing one's career, which, in the extreme case, can be at the expense of personal integrity (intentional or inadvertent). When someone becomes heavily invested in success in a narrow area, his livelihood and professional identity cannot be untethered from his mission. He, therefore, cannot be an objective observer of his own work.

Now, it is natural for someone to believe in, and promote, his own work; that does not necessarily invalidate it. However, approach such claims with healthy skepticism, carefully evaluating any limitations in the presented arguments. Remember: it is easy for anyone, especially novice trainees, to get too caught up in the message without thinking critically about what the speaker may have to gain.

But this scenario shows us even more. Say Dr. Special's research was funded by several government and industry sources, and he was regularly paid for speaking engagements related to the topics of Tumor X and Silver Bullet. These would be *financial COIs*. While some financial COIs are unavoidable in academic research due to funding requirements, transparency and critical evaluation by the consumer are essential. Additionally, Dr. Special and Dr. Pragmatic seem to have an *interpersonal conflict*, at least on a professional level.

Other Conflicts in Medicine

You will also need to manage many other conflicts of interest in medicine. The main types include misplaced financial incentives, self-referrals, and research study recruitment. Physicians have been described as *double agents* in sub-optimally designed clinical trials, where maximizing enrollment may conflict with patient well-being.[166-168] Still, these factors are not always unethical or avoidable. In these cases, conflicts of interest should be managed with appropriate disclosures and mitigation measures.

Mixed Messaging

Now let's consider another source of conflict that is common in medical training—*mixed messaging*. The call for physician well-being fits well in this category. The AMA supports a Charter calling for physicians to pursue personal well-being and to consider the well-being of their colleagues, but this ideal is not always realistic, as the system may simultaneously place formidable barriers.[169] The pursuit of well-being is further complicated by *time constraint conflict*. Another powerful mixed message you will receive is whether you are a *student* or an *early physician*, which creates role confusion.

For example, during residency, you may be treated more like a student by day and an early physician by night (on call). This ambiguous role can leave trainees uncertain about appropriate behavior. Mixed messaging can create internal confusion and strife, simultaneously tugging your efforts toward two mutually exclusive ideals.

In general, to manage conflicts of mixed messaging, your best bet may be to acknowledge them, maintain an appropriately flexible mindset, and grant yourself grace when you are unable to meet both the stated and tacit expectations simultaneously. Other measures may depend on the type of mixed messaging. For well-being, this may mean finding ways to reduce barriers (time, physical, motivational) to well-being practices.

To manage the student-young physician identity conflict, realize that this is a normal part of the process, and at times you will be treated like, feel like, and act like a student and at other times a physician. In addition, to reduce your role ambiguity, proactively seek clear expectations on clinical rotations.[42]

Time

A critical conflict you must manage well for optimal performance centers on *time*. One study found that if one were to follow all evidence-based guidelines, it would take 27 hours each day to practice medicine.[170] This estimate did not factor in all professional demands on physicians and certainly did not consider the time it would take to follow their own lifestyle recommendations for patients such as fitting in 150 minutes of moderate intensity exercise each week.[171] As with many issues in this book, there's no perfect solution. The most practical approach involves prioritizing personal and professional demands and optimizing productivity.

More broadly, the underlying force behind time conflicts is a *supply-demand mismatch* and must navigate many of these in training. Other examples include limited slots for chief residents, fellows, and future staff. It is useful to keep the impact of the major conflicts that you face in mind, realizing that these can drain your emotional and physical energy. Think, are you prioritizing a research project to build your CV or learning material for clinical practice? Are you prioritizing moonlighting to boost your finances or rest to boost your well-being? Are you ordering a costly test to protect yourself from litigation or to help the patient? By identifying conflicts, you can construct tailored ways to mitigate the effects.

While the preceding conflicts are largely internal, interpersonal conflict warrants further exploration.

Interpersonal Conflict Style and Resolution

Occasional interpersonal conflicts are inevitable in medicine as in any career. We'll introduce strategies for working with a wide range of difficult people in Chapter 32, but for now, we'll introduce a general model that can be helpful in dealing with conflict resolution. These skills are essential for physicians to learn. It is important to acknowledge that most of us are uncomfortable with conflict, but experts tell us that it is useful to become more comfortable addressing conflict head-on when it arises, rather than taking a conflict-avoidant stance.[172,173] For many of us, this takes practice.

The Thomas–Killman Model of Conflict Resolution

The *Thomas–Killman Conflict Mode Instrument* defines five styles based on assertiveness (agenda) and cooperativeness (relationship-preserving; Table 9.1). A *collaborating style* is both

Table 9.1 Emphasis on Agenda (Assertiveness) (Y-Axis). Emphasis on Relationship (Cooperativeness) (X-Axis).

Competing	Collaborating
Avoiding	Accommodating

assertive and cooperative, whereas an *avoiding style* is neither. A *competing style* results from high assertiveness without cooperation, whereas *accommodating style* results from high cooperativeness with low assertiveness. Equal moderate emphasis on assertiveness and cooperativeness results in a *compromising style*.

You might use any of the five modes in certain circumstances, though you may inherently tend toward one of them over the others. Certain styles may be more suited for a given circumstance. When faced with conflict, be conscious of your mode to be sure you are using the one that best fits the situation. For example, for high-stakes conflicts like hostage negotiations, it is sometimes best to preserve a relationship because the entire thing may fall through with severe consequences if you do not,[173] though for some high-stakes conflicts at work it may be best to go all-out for the objective even if it jeopardizes the relationship.

For conflicts that involve a low-stakes topic and relationship, or when dealing with a psychopathic or Machiavellian colleague (Chapter 32), some experts suggest using an avoiding style.[174] Given the impracticality of memorizing five distinct styles, focusing on the primary dimensions of agenda and relationship is more useful.

Additional Considerations for Conflict Resolution

Most conflicts are best settled with conversations only after emotions have cooled, using techniques like those described in *Crucial Conversations*.[175] Successful implementation hinges on strong *emotional competence* (discussed in Chapter 11). Given the potential for misinterpretation, email or other electronic communication for conflict resolution is best reserved for times when there is no viable alternative or when a written record is needed.

There are various other views on conflict resolution. While Dale Carnegie mostly suggested a conflict-avoidant strategy in his book *How to Win Friends and Influence People*, other resources remind us that some forms of conflict can be a good thing if addressed in a productive way to solve problems.[172,176] A healthy dose of conflict can even enhance teamwork by reducing complacency and persistence of stale ideas. Organizational Psychologist Adam Grant has called conflict of topics (as opposed to conflict of relationships) within teams "the good fight."[177]

These diverse perspectives and strategies offer complementary approaches. In sum, learn to manage, and even embrace (though not instigate), workplace conflict—it's nearly inevitable. Furthermore, some workplace conflict can be harnessed for positive change.

Intractable Conflict

You may eventually become embroiled in a prolonged and seemingly irreconcilable conflict. In fact, around 5% of conflicts are intractable.[178] Such conflicts are often multifaceted, cannot be fixed with simple solutions,[179] and often arise in scenarios invoking strong emotions or tied to one's personal identity.[179]

Oversimplification of intractable conflicts can create problems, like reinforcing deeply entrenched black-and-white and in-group versus out-group thinking.[178] Thus, one approach to achieve resolution is to reintroduce complexity, which helps both sides see the conflict nuances from various viewpoints.[178] As difficult as it can be, it is also important to try to see the other viewpoint and to realize that resolution can become a long process. Thus, if you approach an ongoing conflict with a binary mindset of "I'm right, they're wrong, and I'll show them why," it will likely go unresolved.

Although you should understand these general concepts of intractable conflict management, there are also practical considerations for real-life medical training. After direct face-to-face attempts at resolution have failed or are clearly not options, you must either accept the situation as is or escalate it to the appropriate person. This decision depends on the parties involved, your training level, and program specifics.

If intractable conflict with other trainees arises during residency, your first point of contact will often be a senior or chief resident. When this option is available, it is usually preferable rather than escalating the issue directly to a program director (PD). This keeps the issue among the trainees and may be handled in a more effective and less threatening way. It also respects the time and energy of the PD, who will likely not want to be involved in minor squabbles.

Senior/chief residents still have one foot in the training realm and so may empathize with the situation, yet they are also more approachable and closer to being a peer, thereby keeping conflict resolution less formal. When a senior/chief resident is unable to resolve the topic, usually the next person to engage is the PD. For most topics, other individuals such as heads of a Department and Deans would only get involved if absolutely necessary for the most serious of problems.

When a colleague brings one of his conflicts to you, it is important to consider if your role is to lend support and advice as a confidant, to be a mediator, or to simply be a sounding board. When you are a mediator, such as a chief resident, it is important to listen to and learn the facts. However, too much listening and agreeing could be interpreted as taking sides. It is important to get the facts and the perceptions of both sides, find root causes, and work toward a solution once emotions have cooled down.

When helping others to a resolution, it is useful to help each party assess the importance of both the relationship and the agenda item. Uncovering misunderstandings stemming from communication style or format (e.g., misinterpreting email tone) is also crucial. There may also be perceptions of inequity or unfairness that need to be addressed.[174] Tactful questions that assume good intentions on the other side to unveil potential false assumptions such as, "Is it possible the other party intended something else instead or had a different set of facts?" can be useful. You should also focus on behavior and actions instead of assumed intentions or *ad hominem* arguments. Finally, maintain consistent messaging and approach.

Hidden Hostility

Some of your colleagues will take a *passive-aggressive approach*.[1] This method of handling conflict brings indirect expression of negative feelings and covert hostility. Their words will be discordant with their actions, though the hostile intent may be carefully veiled. Clues you are facing passive-aggressive opposition include regular delays in response relating to the topic, feigned forgetfulness, resistance to cooperation, stonewalling, and other behind-the-scenes obstruction of progress.

Triggers

Most of us have certain topics or scenarios that, when raised, can trigger fury and interpersonal conflict. Every younger sibling knows what this is: that one thing you can do or say that is sure to get under your older sibling's skin. A colleague's trigger may be unknown and may reflect insecurities, grievances, perceived past injustices, and the like. I've learned these can be difficult to predict, but when a trigger occurs, you can usually tell through subtle or overt body language and verbal clues.

Thus, it is useful to learn the trigger topics of those you work with so you can prevent fruitless angst. It is also important to understand and manage your own triggers. This does not mean trigger topics are forbidden, but if you need to bring one up, do so with care and sensitivity. Otherwise, one seemingly innocent email or comment could cascade into tension and conflict. In addition, you should seek to gain insight into your own triggers and suppress the urge to act responsively when you encounter them.

Key Takeaways

Conflict is an inevitable part of medical training, but by understanding the different types of conflicts, conflict resolution styles, and strategies for managing intractable conflicts, trainees can navigate these challenges more effectively. We'll now turn to another theme that is associated with many potential challenges during training: change.

Note

1 While no longer a formal psychiatric diagnosis (as of *DSM-IV*), passive-aggressive behavior can still warrant attention and, in some cases, treatment.

10

Change

Vance T. Lehman

Medical Training Is a Confluence of Many Changes

Personal Change

Although medical trainees come from all walks of life, as is the case for many, your life has been fairly simple prior to training—a student's life. On a personal level, this often means a life of relatively few personal belongings, no worries of homeownership, simple tax forms, no spouse, and no children. Many of your weekends are free, or at the very least, activities are optional (like sports) or flexible (like studying). You might have some concerns about budget and finance, but living off student loans and the realities of personal finance and debt have not entirely hit home just yet. You may have worked in temporary positions here and there, but these were positions with low professional responsibility.

By the end of training, many or all of these personal situations have reversed. Thus, many critical life changes arrive as a sudden surge during training, in part because medical education often coincides with the time when many people start living like an independent adult instead of a student. These changes alone, notwithstanding the additional demands of medical training, are overwhelming. Thus, you should not underestimate the impact of this convergence of major personal life changes. Some of these will be in your control, and you may want to carefully consider how you manage them, but many will be entirely out of your hands.

Academic Change

On an academic level, school has had its challenges, but the volume of material has usually been manageable with enough effort. There was no need to identify and fill in curriculum gaps to meet professional goals. The curriculum has been tailored to treat you like a student who is at the center of the educational world. Evaluations have been mostly objective, and you may have been able to get by mostly on test performance without having to consider how you are being perceived by others. Previously top students may now feel like just one of many. You have been mostly a learner rather than a teacher.

Throughout training, most of the academic circumstances will reverse as well. The formal curriculum becomes less prescriptive and self-directed study dominates. Test scores become less important. Many of your most important evaluations are subjective, at least in part. Teaching responsibilities increase. You must transition to acting like, and being judged as, a professional. Like any workplace, the environment is more authoritarian rather than

DOI: 10.1201/9781003633389-12

democratic at its core, which can take some getting used to.[152] At times, you feel peripheral to the educational system instead of its focus. Now consider that you must manage all of this in addition to the personal life changes.

But there is even more. Training is punctuated by abrupt transitions, especially the start of medical school, clinical rotations, internship, residency, and fellowship. Many transitions involve relocating to a new city and institution, both significant changes. The third year of medical school and some residencies involve frequent shifts in workload and focus.

Layers of Change from Personal to Societal

Like several other themes, such as culture and expectations, there are many relevant layers of change, too, including those at the personal, institutional, professional, and societal levels. Consider that medical education at large is rapidly changing, as outlined in Chapter 6, making it impossible to rely solely on the experiences of previous generations.

The medical field is also rapidly evolving, both in terms of knowledge and the role of technology. As soon as you learn a medical concept it is at risk of becoming outdated. Finally, society at large is dynamic, and changing societal forces (political, ideological, financial, expectations, etc.) will impact you in many ways, such as the cost and effort required for parenting.

Overall, effective change management is crucial for success in medical training. One way to manage some of the major points of change like the start of clinical rotations is by being proactive, anticipating your needs and getting ready during the off-season. The next section will provide some tips for preparation for your first transition to clinical rotations, although the general principles can be adapted to other major points of transition such as starting an internship and so on.

Before You Start: Preparing for Clinical Rotations

The transition to clinical rotations starts before you might think. It is critical to prepare as much as you can ahead of time since it can be difficult to work it in during or after long workdays. This requires proactive organization in both personal and professional spheres. This section is geared toward medical students who are starting their clinical rotations, but many of the same principles continue to apply ahead of busy times going forward.

Academic Preparation

- Study ahead for basic rotation/shelf material starting with the first rotation as part of a learning plan (i.e., plan to use the off-season).
- Practice basic patient interviewing and physical exams on simulation patients (friends, family, or even pretend patients).
- Review the main concepts of key interpersonal relationship books like *Crucial Conversations*.[175]
- Review a concise resource on key cognitive biases, logical fallacies, and decision-making processes.
- Read through the online AMA code of ethical conduct (found at https://code-medical-ethics.ama-assn.org/). This code provides a framework for ethical decision-making in clinical practice and can help you navigate challenging situations.

- Practice using major clinical resources of medical literature and practice, like PubMed, UpToDate, Cochrane Reviews, and Micromedex. Try a variety of topics but focus on those relevant to the first few rotations.
- Identify and create learning material that you can use for 5- to 10-minute segments of downtime during the day.

Personal Preparation

- Revisit your basic organization strategies such as to-do lists, calendar-approaches, and methods of prioritization.
- Organize your life to allow exercise and healthy eating while also acknowledging that you will be working some very long days without breaks.
  - Learn recipes for one or two new meals that are healthful and easy to prepare.
  - Purchase basic home equipment if you must like a jump rope, adjustable dumbbell set, exercise mat and bench, treadmill etc.
  - Integrate well-being exercises into your routine.
- Be sure your professional attire is set.
- Clear any clutter from your home and your mind.
- Get all routine appointments out of the way: haircut, dentist, eye-doctor, oil change and vehicle tune-up, passport and driver's license renewals, etc.
- Stock up on nonperishable essentials in-house, like toothpaste, toilet paper, paper towels, stamps, checkbooks, etc., so you do not have to make special trips when you should be resting.
- Sleep well and rest.
- Nurture your relationships and ensure expectations are aligned. Communicate your needs and limitations to your loved ones so they understand the demands of your training.
- Update your personal calendar and consider buying any holiday or birthday gifts you will need well ahead of time.
- Find an inspiration (person, quote, etc.) and post it prominently in your bedroom. Find something else you find humorous and do the same.
- Regardless of whether you are a snacker or not, consider finding some relatively nonperishable snacks like protein bars or trail mix with nuts to avoid succumbing to fast food too frequently.

Key Takeaways

Medical training is a confluence of myriad personal and professional changes. Managing these changes well is critical for success. When you prepare for a major transition, such as starting a round of busy clinical rotations, it is a good time to reconsider your short-term life priorities and methods of personal organization and preparation.

11

Psychology

Vance T. Lehman

Overview

This chapter bridges the evolutionary basis of human behavior with subsequent discussions of communication, well-being, and interpersonal dynamics. Thus, understanding basic psychological principles (Table 11.1) is crucial for several reasons, yet medical training often underemphasizes them. This stems partly from the *Flexner Report's* emphasis on scientific rigor, which prioritized basic sciences over behavioral sciences.[180] Importantly, understanding how others think—a key strategy for navigating the hidden curriculum—is central to psychology. Its relevance to patient care is also often overlooked.

This chapter focuses on the roles of different theories in psychology in medicine and the hidden curriculum, emotions, personality, and motivation.

Roles of Psychological Theories

While the latter half of the 20th century saw advancements in psychology's scientific foundation (including the *DSM*), medical trainees often struggle to integrate psychoanalytic, cognitive, behavioral, and biomedical approaches to similar conditions.[181] Clarifying the purpose and interrelationship of these approaches can alleviate this confusion. Most psychologists and psychiatrists now adopt an eclectic approach, recognizing the distinct roles of behavioral, cognitive, and other perspectives in various clinical contexts.[182] These diverse perspectives also illuminate different aspects of the hidden curriculum (Table 11.2).

Emotions

The Importance of Understanding Emotions

Emotions are powerful forces that shape our thoughts and actions.[181] Medical training often fails to prepare trainees for the intense emotional demands of the profession. Trainees experience a wide range of intense emotions—happiness, sadness, anger, anxiety, guilt, and more—often surfacing during crucial conversations or challenging encounters. While emotions can aid decision-making when managed effectively, uncontrolled emotions can impair judgment.[47]

For example, recognizing, examining, accepting (while modulating), and allowing anger to subside can prevent disastrous overreactions. Understanding emotions is crucial for effective decision-making, motivation, leadership, navigating subjective evaluations, habit formation, and patient care.

DOI: 10.1201/9781003633389-13

Table 11.1 Key Areas of Psychology That Are Relevant to Medicine

Abnormal psychology diagnoses
Psychological and psychiatric treatments
Approaches to patient education and counseling
EQ
Personality types
Motivation
Stress management and well-being
Cognitive biases
Leadership and management principles
Negotiation skills

Table 11.2 Different Perspectives in Psychology Relevant to the Hidden Curriculum[182]

Type	Examples in the Hidden Curriculum
Psychoanalytic	The hidden curriculum effects are mediated in part by unconscious factors and defense mechanisms
Biopsychological (or Neuroscience)	Psychological traits like personality are influenced by genetic factors
Evolutionary	Many emotional, cognitive, social psychology principles of workplace behavior reflect selected traits
Behavioral	Classical conditioning impacts aspects of medical learning
Cognitive	The study of effective learning strategies and models of cognitive reasoning is often based in this category
Sociocultural	Individualism in Western education compared to collectivism in Eastern education
Biopsychosocial	Trainees may become frustrated if they do not learn methods to address social determinants of health in practice and may depersonalize patients with unmet social needs

Nonetheless, medical trainees often receive insufficient training on this topic. Overall, it is wise to supplement your education with resources like *Emotional Intelligence* (EQ).[47] Additionally, investing time to become more attuned to your emotions pays large dividends. Self-awareness will help you optimize your own well-being, ability to learn, interactions with colleagues, and ability to treat patients. Although we cannot cover this entire topic here, it is useful to discuss a few essential concepts that are particularly helpful for medical trainees to understand.

The Anatomy of Emotion

Emotions arise from many stimuli including sensory input (visual, auditory, olfactory, taste, somatosensory), as well as thoughts and elicit physiologic responses via limbic system activation. The supratentorial human brain comprises a primitive limbic system and a more evolved rational cortex, which interact closely to inform decisions based on both emotion and reason. The limbic system's rapid processing of sensory input often precedes conscious awareness, explaining the close link between emotions, thoughts, and physiology, and the primacy of emotional responses.

Primary Versus Secondary Emotions

Emotions are either primary (basic, automatic, rapid, and short-lived) or secondary (more complex, arising from primary emotions). Distinguishing between these is helpful in managing emotionally challenging situations. *Basic emotion theory* posits a limited number of primary emotions (happiness, sadness, anger, disgust, surprise).[183-187] Emotions are cross-cultural, evidenced by shared facial expressions despite cultural variations.[188] While some resources promote reading facial expressions as an EQ skill, the reliability of this method is debated.[189]

Variations in Emotional Experience

Individual responses to similar situations vary widely, even among colleagues and patients. Some experience intense emotions, while others have blunted emotional responses or, in extreme cases, *alexithymia* (emotional blindness).[190] This helps explain differing responses to similar circumstances. Table 11.3 summarizes key concepts.

Emotional Intelligence

EQ significantly impacts various aspects of the hidden curriculum, including formal and social learning, understanding hierarchy, crucial conversations, mindfulness, interpersonal effectiveness, and core healing virtues like hope.

Table 11.3 Key Concepts of Emotions

1. Basic emotions seem to be shared across cultures[a]
2. Related to thoughts and physiology
3. Drive one to respond
4. More fleeting and variable than mood or temperament
5. An initial emotion is a primary emotion
6. A secondary emotion is a response to another emotion
7. Vary in intensity by situation and person
8. Are predominantly communicated with body language
9. Experts do not fully agree on the definition or neurologic underpinnings of emotions

[a] This concept is debated by some researchers.

Daniel Goleman identifies four main domains of EQ: self-awareness, self-management, social awareness, and relationship management.[47] Self-awareness is foundational because recognizing and naming emotions aligns the rational and emotional brain, enabling objective examination and effective responses. Develop your ability to recognize primary and secondary emotions, subconscious emotions, the interplay between thoughts and emotions, and physical manifestations of emotion.

EQ becomes *emotional competence* (EC) through practice.[47] EQ is the potential, and EC is the realization as a learned skill. Effective emotion management is crucial in medicine, yet challenges in the modern environment exist. The prevalence of smartphones may hinder self-awareness of emotions in both trainees and patients, replacing reflective processing with immediate access to social media[191].

Managing your emotions is a critical survival skill and expectation in medicine, but we face some modern-day challenges. As a native of the smartphone era, you should consider the possibility that these devices have hampered self-recognition of emotions for both you and your patients. Instead of taking time to reflect and manage emotions during formative years, teenagers these days may learn to instantly turn to phones and social media outlets.[191]

While EQ has been critiqued as being difficult to define or measure and for having mixed data on the importance in post-secondary education settings, understanding emotions and EQ and working to improve EC remain critical skills for medical trainees. By developing EC, you can improve your interpersonal interactions and your well-being.

Personality

The American Psychological Association defines personality as "characteristics and behaviors comprising an individual's unique adjustment to life, including traits, interests, drives, values, self-concept, abilities, and emotional patterns."[192] Core personality traits are basically inherent and stable, yet influenced by cultural values.[192] The concept is, therefore, a complex synthesis of traits, emotions, behaviors, and other factors.

Effective interpersonal interaction begins with self-awareness, fostering authenticity and self-confidence. This enhances preparation for presentations, meetings, and leadership roles, and cultivates a *theory of mind*—understanding others' perspectives. However, self-insight can be challenging.

Begin by identifying your personality type using a common model (discussed in the following section), and then explore how your type generally perceives situations and interacts with others. Seek candid feedback from trusted confidants and practice regular self-reflection. Finally, understand how your personality interacts with others.

Personality Pitfalls

A common pitfall is unconsciously assuming others share your personality traits.[173,193] This often goes unnoticed. For example, as an introvert, I tend to avoid improvisation, viewing it as shooting from the hip or even reckless, and prefer thoughtful consideration before responding. However, I've learned that other approaches, common among extroverts, also possess strengths. Likewise, extroverts should recognize common approaches of introverts to leverage their strengths, such as generating thoughtful analyses.

Similarly, my high conscientiousness has taught me flexibility when working with less conscientious individuals. If you're less conscientious and work for someone highly conscientious, he will expect precise and timely execution of all requests, regardless of your more flexible approach. To a highly conscientious person, requests are not casual suggestions. Make a conscious effort to be organized and detail-oriented. Understanding colleagues' personalities is key to understanding their perspectives.

Personality Models

Uncovering the personality traits of those you work with is a key component to learning how those around you think. Two common personality models are the *Myers–Briggs Type Indicator* (MBTI) and the *Big Five Model (Five-Factor Model)*. The MBTI categorizes preferences into 4 dichotomies, yielding 16 combinations, but it has faced criticism.[194]

The Big Five (Five-Factor Model) has gained prominence among personality experts. This model uses five continuous dimensions (Table 11.4),[195] predicated on methodological rigor, reliability, predictive validity, and integration with other measures like fMRI.[194] Compared to the MBTI, it offers greater comprehensiveness, better captures conscientiousness, and avoids the false dichotomy of thinking versus feeling. The Big Five Model finds application across various fields, from psychology and popular writing to political analysis and social media (use the mnemonic OCEAN).[193,196,197]

However, these models don't encompass all personality traits. Some colleagues remain unflappable, while others react strongly to minor provocations. Some are exceptionally honest, others less so.

Introversion and Shyness

Finally, Western society often favors extroversion, a concept known as the *extrovert ideal*.[198] It is commonly said that introverted, and especially shy, trainees may receive lower subjective evaluations. Outspoken individuals, even without deeper analysis, may be perceived as more intelligent and engaged, particularly if attendings don't actively solicit thoughtful input. Introverts, conversely, reflect before speaking, taking time to process information.[199]

Some advisors steer introverts toward specialties like pathology or radiology, despite the inaccuracy of such stereotypes. This advice aligns with person-environment fit theory.[200] However, avoid limiting specialty choices based solely on perceived personality fit. Many introverts excel in direct patient care, and many extroverts thrive in pathology or radiology. Introverts may be wrongly perceived as lacking interpersonal skills, despite often demonstrating excellent one-on-one communication.

Table 11.4 The Big Five Personality Model

Trait	Description
Openness	Intellectual curiosity, inventive, imaginative, likes novelty
Conscientiousness	Organization, responsibility, dependable, detail-oriented
Extroversion	Sociability, outgoing, and assertiveness
Agreeableness	Compassion, cooperative, trusting, respectful
Neuroticism	Tendency for unstable or negative emotions or states like anxiety, depression, or anger

While the stigma of introversion has lessened, misperceptions persist, and extroversion remains favored in many contexts.[198] For instance, U.S. business schools often emphasize assertive responses as a sign of competence, contrasting with introverts' thoughtful, though slower, responses.[198] This extrovert ideal also persists in medicine.

Introversion is often confused with shyness. Shyness, unlike introversion, involves discomfort, anxiety, and fear of humiliation.[198,199] In medicine, significant shyness can negatively impact evaluations, but so can excessive talking.

Many attendings are introverts, potentially aware of the extrovert bias. Experienced attendings often look beyond personality to assess skills and knowledge. Shy individuals may need extra effort to be proactive.[42] Shy trainees should prioritize rest, proactivity, and engagement during rotations. Some shy individuals may appear standoffish or gruff; Halsted's demeanor, for example, reportedly masked significant shyness.[201] Halsted was also described as shy, reclusive, and contemplative.[202] In sum, understanding personality is essential for effective communication, collaboration, and performance.

Motivation

Motivating oneself, colleagues, and patients is a critical, yet challenging, task in medicine. This is a significant challenge. The *Harvard Business Review* notes that organizational influence on employee motivation is limited.[203] However, organizational culture, shaped by founders and leaders, plays a significant role, though our influence may be limited. Even so, understanding individual motivation beyond cultural factors is crucial. Motivational theories include drive theories (biological needs), evolutionary theories (social behavior), and incentive theories (external rewards; 181).

Theories and Sources of Motivation

Consider there are many different theories and perspectives on motivation. Motivational theories include drive theories (biological needs), evolutionary theories (social behavior), and incentive theories (external rewards).[181] These theories manifest in clinical practice: drive theories in fatigued trainees, evolutionary theories in teamwork, and incentive theories in exam preparation. Other motivational factors include happiness, pleasure, power, belonging, delayed gratification, meaning, guilt, insecurity, empathy, and the need to feel important.[43,47,161,176, 204–206]

Motivation can also be categorized as intrinsic/extrinsic or controlled/self-directed,[207] though these distinctions may lack practical value.[208] As Dale Carnegie stated, "The only way to get someone to do something is to make them want to do it."[176] This underscores the importance of understanding individual perspectives and motivations.

Motivating Others

Motivating colleagues and patients is essential. As a trainee and physician, you will have many informal leadership roles. These leadership roles require collaboration toward common goals, involving diverse team members. While we can't directly know others' motivations, we can infer them from their expressed desires, enjoyment, and reasons for acting.[209]

Further, various behavior-change techniques used by physicians, including motivational interviewing (discussed elsewhere), can be applied broadly.[49,210] These principles are similar to those used in negotiation (discussed later).

Limitations of Motivation

All that said, motivation may be overrated.[208,211] Motivation is capricious; high motivation today may be absent tomorrow. Habit formation emphasizes cues and ease of action, supporting the expression that *action precedes motivation*. What's more, establishing habits can foster motivation.[212]

For example, effective routines for studying and wellness are more important than sustained motivation. Intention is a poor predictor of action (30%-40% correlation), highlighting the intention-action gap.[209] Consider New Year's resolutions. That is, even if you know what you need to do to accomplish a goal, you can still fall short.

The take-home point is that understanding the many sources of motivation and other factors that drive behavior can help you create effective strategies for achieving your goals and helping patients achieve theirs.

12

Gender-Related Topics

Vance T. Lehman, Ariela Marshall

Introduction

We'll now turn to a frequently overlooked yet crucial theme in medical training: the impact of gender. Gender biases, expectations, and power imbalances, deeply rooted in societal history, continue to significantly impact medical training.[127] These forces underpin many complex structural issues within medical training.

Despite modernization, the medical system lags behind evolving gender roles. The past century has witnessed rapid societal shifts in gender roles;[213] for example, women now outnumber men in medical school.[214] The traditional model of the male breadwinner physician is outdated, no longer reflecting the typical physician demographic or family structure.

This chapter focuses on the resulting gender-based expectations, perceptions, assumptions, and biases in medicine, while acknowledging other contributing structural factors. Specifically, we'll examine the impact on trainees, including challenges related to personal obligations, workplace dynamics, academic opportunities, specialty selection, health, family planning, income, and career advancement.

System and Peer Influences in Medical Education

Premedical Settings

Early educational experiences significantly shape perceptions of gender roles and abilities.[215–235] Premedical women experience higher attrition rates, partly due to interpretations of setbacks as indicating a poor fit for medicine and negative interactions with faculty.[236,237]

Medical Training

The hidden curriculum also influences trainees' perceptions of patients, clinical scenarios, and their roles.[238–240] For instance, clinical vignettes often portray gendered roles (e.g., female caregiver, male provider).[238,241] These subtle structural influences shape perceptions of both colleagues and patients.

One study found that medical students valued male attendings for authority and knowledge, while female attendings were seen as role models for "human" attributes like integrity.[242] Medical students also underestimate pain in female patients, reflecting societal influences, curricular gaps, and attending physician beliefs.[243,244] Gender-based assumptions

DOI: 10.1201/9781003633389-14

are prevalent among trainees, some stemming from the educational system itself. Gender biases subtly influence perceptions of patients, colleagues, and self throughout medical education. The remainder of this chapter focuses on the effects of these biases on trainees.

In summary, gender biases can be subtly introduced during medical education, influencing perceptions of patients, colleagues, and self. Recognizing these influences is crucial for mitigating their impact.

Different Expectations, Roles, and Experiences

Let's now take a moment to look more broadly than medical training. Men and women report differing personal and professional experiences, including evaluations, interpersonal interactions, perceptions, and recognition. Societal data reveal these differences in public perceptions, interactions, role segregation, legislation (e.g., Selective Service), and the gender pay gap.[213,245–249] A common perception is that women are more *communal*, while men are more *agentic* (task-oriented).[250]

Societal Expectations

These societal expectations extend to physicians' personal lives. Women physicians spend an average of 100 minutes more per day on household chores than their male counterparts, reflecting broader societal trends.[251,252] Among physicians with partners and children, women dedicate 12 more hours per week to household tasks and childcare.[253] However, this varies; some studies show male partners of full-time female physicians taking on the lion's share of household responsibilities.[254]

Workplace Expectations

General societal expectations can also impact workplace gender roles, which are reinforced by descriptive and prescriptive stereotypes.[255] Clerkship evaluations, MSPEs, and letters of recommendation all show significant differences in agentic versus communal descriptors of performance and personality.[256–262] There is evidence that masculine norms in medical school negatively impact women and LGBTQ+ students.[239,263] Men are more often perceived as leaders, and their work is more frequently cited.[264,265] Healthcare professionals associate men with career and women with family, and men with surgical specialties and women with family medicine.[266]

Formal settings (meetings, rounds, patient encounters) also reveal differing interaction patterns.[267,268] For example, female physicians are interrupted more frequently in meetings. Studies show that while both genders interrupt, men interrupt more often, and women are more likely to interrupt other women.[268]

Female physicians are more often addressed by their first names in formal settings than male physicians.[269–272] This varies by specialty and context; a first-name bias in speaker introductions at national meetings has been observed in some, but not all, specialties.[273–276] Overall, men tend to use informal introductions, while women favor formal titles.[277] Patients increasingly use first names in electronic communication, more so with female physicians.[277]

Patients can also view male and female physicians differently. Female residents and attendings receive more electronic in-box messages and spend more time responding to them.[278,279] Further, female physicians are more likely to be confused for nurses,[280] though this can happen with male physicians as well.[281]

Academic Opportunities

Furthermore, gender disparities exist in academic opportunities and recognition. Male academic physicians generally have higher publication and citation rates, though this varies by field, journal, region, and career stage.[282–292] One notable observation is that male authors are less likely to include female co-authors.[286,293] While female residents and attendings are similarly represented as first authors, they are less often listed as middle authors.[286,294] Beyond publications, women are less likely to win academic awards than men in a variety of settings.[295–300]

Addressing the Gender-Based Experiences

You might wonder, "What can I do about differences in expectations, roles, and experiences?" At home, personal efforts toward equitable home environments are crucial. At work, while you can't control others' actions, you can mitigate your own biases, use formal titles consistently, support colleagues facing bias, and promote inclusivity in academic projects.

Specialty Segregation

Specialty segregation by gender is another critical consideration. Occupational segregation by sex is widespread, affecting various fields, including medicine, both domestically and internationally.[4,301] For example, surgical fields remain predominantly male-dominated globally, even with gender parity or female predominance in training.[4] We do not fully understand the reasons for specialty segregation, but these seem to fall into two broad categories: gendered socialization and structural barriers.[4]

Socialization Factors

Gendered socialization influences specialty choices based on gender roles and preferences. One study found that about a quarter of female physicians with children chose their specialty with parenting in mind.[302] Some attendings advise female students that general practice is a default choice for those wanting children.[303] Still, it is difficult, if not impossible, to ascertain if men and women would tend to have preferences for certain specialties if the socialization factors could be subtracted.

Structural Factors

On the other hand, structural barriers include the effects of mentoring and role models, rotation evaluations, verbal comments to trainees, and practice culture. Trainees in gender-imbalanced specialties face limited access to mentors and role models, hindering guidance and work-life integration. Even male trainees in OB/GYN have reported discrimination, described in the United Kingdom as an "anti-male environment," impacting educational performance.[4] This highlights that gender bias affects both genders. Structural factors create feedback loops, resulting in lower prestige and earnings in female-dominated specialties (e.g., pediatrics).[301]

Surgical specialties often perpetuate a masculine culture valuing aggressiveness and technical skills over analytical skills.[4,304] This reflects an extreme example of how women in general must negotiate a double standard of how assertive behavior is viewed in the workplace.[255] Some women surgeons report adopting a more masculine persona to fit in.[304–306]

Regional Differences

There are also regional variations in specialty segregation, reflecting differing socialization and structural factors. For example, consider that radiology recruits more men than women in most countries but is the lowest in the United States where women comprise just over a quarter of radiology residents each year.[307] In contrast, Taiwan shows a high percentage of women in radiology (85%), suggesting the influence of cultural factors.[307]

Remain Open-Minded

Regardless of the reasons for specialty segregation, remain open-minded about specialty choices, looking beyond societal expectations. Proactively seek mentors and role models, and support colleagues challenging stereotypes. Specialty segregation is a complex issue influenced by socialization and structural factors.

In sum, specialty segregation is a persistent and complex issue in medicine, influenced by both gendered socialization and structural factors. Challenging these stereotypes, finding confidence and freedom to explore your true personal goals, and seeking diverse mentorship can help you make informed career choices.

Health Topics

Let's turn now to a couple health topics that are crucial considerations for trainees that are closely related to several other topics in this chapter, especially specialty choice, family planning, income, and burnout. That is, gender and sex affect many medical conditions directly or indirectly, for both the trainee and her patients. This chapter focuses on two examples that have profound effects on trainees—infertility and suicide.

Infertility

Infertility is an important topic for medical trainees to understand. It is common, relevant to career development, and critically impacts family and life planning. Infertility affects a high percentage of female physicians, disproportionately affecting female trainees and their partners. Female physicians often delay childbearing, experience infertility, and utilize assisted reproductive technology.

Around three-quarters of female physicians delay childbearing, and about 1 in 4 experience infertility.[302,308,309] In contrast, the infertility rate in general is about 50 percent lower (1 in 6).[310] Female physicians have their first child at an average age of 32, compared to 27 for the general population.[311] Up to a quarter seek assisted reproductive technology, but insurance coverage is often inadequate.[308,312]

Many female physicians regret delayed family planning, and some would choose different specialties or cryopreservation.[309,311] Fertility challenges negatively impact well-being and relationships.[311] Given the far-reaching impact on well-being and life trajectory for trainees, early awareness and advocacy for physical, financial, and emotional support are crucial.[313]

Suicidal Ideation

Suicidal ideation, on the other hand, disproportionately affects male physicians, exceeding that of the public.[314] The suicide rate in the United States reached a record high in 2022 at about 24 per 100,000 males and 6 per 100,000 females (despite similar attempt rates).[315] Specific risk factors for physician suicide though include burnout, depression, and medical errors.[314,316,317]

Men also face an increased risk for loneliness (which may be better characterized as social isolation and low interpersonal connectedness), which can be exacerbated during training, as discussed in Chapter 17.[318] Maintaining social connections, seeking early help, and supporting colleagues are crucial.

To summarize, gender and sex significantly impact trainee health, as illustrated by infertility and suicidal ideation. Understanding these differences, seeking appropriate support, and engaging in advocacy are important for trainee well-being.

Workplace Violence

Workplace violence is another major concern, with women facing a disproportionately high risk.[319–321] Workplace violence, defined by the WHO as "incidents where staff are abused, threatened, or assaulted in work-related circumstances,"[321] includes sexual harassment and physical violence, particularly impacting women; these are risk factors for decreased professional performance, depression, and suicidality.[320,322,323] Additionally, spillover psychological effects can impact physicians' family members and social circle.[320]

In sum, it is important to recognize the various forms of harassment and violence, utilize institutional resources, report incidents, support colleagues, and seek support when needed.[324]

The Gender Pay Gap in Medicine

Another significant issue in medicine linked to societal gender roles and the motherhood penalty is the gender pay gap. This section explores the fundamental underlying factors.

In 2023, the overall U.S. gender pay gap was approximately 81 cents on the dollar.[213] Female physicians earn 67 cents for every dollar earned by male physicians, increasing to 82 cents when accounting for specialty, hours, and experience.[213] The Bureau of Labor Statistics identifies occupational segregation as the largest measurable factor, but 70% remains unexplained.[325] Claudia Goldin's Nobel Prize–winning work sheds light on this. Goldin argues that the current pay gap is not primarily due to historically cited factors (discrimination, segregation, mentoring gaps, etc.)[1] but rather a career gap arising after childbirth.

The Career Gap

Two main factors contribute to this career gap.[213] First, higher pay is associated with long, irregular (or "greedy") jobs. Child-rearing often leads to one parent prioritizing family (usually the mother) and the other prioritizing work (usually the father). Unless there is considerable outsourcing, this arrangement is a rational way to optimize income and child-rearing within the confines of the current system.

Data support the notion that there are gender differences in work hours between male and female physicians. Early-to-mid-career male physicians historically worked about ten more hours per week than female physicians,[213,326] though this gap is narrowing. However, even brief career interruptions or part-time work result in lasting lower hourly pay. This leads to the career gap where women are more likely to have flexible and regular, but lower-paying, positions.

The Role of Career Interruptions and Part-Time Status

Career interruptions during early career development, common in medicine, are particularly detrimental, coinciding with child-rearing years. Early career interruptions, often related to childbirth, result in lasting pay disparities.[213]

One study found that nearly 40% of female physicians worked part-time or left the workforce six years post-training, compared to zero male physicians.[327] Furthermore, 75% were working part-time or considering it.[327] Partners of male physicians are four times more likely to work part-time or not at all.[253]

Making Informed Decisions

Thus, much well-intentioned advice to mitigate this gender pay gap, including the recommendations to lean-in and self-advocate, puts the onus on women to solve a systematic problem that would really require more fundamental societal change. For further information, see Claudia Goldin's work, including *Career and Family*.[213] While you can't change systemic issues, use this information to make informed decisions.

Parenting

Parental Expectations by Gender

Beyond decreased pay for female physicians, parenthood can have other substantial ramifications for physicians. For example, different societal roles and expectations exist for parents by gender. Women significantly outnumber men as stay-at-home parents.[252] Cultural and structural factors contribute to maternal discrimination in medicine.[328,329] including higher expectations, false assumptions, fewer leadership opportunities, and lack of support for maternity leave or other activities like pumping.[329]

Maternal discrimination has significant psychological, professional, and financial consequences.[329] Many women work part-time after training due to childcare demands, which is often not a choice but rather required,[329] contributing to the motherhood penalty and career gap described by Goldin. This disproportionately affects early career women, exacerbated by the COVID-19 pandemic.[213,330–332]

Addressing the structural issues underlying the pay gap and motherhood penalty is beyond this book's scope. As a trainee, understand your personal circumstances, recognize systemic factors, and communicate openly with your partner. Support new parents, offering both emotional and practical assistance.

Making Informed Decisions

Consider the joys and challenges of parenthood. The demands can seem daunting during training, and the timing is rarely ideal. There's no perfect time, and planning is essential. Professional demands and sleep deprivation are inevitable. The decision is personal, but delaying parenthood too long can be detrimental. Planning and organization are key.

Also, it is often useful to find assistance for day-to-day tasks like housecleaning or yardwork and, of course, childcare. Overall, parenthood can be a rewarding but challenging experience for medical trainees. Understanding systemic factors and planning effectively will ease the transition.

Women in Leadership

Finally, in addition to the many barriers women can face in the workplace discussed in this chapter, those aspiring to leadership in medicine face numerous other challenges. These, in part, build on several others such as the consequences of the motherhood penalty and career gaps. Career gaps reduce *career capital*, contributing to the *leaky pipeline* and fewer women in leadership positions.[213,250]

Julia Gillard, the first female prime minister of Australia (2010–2013), highlights the insufficient pipeline and challenges faced by women leaders, including sexism, the need to prove competence, and promotion during crises.[333] She also cites recent evidence that young men and women have diverged on several fronts with a resurgent push toward traditional masculinity and conservatism among many young men, which could promote a trend toward maintaining traditional masculine leaders.[334]

These factors affect training-level leadership opportunities (chief residencies, medical societies). Many effective leaders are women; consider these roles and support qualified female colleagues.

Throughout your career, it is best to avoid assumptions about leadership ability or ambition based on motherhood status, avoid writing off others for leadership positions based on part-time status, favor positions that set yourself and others up to succeed, and rethink the notion that traditional masculine traits are always desirable or required for leadership positions.

Key Takeaways

Gender-based considerations can significantly affect trainees' experience on multiple levels, at home and at work. Many of the underlying forces are hidden and can be managed more effectively when recognized and understood. Next, we consider another important demographic consideration in the hidden curriculum: generational trends.

Note

1   These may still play partial roles and potentially a major role in individual cases.

13

Generational Trends

Vance T. Lehman

When the Students Flunk the Teacher

Professor Maitland Jones, a renowned organic chemistry professor with decades of experience and author of an acclaimed textbook, was abruptly fired from New York University in 2022 at age 84. Negative student reviews cited excessive workload, difficult exams, inflexibility, lack of empathy, and limited extra credit opportunities. Jones's dismissal sparked controversy, prompting criticism of university priorities and reinforcing stereotypes about entitled younger generations. The incident highlighted concerns about student mental health, the commodification of education, and intergenerational challenges.

Perceived generational difference is a hotly debated issue affecting medical trainees. Understanding generational perspectives is crucial for navigating the training environment and for effective leadership. This chapter explores whether perceived generational shortcomings are genuine or simply age-old recurring biases. Additionally, it provides some strategies to mitigate these challenges.

The Avocado Toast Generation

Contemporary young adults are often characterized as privileged, entitled, and lacking a strong work ethic, observations that are exemplified by terms like *avocado toast generation*.[335] News articles frequently describe how the younger generations want work-life balance, flexible work hours and locations, "cool bosses," and more, having been influenced by observing overworked parents and new social media–driven entrepreneurial opportunities.[336]

The Maitland Jones case, news reports, books, and medical literature highlight the significance of this issue.[337–342] Many attendings discuss this only behind closed doors, fearing reprisal or misinterpretation.[339,341] Though a nuanced topic, generational bias among attendings is a reality. These biases may be unfounded yet difficult to challenge. However, understanding and mitigating these biases is possible.

Purported Traits of "The Younger Generation"

Now, let's consider some common perceptions of "the Younger Generation":[1]

Work Ethic and Values:

- Value personal well-being, balance, and autonomy, and request greater time off[339,344,345]
- Want jobs that both pay well and align with their personal and societal (e.g., environmental and social justice awareness) priorities[344]

DOI: 10.1201/9781003633389-15

- More likely to value diversity, equity, and inclusion commitment in their employer[345]
- Want to live in a location that is both affordable and offers nightlife opportunities
- Less trusting of their employer,[346] lower loyalty,[345] and low threshold to look for a new job[344,346]

Learning and Communication Style:

- Prefer consuming curated, high-yield information, with a low threshold to miss lectures or seminars or skip reading books that are perceived as not useful or important[343]
- Appreciate being given clearly spelled-out curricula
- Are more accustomed to multiple-choice tests of rote information than tests requiring written or verbal explanation of understanding
- Comfortable with, and often prefer, video communication[345]
- Have less fear of mistakes than generations past and spend more time in the righthand side of the inverted U learning curve (Chapter 3, low stress region)

Attitude and Expectations:

- Increased tendency to place responsibility on a teacher for performance
- Increased reliance on parents to advocate for them in college[337]
- More likely to have a sense of entitlement, such as fast-track advancements[345]
- Desire abundant feedback, but want emphasis on the positive and praise[345]
- Value abundant employer-provided career development programs and opportunities[345]
- Resistant to hierarchical organizational structures perceived as arbitrary,[344] including the needs to "pay dues," and cultural norms, such as professional attire, titles, etc.
- Prefer hybrid, but often not exclusively remote, careers
- Value work-life integration with reduction of work-related obligations when off the clock[344,345]

This compilation of subjective perceptions and survey results are inherently stereotypes and may even reflect intergenerational bias itself.[347] Younger generations feel as though the perception that they are "less capable, more opinionated, and more selfish" is unfair.[347] Internalization of negative perceptions can even harm long-term health.[348] However, are some of these perceptions accurate?

Are Generational Trends Real?

Claims of generational differences are longstanding; Hesiod criticized youth in 700 BC, while some labeled Baby Boomers as the "Me Generation" in the mid-1900s.[349] Similarly, student absenteeism is not new; the influential surgeon (and Halsted mentor) Theodor Billroth lamented poor student attendance in 1872.[350] A 1960 editorial about medical school applicants warned that "the disturbing element, however, is not only in the lessening of the quantity, but in the lower quality (intellectual ability) of the individual applicant," "only a certain percentage of high-grade persons will enter the field of medicine," and that there was a risk of that new trainees will be "of such low aptitude as to be incapable of making progress in the treatment of disease."[351]

Though each generation appears to perceive that which follows to be different, evidence suggests more recent increases in narcissistic traits, overconfidence, and entitlement, alongside a decline in empathy.[123,352,353] These ideas are prevalent in popular discourse, often reinforcing pre-existing biases. Still, interpretations vary, with some authors cautioning against *generational mythmaking*.[354]

Limitations of Generational Labels

The practice of broadly categorizing generations is controversial. Debate exists regarding whether generational differences reflect life-stage or fixed traits, but evidence suggests the former.[355] Generational differences are often attributed to biases (in-group/out-group, hindsight, attribution, illusion of moral decline), leading organizations like the Pew Research Center to abandon generational labels.[356] Experts consider these labels arbitrary, stereotype-perpetuating, and inaccurate reflections of fixed attitudes.

Understanding Generational Differences

If we accept for a moment that there is at least a grain of truth to the differences noted in the younger generation entering medicine nowadays, we should take some time to explore how these differences may have come to be. Several societal changes may have contributed to the traits of the Younger Generation.

For example, it is known that grade inflation affects pre-medical and medical education. In 2022, approximately 80% of Yale and Harvard undergraduates received A's or A–'s.[338] Mean USMLE Step 1 scores increased from 200 to around 230 between 1992 and 2018. Other contextual factors include technology, loneliness, climate change concerns, remote work, AI, student loan debt, job mobility, nonphysician providers, and trainee protections.[357] These factors may have led to the next generation's perceived need for guided learning and regular validation, a phenomenon we will explore in greater detail in the next sections.

Potential Reasons for Decreasing Initiative and Resilience

In the 1980s, concerns that U.S. children were falling behind academically led to the rise of teaching to standardized tests while concerns over abduction and changing family work structures led to *helicopter parents* and replaced free-range kid play with *structured play dates*.[337,358] In the 1990s and early 2000s, parental oversight of college activities skyrocketed, and young adults seemed to navigate college less autonomously than in the past.[337] While past generations faced accusations of rebellion, current youth are perceived as complacent and require more guidance.[349]

Interestingly, many in younger generations acknowledge a desire for more structured guidance. Modern trainees often prefer detailed learning objectives and guidelines. Still, this can reinforce the perception of fact-focused memorization and need for handholding among attendings. Experienced clinicians and other medical educators know that many aspects of medical training cannot be easily prescribed. That is, the complexity of medicine necessitates proactive learning rather than expecting explicit guidance for every conceivable scenario.[337,358]

The Self-Esteem Movement

Another factor that has been implicated in the decreasing initiative and resilience is the *self-esteem movement* that started in the 1980s.[359] While undoubtedly well-intended, some contend that it has fostered superficial and fragile self-confidence based on external rewards and praise instead of true confidence founded on experience of overcoming challenges.[360] Although controversial, this viewpoint could help explain the recent student response to

Maitland Jones and why medical attendings have become increasingly reluctant to provide constructive feedback.

Commodification of Education

The Maitland Jones case, grade inflation, and increased parental involvement also reflect the commodification of education, treating it as a consumer product. It is critical to recognize the consequences of this commodification, where enrollment, experiences, and grading prioritize student satisfaction.

For example, institutions may prioritize reputation and student satisfaction, over educational rigor or truly working in the best interest of the student's education. Student satisfaction surveys may exacerbate trainees' overconfidence bias in their ability to assess their own educational needs. Educational institutions now seek prominence in ranking systems, in part to recruit learners, but these have recently come under scrutiny as high-profile institutions have played games to rig the score and even submitted false data.[361]

Fearing Maitland Jones-like repercussions, teachers may be hesitant to provide corrective feedback. Since you ultimately will benefit from being pushed to your limits (to a safe degree and in a respectful manner), you may need to take extra measures to show you truly welcome constructive criticism.

First of all, you need to adopt a mindset that would be truly prepared to receive it; remember that honest feedback is one of the greatest gifts you can be given. Next, it is always fair to ask your teachers for feedback on what could be done better, once you establish that it is a convenient time to have such a discussion. It is important to emphasize that you really want to grow and are not just looking for compliments. It can be helpful to your mentors if you can ask about specific aspects you are trying to improve upon, such that they can direct their suggestions accordingly.

Generational Viewpoints on Duty-Hour Reform

The topic of duty-hour reform can be a source of intergenerational tensions and misalignment within medical training culture. Understanding generational viewpoints on this topic is crucial. In the past, there was a sense that living in the hospital during residency was simply *part of the deal*. Residents paid their dues while treating patients and benefiting from an experiential education. Trainees' perceptions of residency may be more influenced by duty-hour expectations than by total hours. Generational differences in expectations shape perceptions.

Prior generations may defend the legacy model for reasons that may include cognitive dissonance, rationalization, jealousy, hindsight bias, and/or inculcation into the medical culture. One longitudinal study found that attendings have a much rosier view of residency 5 years out from training compared to what they reported during training.[136] Many also truly believe that trainees and patients are being short-changed by reduced exposure to educational experiences and even propose that training should be lengthened to compensate.

Newer generations may resist marathon work weeks for an assortment of reasons, such as increased focus on well-being, concern for patient safety, overestimation of ability and/or experience, rise of individualism over hierarchy, citation of the support offered by accrediting bodies and graduate schools (who are also supportive of work-hour restrictions), resentment regarding the increasing percentage of worktime spent on clerical tasks rather than direct patient care, and/or diminished promise of prestige for the time investment or opportunity cost.[362]

Despite recent regulations aiming to protect residents from being overworked, the work-hour reform debate has, if anything, heated up. A recent commentary by cardiologist Dr. Lisa Rosenbaum in the *NEJM* directly addresses the broader training situation.[339] The overall message is that "once-routine aspects of training are now deemed potentially harmful."[339]

For many reasons, some trainees exceed official duty-hour limits, skip wellness days to get in more OR time, etc., and these actions potentially create inter-trainee conflict. In response, other attendings and trainees express alternative perspectives, such as a continued need to counter trainee exploitation.[363,364]

Navigating Generational Perceptions

What is the reality? Even with evidence of intergenerational bias, many attendings maintain that significant generational differences exist. You should seek to understand attending perspectives and employ impression management strategies.

Among the most critical perceptions to manage—and ones that are under your control—relate to punctuality and commitment. That is, demonstrate equal or greater commitment to patient care and your education than your attending. Make a reasonable effort to arrive on time and avoid leaving early (typically when there are ongoing clinical tasks and the attending or senior resident is still present). It is especially important to avoid asking to leave early for optional personal reasons—such as group exercise classes, desire to beat rush hour traffic, ordinary pet care, routine appointments, or because it is a nice day outside. Doing so almost ensures that the episode will be discussed in an unfavorable light and reinforces generational stereotypes.

In summary, regardless of the reality of generational differences, managing perceptions is crucial for success in medical training. It is critical to demonstrate commitment, responsibility, and a strong work ethic to help mitigate the effects of generational perceptions and bias.

Note

1 While younger professionals (essentially millennials and members of Generation Z) are grouped here for simplicity, there are some differences between reported trends between these groups.

14

Expectations

Vance T. Lehman

Introduction

Consider the profound and widespread expectations placed upon you. Effective management is crucial for optimal performance in training. These expectations shape perceptions and outcomes. While some are universal, others are specific to the medical profession. Expectations seem abstract but have tangible physiological effects. They influence brain activity and neurotransmitter release; for instance, positive situations trigger dopamine release, creating expectations of future positive feelings (such as in habit formation, Chapter 23).[208]

Previous chapters explored the impact of expectations on training, including basic, gender-related, and generational factors. This chapter broadens the scope to a theme, examining expectations from various sources. Expectations from the broadest to narrowest sources—the government and society at large, governing bodies in medicine, our profession, our family, and ourselves—compete for our limited time and energy.

Broader Expectations

Societal Expectations

Starting broadly, society has long petitioned physicians to uphold near-universal professional etiquette and to be pillars of their community.[365] This includes being stewards of community health and philanthropy, having appropriate public (or social media) presentation, demonstrating the social savvy to avoid politics and religion during public conversation, and showing basic social graces. These societal forces have profound effects on our daily lives and, by extension, on our professional experience.

Managing Personal Administrative Tasks

We must also manage many other societal demands that tend to increase during medical training. These range from tax filings to medical license renewals. Electronic communication blurs work-life boundaries, increasing expectations of immediate availability. Numerous other examples exist. The goal here is not to list them all, but to call attention to the fact that these tasks will probably consume a higher percentage of your time and energy than you would predict, so you should plan accordingly. These are also good reasons to favor a simple/minimalist lifestyle in medical training.

DOI: 10.1201/9781003633389-16

Societal Expectations of Parents

Building off the discussion of parenthood in training from Chapter 12, heightened societal expectations on modern parents, particularly physician parents, warrant attention. Remember, there's no ideal time for parenthood, regardless of training status. There will always be professional obligations vying for your attention, and newborns in the house will (nearly) always lead to sleep-deprived nights. Professional demands and sleep deprivation are inevitable.

Nowadays, the organization of family activity calendars alone, particularly in homes with busy school-aged children, could be a full-time job. The numerous strains on parents from these realities and other developments like social comparisons on social media even prompted a surgeon general advisory on parenting stress in 2024.[366]

In summary, modern societal expectations place a wide range of demands on medical trainees, requiring careful time management and prioritization. It is critical to recognize these expectations and plan accordingly to both serve the greater demands of society and to maintain a healthy work-life balance.

Profession-Level Expectations

Now, let's examine the expectations and requirements that come from the medical establishment. The online AMA article "The Premed Competencies for Entering Medical Students" outlines 17 skills expected of ideal students.[367] These competencies encompass preprofessional skills, living systems knowledge, and critical thinking abilities.[367] However, this list doesn't align with premedical coursework, highlighting a disconnect between stated expectations and formal preparation.

Instead, the emphasis is on traits like "ethical responsibility" and "resilience and adaptability," raising questions about the lack of formal preparation for these acknowledged skills.[367] Although this list makes important inroads, it doesn't fully capture the hidden curriculum's expectations.

As your career progresses, you will face many other professional-level expectations—like becoming a member of a specialty board, taking an initial and re-certification examination, and paying state licensing and various medical society dues. For example, a joint commission requirement for outlier radiologist performance screening cost over a billion dollars over 15 years, yielded minimal results, and negatively impacted safety culture.[368]

Daily Expectations at Work

Attending-Level Expectations

Now, let's consider trainee expectations that arise daily, starting with those from attendings. There are as many sets of expectations as there are attendings, often diverging from those of the formal objectives or other attendings. Complicating matters further, attendings do not always reveal their true expectations. Instead, they might complain straight to the education leadership, only mark it down on your evaluation after the fact, or say nothing at all.

Several factors contribute to this: perceived effort, an "adult learning" philosophy, or the belief that expectations are self-evident. They may also believe that if they must tell you, it is already too late. Finally, the attending might blame the education leadership/committee for unclear instructions (which still doesn't get you off the hook). Therefore, actively discern each attending's expectations. Failure to do so can lead to poor performance, potentially creating a negative feedback loop between a trainee and an attending resulting in a *set-up-to-fail syndrome*.[203]

In addition, subjective grading on clerkships has been criticized but remains a reality.[369] While we have limited ability to solve the underlying structural limitations, we can tilt the subjective component in our favor by understanding expectations. Overall, meeting attendings' expectations requires proactive feedback, seeking and adapting to individual preferences. Beyond aiming for positive evaluations, uncovering attending-level expectations can help ensure a smooth and productive educational experience.

Patient-Level Expectations

Patients also rightfully have high expectations of physicians (and trainees). One challenge with this is that sometimes it seems that patients expect that physicians know everything medicine related. This is not to say that patients do not understand physicians have limitations. Mostly they do, but patients sometimes need clarification regarding physician expertise. Meeting or managing such patient expectations is a key skill. When faced with a question that is better posed for someone else or one you simply do not know, a polite reminder of your scope of expertise and an offer of an alternative source will usually suffice.

Additionally, there has been increased focus on patient expectations regarding medical care and physician interactions during the past couple decades.[370] Some expectations are near universal, such as being empathic and trustworthy.[370] Most patients prefer physicians in formal attire, especially scrubs and white coats.[371] Other expectations, though, vary by patient traits such as anxiety level or personality.[370] Thus, "personalized communication will be needed as well as personalized health care."[370] Furthermore, patient expectations has become a larger consideration with increasing use of patient satisfaction surveys after clinical visits.

Other patient expectations are not emphasized in medical training. Here is just one example: happiness. One *Huffington Post* article asks, "When was the last time a doctor asked you if you are feeling happy and satisfied with your life?" The same article explains this by the fact that "happiness does not have a drug rep."[372] So, shouldn't we understand what happiness is and how it impacts physician and patient well-being? It turns out that there are many important things we should be exploring about happiness like 'has humanism inadvertently pathologized (un)happiness?' and "who bears responsibility for trainee happiness" that are considered in other resources.[341]

How can you possibly learn about all the side topics like happiness on top of the formal curriculum? It is a major challenge and takes time. To start though, simply being aware of the expectations will help you soak in information as you come across it.

In sum, patients have diverse expectations, many beyond formal training, requiring effective communication and personalized care. Understanding and managing these expectations is essential for strong patient-physician relationships.

Colleague Expectations

Your colleagues will also have expectations for you at every level in medical training and beyond. These include teamwork, fair workload distribution, competent patient care, and responsible work attendance. Reliable colleagues are valued, as are fair work practices and transparent decision-making. Further, our tendency to overestimate our own contributions can hinder meeting peer expectations.

Personal Expectations

Significant Other Expectations

Another crucial consideration is your significant other's expectations. Unmet expectations can cause significant relationship stress during training. This includes discussion of possible career trajectories, work hours, at-home work, other time-consuming activities, domestic duties, family planning (or pet adoption planning), finances, together time, and a plan for managing stressful times as a team. There is no one-size-fits-all solution, but periodic check-ins and agreement for reasonable flexibility are essential.

Self-Expectations

One source of expectations *always* lurks in your shadows—those from within. High expectations for personal achievement can be functional or, if unrealistic, detrimental (further discussed in Chapter 24). Focus on effort and dedication that are entirely in your control rather than things that are not—grades and accolades. In fact, the greatest rewards come from patient care, even if often unacknowledged beyond the patient and family.

However, self-expectation adjustments may be necessary. For example, balancing extensive leisure activities with academic success requires prioritization. Competitive residencies demand significant commitment and prioritization. Entering a competitive program without sufficient effort can lead to disappointment.

You should also consider whether your expectations are your own or imposed by others. For example, unrealistic parental expectations can cause anxiety and impair performance,[373] increasing burnout risk and negative perceptions of medical practice.[373,374]

Finally, consider that your satisfaction is relative to your expectations. Increased vacation time or number of wellness days compared to past generations of trainees, for example, quickly becomes viewed as the norm rather than a bonus benefit. Overall, setting realistic and healthy self-expectations is crucial for maintaining well-being (Chapter 17), avoiding burnout (Chapter 17), and forming habits (Chapter 23). Focusing on effort, dedication, and the rewards of patient care can help you stay motivated and fulfilled.

Your Expectations of Others

Beyond self-expectations, consider your expectations of others. Avoid creating counterproductive expectations for those you supervise. Clear expectations are essential for effective leadership and feedback. Remember that your expectations and appraisal of others are unique and probably differ from each of your colleagues.

Unclear expectations hinder your ability to provide effective feedback. Others may be meeting their own expectations, unaware of yours. Negative feedback over unspoken expectations leads to confusion and frustration. The outcomes will be much more positive when expectations are casually, but clearly, set ahead of time. People will tend to live up to realistic expectations, and when you provide positive feedback for the expectations they meet, a positive feedback loop results.[160]

Key Takeaways

This chapter highlights both universal and physician-specific expectations, both overt and covert. Hidden expectations in training directly contribute to the hidden curriculum.
A myriad of broader expectations also create significant challenges, competing for time and energy and substantially impacting the training experience. Thus, recognizing and managing expectations effectively is critical for success in medical training.

15

Communication

Vance T. Lehman

The Importance of Communication Skills

Effective communication skills are a key differentiating factor for a successful medical trainee. Two of the AAMC's top 17 competencies expected of incoming medical students relate directly to communication—oral and written.[367] However, no new medical student is already an outstanding communicator in all professional situations. While we can expect a college graduate to have basic communication skills, mastery of medical writing and oral presentation usually takes many additional years of refinement. Still, I find that many, if not most, trainees underestimate their need to work on their communication skills.

The First Step: Know Your Audience

The first step to effective communication taught in an introductory communications class is simple: knowing your audience. Failure of messaging has brought down politicians, university presidents, and CEOs at the highest levels, so it is important for the rest of us too. Therefore, be sure to tailor your communication to your audience, whether it's a patient, peer, attending, student, insurance company representative, or anyone else.

An Overarching Principle: Be Clear and Concise

Second, for all forms of communication, you should be clear and concise. We'll see why it is a mistake to garnish communication with excess jargon, filler words, and verbosity.

Effective Communication Takes Practice

Third, communication is a modifiable skill set that requires preparation, execution, and reflection. Too often, we focus on the execution phase without adequate preparation or reflection. A professional actor does not show up on set and then learn how to get into character while filming. He practices the character and lines at home first. If professional actors cannot do it, neither can we. So, whether it is for a formal lecture, presentation on rounds, progress notes, a crucial conversation, or sending out an official email, it is useful to plan it out and practice. Internal debriefings, self-reflection, and seeking feedback are useful after an event.

 DOI: 10.1201/9781003633389-17

The Importance of Active Listening

Fourth, active listening is one of the most important skills in all areas of medical practice, including listening to patients, superiors, and colleagues. Many trainees fall short here, so remember that it requires unfettered attention, an open clear mind, appropriate reflection, and summarization. In contrast, selective listening confirms prior beliefs, and unrequited monologues can fail to reveal vital information.

Other General Considerations

Other key general topics include body language, timing, clarity, listening, checking for understanding, and mutual respect. Remember that emotions are largely conveyed through body language and tone. Additionally, we continuously transmit body language signals, even when just tagging along on rounds.

Finally, a key concept of persuasion and negotiation in medicine is conveying that your stance is for the greater good rather than any self-serving purpose—and to practice regular self-reflection to ensure that your motivations remain true to this purpose. This approach to interpersonal communication is most likely to resonate and gain support and typically requires putting the needs of patient care and the true professional missions first.

Interpersonal Space

In Western culture, we have four zones of interpersonal space: intimate (up to 18 inches), personal (18-48 inches), social (48 inches to 12 feet), and public (greater than 12 feet).[375] [1] These descriptions of zones are overly simplistic in that they ignore other aspects of interactions such as the direction of eye gaze, mood, type of occasion, and physical layout of the environment.[376] Nonetheless, the zone concept is useful for you to know for several reasons.

Above all, you must avoid intimate zone violations. One inadvertent intimate zone violation occurs with electronic meetings, when someone leans in too close to the camera. Instead, set your position relative to the camera to simulate a personal zone, especially on calls with people you do not know well. If you are a highly social extrovert, be aware that you may be more likely to encroach the intimate zone on camera or in person, which may make others, particularly more reserved introverts, uncomfortable.

For public speaking, it is useful to understand that details of facial expression and subtle gestures are lost in the public zone, especially at distances greater than 30 feet.[375] Therefore, public speakers benefit from optimizing larger gestures and body stance.[375]

That said, interpersonal space is relative and situational. For example, it is more acceptable to come within an intimate zone in crowded situations. In medical settings, operating room (OR) staff work very closely in a tight area for hours at a time. This proximity is necessary, given the need for multiple individuals to work on one area of the patient's body. Additionally, the concept of space and personal zones varies by culture, so we may need to allow some flexibility in medicine when interacting with people of all backgrounds.[376]

Nonverbal and Paralinguistic Communication

Charles Darwin's *On the Expressions of the Emotions in Man and Animal* ushered in the modern study of nonverbal communication. Nowadays, a classic teaching in communication is that the meaning of communication is 7% words, 38% vocal tone, and 55% body language. However, this data originates from two heavily critiqued 1967 papers,[377,378] and best applies to situations where words and other communication are discordant.[379] Nonetheless, body language and tone are still important even if less impactful than traditionally taught.

Body Language

The formal medical school curriculum includes training on patient interactions and interviewing but may shortchange useful concepts in nonverbal communication. I have found that this is more important than I initially realized because we are constantly transmitting messages, and some may be very different than what we intend. There are, fortunately, a variety of resources with various perspectives at your disposal.[176,193,380]

Common themes of these resources include using body language in a way that builds trust, warmth, and connection. Various techniques such as appropriate eye contact, keeping your hands visible, keeping confident posture, using a genuine smile, pointing feet toward the person you are talking to, and being relaxed instead of catatonic or fidgety. In addition, you must seek feedback, indicate vulnerability to feedback, and remain cognizant of how you are feeling and acting.

For example, hand visibility is an important indicator of trust. This holds true with in-person interactions, on a podium, or even video calls. In each scenario, your hands should be out of your pockets. Formal podium presentations are delivered at the public zone, where body language counts a lot and hand visibility is important for communication and trust. Too often, speakers hide their hands or continuously clutch the podium or computer mouse. Hands should even be visible on video calls from time to time through minor hand gestures or a friendly upfront wave.

Eye Contact

Another important concept is eye contact, which fosters trust, warmth, and connection.[193,380] Experts believe that the human eye evolved with a relatively large amount of exposed white sclera to help us gauge where others are looking.[381] In fact, in the public zone, we mostly discern the white sclera rather than eye color.[375] Regarding the optimal amount of eye contact in a conversation, the communications company Quantified suggests a rate around 60%–70%, slightly more so when listening than when talking.[382] Functional brain imaging studies are starting to unravel neuronal pathways that are activated with eye contact, suggesting the effects require real-time interaction and may not transfer to video calls.[383,384]

However, sustained direct eye contact (especially greater than ten seconds) could be seen as aggressive or even threatening.[382] Further, some data find that true eye-to-eye contact is infrequent, while general eye-to-face gaze is more common, suggesting it may be more natural to look at someone but to limit duration of locked deep eye gaze.[385] True direct eye contact also requires mental effort and may lower ability to think critically.[386]

In her book *How to Improve Doctor Patient Connection*, Dr. Christine Ko suggests making a mental note of a patient's eye color at the beginning of patient encounters to ensure eye contact.[387] Lowndes introduces a concept called "sticky eyes," suggesting we think of our eyes as glued to another's (with some caveats) and do not turn away too rapidly.[380] When using these techniques, however, keep differences in cultural norms in mind.

The Smile

Many resources suggest enhanced connection through a genuine, instead of a feigned smile. It is said you can see a real smile (aka Duchenne smile) in one's eyes, with slight wrinkling of the skin along the lateral margin (crow's feet).[388] Though this seems to hold up in real life, there is also evidence that these features are mostly indicators of smile intensity.[388,389] Either way, overdoing a smile could be perceived as disingenuous, so some recommend a slight pause before smiling so that it looks like a genuine reaction.[380] Perhaps the best advice is to have a genuinely open attitude toward the conversation partner so authentic and appropriately timed smiles come naturally.

Since Darwin's book, the preponderance of research on emotional expression has focused on facial expressions. We have in-born mechanisms to mirror the facial expressions and mannerisms of others, the *chameleon effect*.[390,391] Mimicking may be an empathy catalyst, as suggested by video-monitored fMRI and psychosocial studies that have found that facial expressions and emotions are "contagious."[391] This means your aura may not only be noticed by others but also felt in physical and physiological ways.[193,391]

Paralinguistic Factors

It is also useful to fine-tune paralinguistic factors like voice tone, pitch, speed, and volume. In general, with patient interactions it is best to error on the slower pace and deeper range of your natural pitch range. You may need to adjust your volume if a patient has hearing impairment, but in general a moderate volume works well. Speaking too softly can be misinterpreted as lack of confidence, though occasionally patients are annoyed if their physician talks too loudly. Finally, when talking to patients or colleagues, avoid ending sentences with upward pitch unless you are intentionally trying to convey lack of confidence or to ask a question.

Caveats

While there is no doubt that the concepts of nonverbal communication are important, we must be cautious not to over-interpret the conclusions and advice from popular resources. Some experts believe that common teachings are not well-supported by evidence. For example, they point out that body language lacks syntax and consistent meaning.[376] They also question the teachings that facial expressions are true indicators of inner emotions and are universal across cultures.[376]

The main practical implication is that we should not read too much into our perceptions of the body language of others but be aware that our own body language does send signals, perhaps some we do not intend, to others.

Introductions and First Impressions

Introductions and first impressions carry such importance that these topics receive extra attention in books on interpersonal skills and communication. The impact of first impressions are also reinforced elsewhere in this book. We already saw how first impressions can amplify via labeling effects in Chapter 2 and will expand on their importance on clinical rotations in Chapter 36. Here, we'll focus on impression related to introductions.

One common theme is that introductions are an opportunity to highlight interesting or relevant traits and facts of yourself or others.[193,380] For example, when introducing one acquaintance to another, go beyond simply stating names and offer additional background that paints the new person in a positive light. Depending on context, this could mean personal or professional accolades. For example, "Dr. Mason, this is Dr. Lee, one of our star pediatric neurologists on staff. She is doing incredible research on the topic of seizure management, and she was just elected vice president of our national society."

The introduction is also the time to learn a person's name so you can repeat it. Except for situations where a formal title is standard, people generally love the sound of their own first names.[176] Using first names can help two people connect. It can take practice but try to form the habit of paying close attention to the names of new acquaintances. This often means using minor mental tricks like repeating it to yourself, repeating the name out loud as part of the introduction, or visualization tactics (e.g., for Dawn, envision the person's face at dawn). One semiformal situation to keep in mind is meeting a patient for the first time.

Formal Titles

While we usually use first names for pediatric patients and young adults, consider starting with a formal title for anyone else and be sure to get it right. This means you should determine, when possible, if the title is Mr., Ms., Mrs., Dr., reverend, or anything else before you meet the patient. Of these, it is especially important to avoid omitting a doctorate level title or calling someone Mrs. when she goes by Ms.

Whether during an introduction or other setting, there will be times when others get your title wrong or just opt not to use it. Some patients or other colleagues will still call you by your first name even if you introduce yourself formally. It is tempting to ascribe a reason to this thinking: "It is due to my age, my appearance, my gender, or is a lack of acknowledgment of respect." While one of those things *might* be true, this will happen to everyone, and it is counterproductive to dwell on it. Perhaps the person feels at ease working with you, for example. In most cases, it is best just to let it go.

Handshakes

An introduction is a key time to use the all-important handshake. During the COVID-19 pandemic, many predicted a handshake extinction, but it has made a defiant comeback. In medicine, opinions about if or when we should shake hands run the gamut, but regardless of where your personal feelings on this topic lie, this remains a standard business practice. While fist-bumps and elbow taps have been used as hygienic substitutes to the handshake, they are also awkward in their own way and do not bring the same interpersonal connection. Further, applicants with higher quality handshakes during an interview are rated as more employable, and a handshake at the start of a negotiation signals the intention for cooperative deal-making.[392,393]

We can further consider handshakes in the context of routine socialization, patient care, attending interactions, and business interactions. Though data are conflicting, it seems that most patients still prefer to shake hands with their physicians.[394] Conversely, for whatever reason, some attendings do not routinely offer or want a handshake with their trainees. Be aware that the preference varies by situation and person. When making introductions with patients and their families, it is important to read their body language regarding their preferences for a handshake and, when in doubt—ask.

Formal Presentations

There was a societal shift from a *culture of character* to a *culture of personality* during the early 1900s, which placed greater pressure on everyday people to sell themselves with public speaking performances.[198] According to Cain, this was exemplified by Dale Carnegie's rise from a farm boy to public speaking guru.[198] It holds that in modern medicine, as in business and other facets of life, there is a premium on polished, confident oral communication skills.

Some trainees worry that over-rehearsal will lead to a robotic, unnatural oral presentations. This concern is largely overblown. To reduce anxiety about sounding too rehearsed, one can limit the memorization to just a few reminder words for each major concept and vary the dialogue during practice. For neophytes, proper preparation and rehearsal should include attention to expression and intonation but still leave some room for flexibility. Still, a presentation that sounds mildly rehearsed is still far preferable to one that is underprepared.

Written Communication

In medicine, it is critical to master the art of written communication. We'll explore this in greater detail in Chapter 25, including general writing concepts, medical manuscript composition, and clinical notes and reports. For now, we'll introduce a few basic concepts.

The style of written communication makes a tremendous difference in how it is perceived and conveys the intended points. However, certain aspects of this competency have probably been compromised in the era of electronic communication. The tone of a message has a particular risk of misinterpretation with electronic communication. There is no voice volume, speed, pitch, body language, or opportunity for clarification to help convey the message and no human being in front of you to offer verbal or nonverbal feedback—just a screen. Even exclamation marks and emojis, while sometimes helpful to convey tone, must be used judiciously, since these can be misinterpreted as well. One person's genuine smiley face is another's passive-aggressive gesture or emblem of naivety.

Thank You Notes and Cover Letters

Two forms of written communication deserve special attention: thank-you notes and cover letters. During recent years, many applicants omit cover letters for physician job applications when not absolutely required during the application process or skip thank-you letters after interviews (for physician trainee or staff positions). While an absent cover letter or thank-you note may not compromise your chances at a position, it is a missed opportunity to demonstrate your professionalism, attention to detail, elaborate on reasons why you are applying for a job and why it could be a great fit, and expressing your gratitude to the interview team for their effort and consideration.

Not too long ago, medical students wrote personalized thank-you letters and address envelopes in airport lobbies and flights home after in-person residency interviews. While electronic thank-you notes are now entirely acceptable and perhaps even preferable because they can be timelier, even those are nearing extinction. Certainly, you can argue that this is time wasted since thank-you notes may not affect the applicant's position on residency or fellowship rank-order. Still, if there is a position you strongly desire, there is no good reason not to send a thank-you note, and it might help you if you do. It is an easy thing that you ought to get right.

The ideal thank you note will be personalized to the intended recipient (e.g. follow-up on something discussed during the interview). If you decide to cut and paste portions of a note, be sure that all personalized portions are appropriately updated—sometimes they are not! The single exception for never writing thank-you notes would be for programs that explicitly instruct you not to send them. There are many other occasions to send thank-you notes as well; if it even crosses your mind, it is probably a good idea.

Negotiation

We negotiate constantly in medicine and in life. We negotiate with our bosses/supervisors, prospective employers, patients, peers, our family and even ourselves. Negotiation can help us gather information and influence behavior.[173] Sometimes the stakes are paramount—whether to take a critically ill patient to surgery or whether to take a new job in a distant city—and other times, the stakes are minor—who will clean the house this week (though little things can matter a lot, too). We have all seen the good cop/bad cop routine, local union-employer standoffs, and price talks with a car salesperson, but negotiations are often subtler.

Positions and Interests

We cannot cover the entire topic of negotiation here, but we can introduce the critical concepts. Since its publication in 1981, *Getting to Yes* has become the quintessential popular guide to negotiation in business, politics, and life.[395] This book introduced central concepts like distinguishing *interests* and *positions*, predetermining a *best alternative to a negotiated agreement* (BATNA), and separating people from the process.

A position is a formal ask or surface stance. An interest represents what someone really wants—his true underlying motives and goals—but is often cloaked in a different formal ask (the position). Negotiation novices tend to focus too much on the position instead of the interest. A position might be a concrete ask such as a pay raise, when the interest is obtaining more control over one's schedule or receiving respectful treatment, for example.

Uncovering interests, in negotiation or elsewhere, is one way we figure out how others think and what they truly want. This is done by establishing rapport, active listening, searching for underlying motives (e.g. asking why someone has a position), showing empathy, and by deploying other communication tactics like summarizing (note that these are not always appropriate though, depending on the situation). Understanding interests is also needed to find true *common ground*.

However, as a counter example, the book *Never Split the Difference* describes a reaction to the shortcomings of the academic *Getting to Yes* approach in high-stakes real life situations like hostage negotiation. Fifty-fifty compromise is portrayed as a lose-lose proposition. Instead, humans make negotiation decisions based on cognitive biases like anchoring and emotions rather than pure objective calculations. It is often best to let the other side think they are in control of the decision-making and to help guide them with open-ended questions and active listening to arrive at your point of view on their own. Other resources acknowledge the importance of anchoring with an aspirational (but not outrageous) initial ask since the (perceived) concession that follows gives the negotiator leverage and the upper hand.[160]

Negotiating on Uneven Ground

Finally, the general popular guides for negotiation do not factor in instances where there are large differences in expertise between the two parties. In medicine, one party in a negotiation commonly has far greater experience or knowledge than the other (e.g. a physician negotiating the best course of treatment with the patient; a world-expert subspecialist discussing a related diagnosis with a resident). If you are an expert on a topic and open by leveling the playing field and conveying too much humility when negotiating against an overconfident, but less experienced counterpart, the weight of your expertise in the negotiation is compromised.

Key Takeaways

Effective communication is a key way that trainees can show competence, convey ideas, and form relationships, but it requires substantial and sustained work on multiple fronts. It is important to critically examine your own communication style and to seek candid feedback about how your written, oral, and body language communication is perceived by others. The ability to communicate effectively and tactfully is also a component of our next theme: professionalism.

Note

1   Edward T. Hall named the study of interpersonal zones *proxemics*.

16

Professionalism

Vance T. Lehman

Introduction

Matters of professionalism are crucial components of the hidden curriculum in medical training for several reasons. First, it is often said that people are *hired for ability and fired for attitude*, and while professionalism entails more than pure attitude, the general idea still holds. Additionally, a major effect of the hidden curriculum is teaching professional norms, which can have both positive and negative effects. Physicians experience periods of stress, making it easier to slip into unprofessional behavior, but these are the most critical times to maintain professionalism.

There are also societal, professional, patient-level, and peer-level expectations that physicians act professionally, a trait that underlies public trust in the profession.[396] Some professional lapses can jeopardize patient confidentiality and cause great harm. We are hardwired to do what others around us do, often regardless of what we formally have been taught to do,[160] and you will be judged (graded) by your professionalism and appearance in ways that are both conscious and unconscious as well as fair and unfair.[160,397]

However, the concept of professionalism is elusive, defined differently by different institutions and people.[398] It encompasses various aspects, including conduct, intrinsic attributes, ability, presentation, and interactions with others (one article describes 19 dimensions of professionalism, for example).[398] The difficulty in defining professionalism makes it hard to teach. Therefore, even though many professionalism standards are near-universal, it is still useful to seek out unique standards of your environment such as an institutional dress code.

Given the multifaceted nature of this topic, we'll focus on the areas that are most practical and important for medical trainees to know in this chapter, including major and minor lapses in professionalism, being your authentic self, etiquette, potential negative effects on trainees, individuality, and a few ways to manage these topics. Further, since professionalism plays a central role in medicine, related topics are found in many other chapters too and specific considerations for clinical rotations are given a dedicated chapter in Part V.

Lapses in Professionalism

In the long run, trainee professionalism lapses in training predict the likelihood of future professionalism struggles.[399] In the short run, serious infractions can completely curb your career, minor lapses can have substantial cascading effects, and trainees can inadvertently adopt bad practices if they are not careful. While you should try to avoid them, occasional minor lapses in professionalism are a part of normal professional development and should be

DOI: 10.1201/9781003633389-18

viewed as such.[400] If you receive feedback or corrective action for a minor lapse, view it as a growth opportunity rather than a punishment.

Serious Lapses

Above all though, you must avoid *serious* lapses of professionalism. This is where even the most talented trainees typically encounter the most trouble. For example, trainees are skating on thin ice if they lie about factors that impact patient care (e.g. fabricating results, covering up mistakes, etc.), misuse the electronic medical record (EMR), break patient confidentiality, lie about reasons for being away from work, or harass other people. Serious lapses away from the work setting such as posting unwise and offensive items to social media accounts can also have serious ramifications, as we'll see.

Minor Lapses

While serious lapses are the most critical, the less serious (but still problematic) ones are much more common. In addition to the crucial importance of the basic expectations (Chapter 2), remember that general societal norms of professionalism and etiquette also apply to medical training. Public debates or pronouncements of religion, politics, or personal finance are generally taboo at work just as they are at a dinner party. This does not mean that the topics are never appropriate, but consider the audience, purpose, and tone. Be particularly sensitive if you are within earshot of patients, colleagues you do not know well, or individuals with different life circumstances.

Now, we'll take a close look at two other categories that, while not usually serious, deserve some special attention. These are behaviors that can annoy colleagues. Since you rely on those around you for collaboration and evaluations, you want to avoid irritating them or even triggering too many of their pet peeves.

Just Be Your Authentic Self…with a Caveat

The common adage *just be yourself* is found in social settings, negotiation books, and leadership books alike.[173,401] This reflects the idea that people have a sixth sense for real versus inauthentic self-presentation,[1] but is this always sound advice for medical trainees? As is common in medical training, the answer is complicated. That is, trainees should be comfortable in their own skin and not have to constantly second guess their words or actions.

Self-restraint complements our authentic selves. Unfiltered, informal conduct as one would have with family, for example, may not be the best side to show at work. Off-color jokes, boisterous banter or interruptions, complete silliness, negativity, and many other things may be considered unprofessional or strike a nerve with a colleague or attending. Be authentic but always make it your best professional self.

Bad Habits and Etiquette

Little Annoyances

Though the basic expectations form the core group of minimum standards, there is another layer of expectations that, if violated, make your professional life more challenging—common etiquette.

For starters, think of distractions that annoy you when you are trying to concentrate, at a testing center for example. What if an oblivious person sitting next to you were whistling or aggressively smacking gum? What if his phone notifications blurted out a 120-decibel chime? What if she kept sneezing or coughing without covering their face? What if he decides to take a break and starts gossiping to a friend two cubicles over? If these things might bother you, you can rest assured that colleagues in the hospital or clinic will be even more bothered if you do them when they are trying to work.

Balance Socialization with Work and Respect Others' Time

You are in a workspace, not a social scene. Yet, the lines blur, because you spend much of your time, and thus socialize, at work. Still, it is difficult to know what will inadvertently get under the skin of others working alongside you, and it is easy to forget how much our distractions could bother others. Especially in shared workspaces, avoid creating distractions if others are trying to concentrate. Remember that your colleagues may have dramatically different preferences for socializing and desire for a quiet workplace than you do.

Furthermore, always consider your colleagues' time constraints. Even when you have no place better to be, others might. A colleague could have an appointment, deadline, or children who need transport to an activity after work. Any inkling that a colleague is under time pressure should be a clue to limit the interruptions and socialization to essential work-related items and pick up again at a better time.

General Etiquette

General etiquette in public places is also important. People will notice if you let a door slam shut on the person behind you, allow others to exit an elevator before you charge on it, or publicly broadcast a loud video call. Public conversations about income or luxurious lifestyles are generally inappropriate. Overall, these items can be summed up as respecting others' time, comfort, health, dignity, and ability to concentrate.

Training Environment Effects

Detrimental Effects

Ironically, subpar role modeling and counterproductive incentives in the training environment can promote unproductive or unprofessional behavior and impede compassionate care.[136,402,403] In fact, it seems that decrements in professionalism during training are largely related to the hidden curriculum since this is seen even when dedicated lectures about professionalism are provided in the formal curriculum.[403] Compelling data show that our behavior is deeply influenced by that of those around us, including peers and attendings.[43,136,204,402–404]

Counterproductive incentives can include time pressure and rewards for projection of competence or test scores. That is, time pressure can lead to rushed clinical encounters, cutting corners, and avoiding patients. Fault lines in the ideal of a blameless culture and overemphasis on rewarding confidence can lead to lying and coverups. Overemphasis of test scores for grades may shift focus from patient care to information needed to pass examinations.[403]

Word Choices

Also, recall from Chapter 4 that the words we use matter. It turns out that the workplace environment can affect the language we use and our perceptions of patient care situations. A longitudinal study of house staff by Terry Mizrahi around 1980 sums up the situation with the title of her book on the study called *Getting Rid of Patients*.[136] Trainees can also pick up terminology that compares patient care to a combat zone like "being in the trenches." Remember, this may be how it feels in the moment, but it is not what it is.[136]

In addition to normalizing such behavior, exposure to unprofessional role modeling behavior impacts trainee's level of burnout and cynicism.[405] Further, trainee empathy for patients and the poor decreases over the course of medical training.[28,406,407] As we'll see, there are influences in the hidden curriculum that can compel you toward conformity—in either a positive or negative way.

Resisting Negative Influences

Exposure to unprofessional behavior is a clear example of influences that you should recognize and resist, but this is one of the trickiest things in the hidden curriculum to navigate. In general, you can choose to perform a variety of verbal and non-verbal responses of various levels of resistance either in the moment or later depending on the situation.[408] In some cases, this is directly (and tactfully) challenging the action, but more commonly is done by role modeling appropriate verbal and non-verbal behavior yourself.[408] It is also useful to reflect upon your situations, the responses of those around you, and your own response.[408] Confidential discussion in peer support groups can be useful too.[408]

Setting Expectations for Professional Behavior

As you progress to higher ranks, it is also useful to develop skills to help others on your team.[409] To preempt problems, set expectations for professionalism upfront, including clear lines for exemplary and intolerable behavior.[409] If you do need to address a minor lapse, be clear about why the lapse violates standards, how serious it is.[409] For first time offenses, be clear that the intervention is for formative, not summative and punitive, purposes.[409] More serious lapses may need elevation to other resources, however.[409]

Professionalism and Individuality

Some trainees express concern that unstated expectations of professional conformity erode individuality.[410] They feel, for example, that norms of medical professionalism (like professional appearance) are antiquated, diminish individuality, and can even discriminate against those with diverse backgrounds.[410] Underrepresented minorities can even face bias, stereotype threat, and impostor syndrome.[411] They may also have difficulty identifying mentors with similar backgrounds to help them navigate the system.[411] LGBTQ+ trainees can also face discrimination, insufficient mentorship and role modeling, and even hostility.[412] Similarly, the requirements for women to wear pantyhose when donning skirts or dresses have been characterized as outdated or even a symbol of female repression, and many medical centers have lifted this requirement.[413]

If you feel your identity is being compromised, you may need to be proactive in seeking out mentors and other guides. If none are available, you might need to look for them in other environments. Mentors can still have plenty to offer even if they are not directly within your planned career trajectory and may even open your horizons to new viewpoints. Additionally, it is in your best interest to respect your institutional dress code, but this does not mean that you can't look for ways to express individuality within these rules.

Key Takeaways

Striving to achieve high standards of professionalism can positively impact your training experience and professional development. Actively seek out positive role models and advice while consciously avoiding negative influences. While maintaining professionalism is essential, it is also important to preserve your individuality and authenticity. For this, it is important to seek ways to express your unique identity within the bounds of professional norms.

In the next chapter, we'll turn to the final theme: well-Being. This is a fitting final theme since it is central to many other topics in the hidden curriculum. These include effective learning, evolutionary influences, mixed messaging, EQ, gender-related topics, setting reasonable self-expectations, and resilience. It also ties into many topics to come, including organization and productivity, failure management, social media, and more.

Note

1 While this assertion seems to have merit, remember the multiple caveats for interpretation of nonverbal language.[376]

17

Well-Being

Vance T. Lehman

When physician health or wellness is compromised, so may the safety and effectiveness of the medical care provided.

AMA Code of Medical Ethics, Opinion 9.3.1[414]

Overview

Trainee well-being, our final theme, connects many topics we have already discussed and many more to come. Well-being (or wellness), however, can mean different things to different people. This includes various topics such as social support, finance, nutrition, sleep, exercise, alcohol use, anxiety, depression, other psychological conditions, workplace joy, and more. Physician well-being is formally espoused in statements such as the opening quote, and medical schools have implemented various types of well-being programs.[415]

Despite these positive steps, however, a great irony of medical training is that health and well-being of health professionals can suffer from the health professional training process.[416] We could learn something from elite athletes in this realm. While they optimize performance with detailed attention to their sleep, diet, heart rate, and nutrition, medical training can tacitly or overtly impede optimization of these parameters. In addition to the inherent virtue of self-care, role modeling well-being enhances physicians' credibility when discussing these topics with patients and encouraging behavior change.[417,418]

There are many sources of this hidden curriculum theme, both deep and proximate. Deep sources include persistent Halstedian influence on training culture, a historical under-recognition of the importance of many facets of well-being such as sufficient sleep, and financial reasons. Proximate sources include praise for individuals who work overtime at the expense of self-care, subtle comments about commitment, hospital cafeteria offerings, exercise and well-being facility availability, role modeling by attendings, and other influences or mixed messages. In addition, there can be insufficient guidance for trainees for managing the amount of information and workload inherent in medical training.

It is also useful to view well-being through an evolutionary lens of the modern-day forager mismatch. Imagine transporting one of our hunter-gatherer ancestors to modern-day New York City. He grabs fast food between shifts, is short on sleep, rarely exercises, and mainly socializes and finds relaxation with alcohol. The mismatch to his natural environment is stark. With the intensity of a career in medicine, however, this mismatch is magnified. This is why intentional management of many facets of well-being is critical.

DOI: 10.1201/9781003633389-19

Counseling and Treatment

Above all, if you or others think there is any possibility you could have a medical or psychological condition or substance use disorder, seek professional advice. This is often difficult. Medical students often avoid seeking professional help due to *stigma* concern.[419,420] After training, certain licensing questions about mental health and substance abuse can discourage treatment.[421] Here though, we will start by considering several potential challenges to well-being in training, including stress, burnout, fatigue, anxiety, depression, and loneliness.

Stress, Burnout, and Resilience

Stress

Psychological stress can have independent physiological, cognitive, affective and behavioral manifestations.[181] Stress responses can manifest physiologically without conscious awareness, though other combinations are possible. *Burnout* is characterized by three domains – emotional exhaustion, depersonalization, and low personal accomplishment.[422] Considering just 2 of the 22 questions of the gold standard Maslach Burnout Inventory is both practical and meaningful: (1) "I feel burned out from my work" (emotional exhaustion domain), and (2) "I have become more callous toward people since I took this job" (depersonalization domain).[422]

Burnout and Resilience

Medical trainees have a high burnout rate.[423] Trainee burnout and empathy is worsened by mistreatment, higher faculty demands, and poor-quality faculty relationships.[424] One study found that physicians have a higher resilience level than the general population, but burnout remains elevated.[422] Another study found that both a history of *adverse childhood events* (e.g., emotional abuse) and *adverse occupational events* (e.g., making a significant medical error) increase burnout and depression risk.[425,426] A controversial viewpoint suggests that physicians' experiences are better described as *moral injury*, resulting from systemic violations of personal moral boundaries.[427–429]

Thus, if you experience burnout or related distress, you should recognize it as a symptom of a systemic problem, where the demands placed on you exceeded your capacity or were discordant with your values, rather than an intrinsic failure to cope.[430] However, there are steps you can take to address or prevent burnout and enhanced resilience. These include focusing on positive role models of professionalism, practicing compassion, practicing gratitude and mindfulness, nurturing your personal spirituality, maintaining a peer-support group and prioritizing other aspects of your well-being like sleep, nutrition, and exercise.[415,431,432]

Fatigue

Endurance and fatigue are important concepts for medical trainees to know. *Fatigue* implies energy depletion and weariness; however, the definition may simply reflect participant perception in some studies. In distinction, *sleepiness* entails drowsiness and decreased alertness. Residents experiencing fatigue, sleepiness, burnout, or depression report more self-perceived medical errors.[433] To help stave off these deleterious effects, the Institute of Medicine has prioritized fatigue reduction and sleep enhancement with recent recommendations, including duty hour reforms.[433]

It is important to recognize that psychological and physical exertion are related. We can glean lessons from the Minnesota Starvation Experiment conducted at the University of Minnesota Laboratory of Physiological Hygiene. In this study, 36 conscientious World War II objectors were prescribed a control diet, followed by a 24-week semi-starvation diet during which time the subjects lost around 25% of their body weight.[434]

In addition to physical changes, numerous psychological changes ensued. These included fatigue, irritability, preoccupation with food, depressive and anxiety symptoms, reduced positive emotions, social withdrawal, and other behavioral changes.[434] The results inform the treatment of eating disorders even today.[434] Though most of us will never face these extreme conditions, we all have limits and need to recharge mentally and physically.

Nevertheless, sufficient recovery can be tacitly discouraged in training. In medical school, one surgery resident on my inpatient team lamented the drawbacks of the recently implemented "*wimpy* 80-hour work week."

Anxiety and Depression

One study found that about a sixth of medical students show signs of depression.[435] Depression, in turn, is a risk factor for serious effects both on trainees (including suicidal ideation) and on their patients (regarding increased rates of medical errors). The numerous increased demands, responsibilities, and transitions of medical training could contribute to the risk of both anxiety and depression.

Loneliness

Recognizing the loneliness epidemic in American society, U.S. Surgeon General Dr. Vivek Murthy released a public health advisory warning in 2023.[436] This stated that the negative impact of loneliness on health is akin to that of smoking daily.[436] Men, as we learned, are particularly vulnerable to loneliness.

There are many potential reasons for this trend, such as the rapid secularization and breakdown of local community ties (sometimes replaced with social media ties) in the United States over the past couple of decades, leading to a loss of purpose.[437] Medical trainees are susceptible to many risk factors. For example, medical education often requires moving to a new city and allows less time to socialize, while old friends may also move on to busier work or family situations.

Worry, Distress Tolerance, and Relaxation Techniques

You may benefit from *worry journaling*. Worry journaling involves dedicating 10–15 minutes daily to writing down worries and planning how to manage them. If a (nonurgent) worry intrudes into your thoughts during another time of day, you can dispassionately recognize it as a topic you will address during your dedicated journaling time and then nonchalantly move on with your day.

Distress is another state distinct from fatigue and sleepiness. Distress tolerance fortification is another adaptive method to cope with stressors. Specific strategies include using automatic *coping thoughts* in the face of adversity. An example coping thought is "I've overcome challenges before and I can do it again." In addition, it is useful to visualize relaxing or poignant environments that have special meaning. Finally, forms of relaxation are useful, such as guided imagery, progressive muscle relaxation, mindful breathing, and other mindfulness exercises.[438] To learn these, there are various resources at your disposal including YouTube videos, books, or therapy.[438]

Mindfulness

One method to help combat burnout, worry, and distress is mindfulness. Jon Kabat-Zinn introduced the ancient Buddhist meditation-based concept of *mindfulness-based stress reduction* to mainstream medicine and science in 1979.[439] He originally conceptualized the practice as a public health initiative rather than a therapy (though it has since been introduced into some therapies). A core goal was to reduce human suffering resulting from unhealthy mindsets. Today, this practice consists of many techniques for focusing objectively on the moment and diminishing inward and outward judgment. This focus may be internal (e.g., sensations of breathing), on external sensory experiences, or on an external object.

Evidence

The therapeutic effect of mindfulness has a neurological basis that can be demonstrated with functional brain mapping techniques. In brief, a meditator can learn to activate the attention networks in the brain instead of the network of brain regions associated with daydreaming, rumination, and fixation of the past or future.[1]

However, mindfulness research in medicine remains inconclusive, hampered by selective reporting, study limitations, heterogeneity, and hype.[122,440] When well-done, mindfulness can still provide many benefits, but we should understand that there are many different types of mindfulness and meditation, that these require practice, and some forms may be more practical than others.[122]

Practical Considerations

In his book *Mindfulness Redesigned for the Twenty-First Century*, Dr. Amit Sood points out that many traits that provided an evolutionary survival advantage like social comparisons and impulse to keep constant guard by switching attention can work against mindful presence today.[122] Moreover, meditation was developed 2,500 years ago and is not a good fit in original forms for most individuals in industrialized society.

Specifically, dedicated mindfulness sessions focused on clearing the mind may be less effective than integrating mindfulness into daily experiences. Further, working to replace judgmental thoughts with compassionate ones changes our brain from a state of depletion to one of energization and helps keep us grounded in the moment.[122] Incorporating these types of methods into daily habits is also more practical for busy medical trainees than setting aside time for dedicated sessions.

Sleep, Exercise, and Nutrition

Now, let's turn from negative states of well-being to three pillars of health: sleep, exercise, and nutrition. Unfortunately, these are still relatively neglected in general in medical education. With difficult work hours and often high levels of education-related debt, it may seem close to impossible for medical trainees to follow what they may know to be true about the importance of adequate levels of sleep, regular exercise, and high-quality nutrition. Therefore, self-care is crucial for providing optimal patient care.

Sleep

A mountain of data has now shown that high-quality sleep is essential for learning and for a wide range of fundamental health parameters.[90] [2] However, impairment due to sleep deprivation is an "occupational hazard" of medical training and is associated with physician burnout and self-reported medical errors.[425] Though you will have limited ability to control work schedules, and physicians are needed to take care of patients around the clock, there are measures that can be taken to optimize quantity and quality of sleep most nights.

For example, avoid the false economy of sacrificing sleep for study time, which negatively impacts time, energy, and overall productivity. Additionally, take steps to improve sleep hygiene, such as keeping the bedroom reasonably cool, reducing alcohol consumption, minimizing nighttime exposure to blue light (e.g., phone screens), avoiding late meals, and having reasonable exposure to natural light during daytime hours.[90] Finally, consider investing in a wearable sleep (and exercise) monitor to gain insights into your sleep efficiency.

Despite improvements, tacit messages about the virtues of working overnight and sacrificing sleep for work may persist in training. During medical school, one attending told me how his dedication to patient care left him proudly with only four hours of sleep most nights, even after residency.

Exercise

Next, while finding time to exercise can be a challenge, there are several ways you can work it in. Above all, your plan must be enjoyable and accessible, otherwise it will break down. If you do not find exercise enjoyable, try coupling it with something else you like such as music or podcasts. For accessibility, look for realistic home exercise equipment and gyms that are on your commuting route. As we saw, action often comes before motivation, so after you have found something that is both enjoyable and accessible, it is critical to establish it as a habit.

Additionally, some exercise can be built-in at work like walking, taking the stairs, and doing deskwork while standing if the set-up allows. For real benefit, consistency is key but you must also be flexible. For example, even professional athletes have hard days and easy days. If you go hard on your day off and just one other day per week, the rest of the days can be relatively easy.[441] Additionally, small chunks of activity on busy workdays can add up to have beneficial effects.[441]

Additional hidden curriculum challenges in this arena are found when major healthcare facilities do not provide space for exercise and when the topic is not a quintessential part of conversations surrounding well-being and physician identity. To help manage this, remember that your individual identity as a healthcare professional does not need to fully conform to that espoused by the system.

Nutrition

Finally, you may encounter barriers to learning essential nutritional concepts. As mentioned, the transition to an integrative problem-solving rather than traditional didactic curricula risks leaving nutrition by the wayside.[442] The topic is already challenging to learn given the wide range of popular diets with sometimes contradictory recommendations (e.g., animal-based versus plant-based or low fat versus low carbohydrate diets).[443,444] Overall, evidence suggests that most medical professionals ought to know more about nutrition and cooking.[445]

Beyond the formal literature available,[443] the best education though, like elsewhere in medicine, may be experiential; in this case learning about and managing your own nutrition. For this, it is useful to find a couple of basic cooking and nutritional resources and learn to cook during slower periods (the *off-season*). It is useful to learn some easy to prepare but healthful options for the busy times, such as overnight oatmeal, and to keep your most accessible options healthful, like nuts and dark chocolate. Finally, for an excellent overview on how to select, store, and prepare fruits and vegetables for flavor and nutrition, consider reading *Eating on the Wild Side* by Jo Robinson.

Finance

We will finish this chapter by turning to finance, another critical topic for trainee well-being. With modern financial pressures like increasing burden of student loan debt and cost of housing and childcare, financial considerations are as important as ever for a medical trainee's well-being and independence. In the short term, student loan debt can negatively impact your well-being.[446,447] In the long term, financial security can relax barriers to leaving a dissatisfying job situation or reducing work hours to pursue other personal goals.

To counter these effects, the three main things you should seek to understand are the importance of following a personal budget, basic investment principles, and the difference between income and net worth. This section emphasizes the importance of self-education in personal finance.

Personal Budget

The most basic step for personal finance is creating a personal budget, which is more important for physicians than many trainees realize. Budgeting during training mitigates debt and establishes good financial habits. Post-training income increases are often absorbed by taxes, housing, vehicles, and other expenses. Financial security can be elusive, as people often adjust their lifestyles to match income, which rarely feels sufficient.

Investing Basics

Consider contributing to basic retirement funds early on if possible during or early after training. Once your personal budget is in order, you may also be able to pursue additional investments. Fortunately, the essential concepts for investment are readily learned without needing to read endless books about stock picks, options, various real-estate investments, and so on.

The Simple Path to Wealth outlines a practical investment approach for trainees. There are other good resources that are geared specifically toward physicians. For example, whitecoatinvestor.com provides a wealth of information for free, ranging from basic topics to more advanced investment strategies for those who are interested and in a position to apply them.

Income Versus Net Worth

You should understand the difference between income and net worth because newly minted attendings can undermine their own financial security with a top 1% net worth lifestyle when they are really top 1% (or so) of income. Income is a short-term measure, while net worth reflects accumulated assets and liabilities.

Few trainees realize the high threshold for the top 1% net worth in the United States (approximately $11.5 million in 2022).[448] The top percentile is the extreme situation of course and, if achieved, usually comes later in a career; you can have an extraordinarily nice lifestyle with much less. Therefore, high post-training income doesn't guarantee a lavish lifestyle.

Income Guilt

A final personal finance challenge for trainees is the pressure from various sources that can instill income guilt, even pre-emptively. Resist internalizing these counterproductive and unfair messages.[449]

Key Takeaways

Paradoxically, many forces promote a false choice between the well-being of physicians and professional success. Carefully consider your personal priorities, ensuring they align with your values and the advice you provide to patients regarding healthy lifestyles. At times, doing so requires going against the tides of the system.

You may also have to unlearn bad habits picked up in college related to exercise, sleep, alcohol, and nutrition. You can also fall prey to unrealistic *health optimism*, an illusion of control of being healthier and impervious to effects of suboptimal lifestyle choices.[116] Delaying healthy habits often results in never starting them. When you are short on time, even small steps count. I think that health optimism poses an under-recognized threat to trainees. It is also useful to actively seek out positive physician role models who succeed both at work and with well-being.

Now that we have laid the groundwork to understand the hidden curriculum through the foundational concepts of Part I and the 12 themes of Part II, it is time to delve into additional specific topics that help form the hidden curriculum, which we will do in Part III.

Notes

1 Not all default mode network activation is maladaptive; for example, activation can be associated with creativity and help us search for deeper meanings.[122]
2 Note that some online analyses challenge some of the claims or degree of evidence in this book.

Part III

Introduction

In Part III, we'll introduce several special topics as a bridge to the clinical-focused topics in Part IV. We'll first uncover several profound stealth influences that the hidden curriculum casts upon medical trainees, then turn to some special challenges and underutilized skills in medicine and finish up with items related to professional development (Table III.1).

Like the themes, each special topic is critically important, but more focused. Most topics here have close relationships to one or several of the themes from Part II (like medical writing and the theme of communication) and some to the problem-solving topic from Part I (like logical fallacies, cognitive biases, and EBM), but each has a unique flavor. What's more important is that you remember that these topics are all connected.

Table III.1 Categories of Part III Topics

Influences (Chapters 18–22)	Challenges and Skills (Chapters 23–29)	Professional Development (Chapters 30–33)
First-Generation Physicians	Organization, Productivity, and Habit	Social Media
Cadavers, Clinical Anatomy, and Autopsies	Failure	Leadership and Management
White Coat Ceremonies and Oaths	Medical Writing	Meetings, Workplace Politics, and Difficult People
Compassion and Empathy	Research	Mentors, Sponsors, and Role Models
Religion and Spirituality	Statistics	
	Evidence-Based Medicine	
	Logical Fallacies and Cognitive Biases	

DOI: 10.1201/9781003633389-20

We'll start by exploring influences related to first-generation medical trainees, contrasting them to the potential advantages that multigenerational trainees enjoy. In medicine, you will interact with colleagues from many backgrounds and it is useful to understand their experiences, challenges, and viewpoints. Notice that this topic has connections to the themes of history, culture, conflict, change, and well-being.

In the second half of this chapter, we'll consider the generational status of physicians in context of the conflict theory of education; we'll finish by briefly contrasting it with the sociological perspectives of functionalism and symbolic interactionism.

18

First-Generation Physicians

Vance T. Lehman

Secret Societies

Whether you are a first-generational physician or hail from a long line, it is useful to understand how generational status impacts your environment and the training experience. This is nothing new and certainly not limited to medicine. Consider that in 1832, Alphonso Taft was one of two founding members of the Skull and Bones secret society on the Yale Campus. His son William Howard Taft later joined this society, ultimately ascended to the U.S. presidency, and would be followed by other members who would achieve prominence in American government and business (George H. W. Bush, George W. Bush, presidential candidate John Kerry, and many others). Interestingly, though his father was a Skull and Bones member, and despite attending Yale University, Dr. William Halsted was not offered a position.

The number 322 is cast on the society's emblem, thought to represent the year 322 BC, when Greece transitioned from a democracy to a plutocracy under the rule of the wealthy class. Even though many of the society's values, activities, and principles remain secretive, this observation gives some insight into the nature of the society, including the dramatic impact of both generational and other insider privilege. This privilege includes social connections, wealth, access to opportunities, support systems, and a sense of belonging. As we'll discuss next, nearly 200 years after the conception of Skull and Bones, the advantages of insider status and privilege remain ever-present beneath the surface of the pursuit of the American dream.

Structural Advantages Influenced by the Flexner Report

In medicine, insider advantage comes more from generational privilege than from an exclusive society like Skull and Bones, although there are undeniable parallels. Further, the *Flexner Report* (as introduced in Chapter 6) is a key driver of legacy and insider advantage. By shuttering lower tier medical schools, it ushered in an era of preponderance of middle to upper class medical students, particularly from medical families.[450]

Since access to medical-related and other extra-curricular activities increases the odds of admission and the financial means to defer income during a long training period lowers the barrier to entry, a skew toward privilege may have been unavoidable. For a variety of reasons, reports indicate that between 13% and 44% of incoming medical students now have at least one physician parent.[451,452] Regardless, the situation has ripple effects on a personal level and systems/societal level for the modern trainee.

There are potential effects on trainee class mobility and other educational experiences. Admissions to top colleges strongly reflects student family income quartile, even when adjusting for test scores.[453] Medical school admissions are also stratified by income, which is in turn associated with race and ethnicity.[454,455] While it seems unlikely that medical schools today deliberately propagate class stratification, it is worth considering if this is a *de facto* outcome. In the end, first-generation college students are less likely to apply, be accepted, and matriculate to medical school.[60]

Further, the current system presents formidable barriers, both at the point of entry to medical school and then again for certain (often highly compensated) (sub)specialties that require long training routes and other commitments. For those with lower financial means, the benefits of gap year experiences, travel volunteerism, and research years and attending prestigious urban programs are expensive and risky (if not prohibitive).

Beyond finance, first-generation residents in surgical specialties may experience feelings of inferiority, a sense of exclusion, and a paucity of role models and mentors.[456,457] These many barriers may be reflected in the fact that first-generation physicians are more likely to be from groups that are traditionally underrepresented in medicine by race, ethnicity, age, and parental income.[458]

Insider Information

Beyond a smoother journey to medical school admission, there are other potential benefits of being a multigenerational medical family insider. This is not meant to be a slight toward the noble pursuits of multigeneration physicians but rather an acknowledgment of certain challenges more commonly faced by first-generation physicians.

Surprisingly though, there is little information available describing the effect of the hidden curriculum on first-generation physicians, despite the increasing focus of first-generation college students. The AAMC did not recognize the first-generation indicator until 2018; this indicator specifically (as in most places) assessed whether either parent achieved an associate degree or higher degree rather than a medical degree.

Adversity and Challenges for First-Generation Students

There are emerging discussions surrounding this topic, however. One study found that first-generation college graduates in medical school faced unique adversity, requiring heightened grit and resilience.[459] Another report described the need to increase the representation of first-generation physician-scientists, who constitute less than 10% of matriculants.[460]

Additionally, first-generation trainees may experience pressure to *"code switch"* (expressing oneself differently by environment), discouragement from pursuing ambitious professional pathways, increased stress, impostor syndrome, stereotype threat, and financial challenges.[456,461,462] The topic is also explored in editorial pieces, acknowledged in an AAMC resource, and addressed with dedicated resources at some medical schools.[458,463–466]

At the college level, one study investigated the topic of first-generation students entering legacy schools with standardized interviews of 126 first-generational or legacy college students at either Harvard or Georgetown Universities.[8] This found a wide range of effects like adoption of strategies to divert conversations away from socioeconomic background exposure.

The impact on medical students specifically has also been studied. For example, medical students who do not identify as coming from a privileged background often report feeling like they "live in two different worlds."[467] They also report feeling uncomfortable discussing parental occupations or typical weekend trips or vacations, sometimes trying to shrink into the background.[467]

Multigenerational Advantages

Multigenerational medical trainees may be more familiar with medical culture and feel more at ease in a medical environment (or perhaps a country club, for that matter). Parents may have more mobility to move nearby when support (such as child-care) is needed. Even welcome receptions and events, meant to strengthen social connections and well-being, can ironically alienate some students when they are held at traditionally exclusive venues. While we cannot control our family backgrounds, we can stay tuned to the topics and do our best to understand them and mitigate any such untoward effects.

Steps to Mitigate the Systemic Effects

While all the factors presented point to challenges, there are many things that can help first-generation medical students succeed. If you are a first-generation medical trainee, heeding advice in resources like this book can help. This also means proactively seeking financial and well-being education, information about program culture, peer support groups, and mentorship.[457,468,469] Remember that you deserve to be in your position as much as anyone else and your skills and commitment matter most in the end.

While we should acknowledge the effects of privilege, we should not begrudge those who seem to have benefited. First, a tendency to follow in their parents' footsteps is expected and laudable. What's more, they too may have faced hidden adversity, have made a commitment to a noble cause, and, like everyone else, cannot change their background.

For multigenerational medical trainees, it is useful to be mindful of conversation topics that might inadvertently be exclusive to help foster an inclusive and welcoming atmosphere. It is natural to discuss family vacations or other markers of privilege, but if you notice someone is becoming silent or uncomfortable, it is helpful to stay warm and inviting and even redirect the conversation if needed. While this is the right thing to do for others, it is to your benefit as well. Being well-liked and having social connections can open many doors in the future, including the ability to provide better patient care through teamwork, professional collaboration, job opportunities, and more.

Three Perspectives of Education

Generational privilege in medicine is related to the conflict theory of education, which helps us understand the origins and influences of the hidden curriculum.[470] Broadly speaking, the functional effect of education has been considered over centuries by the likes of Marx (who advanced conflict theory) and sociologists. The implication here is that the hidden curriculum helps serve the true purpose(s) of education, which can be described by three main theories of sociology—*conflict theory*, *functionalism*, and *symbolic interactionism* (Table 18.1).

Conflict Theory and Social Stratification

The first two categories look at the global effects of education and how it may be designed to perpetuate class hierarchy and conflict or to be functional to serve societal needs. Both are true, but which is dominant in medicine is up for debate. The basic expectations of training adopted from Emile Durkheim's insight that we introduced in Chapter 2 reflect the functionalist view. In college, the higher education system still plays a demonstrable role in the propagation of privilege.

By the conflict theory of education, a primary effect of education is to instill and perpetuate a social hierarchy as a hidden curriculum. For medical training, one analysis found that even well-intended, but inadequate, efforts to integrate social science and humanities have had the unintended effect of promoting social hierarchy.[141] The data shown in the last section also lends support to this viewpoint. Whether intentional, or as a byproduct, barriers to medical education have long helped perpetuate social stratification.

When a welcome reception is held at an exclusive location, this sends a signal. When interviewers are fascinated by the world travels of *cultured* applicants, this sends a message. When an admissions committee factors in that an applicant really knows that she wants to do medicine because her parent is a physician, this has an effect. While there is nothing wrong with country clubs, travel, and familial physician role models, we cannot deny these have influences. These include the promotion of impostor syndrome, instillation of a sense of not belonging in others, and even molding the demographic makeup of the workforce.

Table 18.1 Three Sociological Perspectives of Education

Theory	Brief Description
Conflict Theory	Education primarily perpetuates and reinforces social hierarchy
Functionalism	Education serves the needs of society, including socialization and skill development
Symbolic Interactionism	Interpersonal interactions re-enforce identities and teacher labels and expectations affect academic success

Functionalism and Symbolic Interactionism

While a deep dive into the relevance of these sociological perspectives about the purpose and effects of education is out of the scope of this book, they both merit brief mention. A broader purpose of medical education, including the stated purpose, aligns with the functionalism perspective. Socializing trainees to act and function as physicians for the broader good of society is a major component of medical training, with the forces sometimes overt and sometimes covert as part of the hidden curriculum.

Finally, medical training, including effects of the hidden curriculum, can be viewed through the symbolic-interactionism lens. This focuses on the direct effects of individual interactions (e.g., trainee-attending interactions) rather than broader societal forces. Examples include trainee labeling, deciphering staff expectations, and formation of a professional identity.

19

Cadavers, Clinical Anatomy, and Autopsies

Vance T. Lehman

Cadavers and Dissection

Now, we'll turn to a different type of privilege, one that has a history of controversies and carries a different set of hidden influences—the relationship between physicians and cadavers. Gross anatomy, a foundational course, holds deeper meaning beyond its stated learning objectives.

Historical Perspective

Consider the stagnation of anatomy discovery during the era of dissection prohibition from the time of Galen to Andreas Vesalius. The legalization of human dissection allowed Vesalius to publish *De humani corporis fabrica*, a landmark work of the scientific revolution. However, access to cadavers remained challenging; grave robbing and even murder were common in 19th-century Scotland, for example. Wealthy individuals like William Halsted gained an advantage by purchasing cadavers, highlighting the privileged access to dissection throughout history.[131]

Sacred Perspective

From a religious and spiritual perspective, cadaver dissection has been compared to religious or shamanistic indoctrination, underscoring the sacred nature of medical practice.[471] From a secular perspective, there has been increased focus on humanism and professionalism in the anatomy lab in recent years.[472] This is why your formal curriculum may include writing assignments or ceremonies to honor and respect the donors.[473,474] Today, a cadaver may be viewed as your "first patient," not merely an object.[475]

Dissection and Habituation

Anatomic dissection also habituates medical trainees to the sight and smell of death. You must reconcile honoring the person who gave their body and objectively dissecting it. This highlights the inherent tension between dispassionate objectivity and empathy in medical practice. One study reported that students can even develop post-traumatic stress, nightmares, and intrusive dreams after an anatomy course.[476] Another study found that over half of students experienced distress at the prospect of dissection, often coping with *dark humor*.[477] A subset, though, believed that such humor is unprofessional.[477]

DOI: 10.1201/9781003633389-22

The appropriateness of dark humor is complex, varying across individuals and contexts. Moderate use of dark humor may be acceptable as a coping mechanism, but excessive use can undermine professionalism. It is also discouraged by some professionals who view the anatomy lab as a crucial setting to develop professional skills.[478]

Is Dissection Necessary?

The value of dissection is increasingly debated. Dissection is resource-intensive, and alternatives exist. As we saw, anatomy topics are being relegated to the null curriculum, even though the need to understand detailed *medical school* anatomy is increasing with advances in medical imaging and understanding of pathophysiology.

Cadaver dissection, while not imperative, remains very beneficial. If your program uses alternatives though, be sure that these incorporate effective learning methods over rote notecard type memorization. For this, remember that anatomy is best learned by correlating it to function, clinical relevance, and cross-sectional imaging. High-quality 3D models may also serve as valuable supplements.

Clinical and Cross-Sectional Anatomy

Beyond cadaver dissection, other methods are useful for learning clinical anatomy. Clinical anatomy takes many forms, such as through a microscope, endoscope, or on cross-sectional imaging. Each method offers unique advantages, but one that is critical and accessible is cross-sectional imaging. Cross-sectional imaging exemplifies the benefits of active, task-specific, experience-based learning over rote memorization.

Radiology residents often use online brain atlases, which offer features like interactive labels and linked information. These atlases have functionality like scrolling and labels that can be turned off and on, and maybe even links to relevant factoids or buzzwords. While these are good supplemental resources, they are ineffective primary learning tools. Here's a more effective approach:

A Radiologist's Brain Anatomy Lesson

A radiologist asks a trainee to turn away from the atlas and look at a real case, let's say a head CT. Head CTs exhibit variations in appearance, scan angle, and patient positioning compared to the atlas. The radiologist then asks the trainee to identify the same structure he just reviewed on the atlas on the live images. Few trainees can accurately and confidently identify basic structures on real images after using atlases alone. This holds true regardless of study time, even with immediate testing.

Then, the radiologist might take a different approach. Instead of just looking at the atlas, he points out several other spatial relationships—how sulci and gyri forms shapes, patterns, and how the orientations matter. This is analogous to identifying constellations rather than individual stars. At the same time, the radiologist might discuss the function and clinical significance of the structures to bring them to life.

Moreover, comparison to examples of pathologically altered anatomy enhances understanding. By directly comparing the appearance of normal and abnormal anatomy, the differences are highlighted, and *normal* starts to be meaningful. Understanding clinical deficits clarifies the function of each structure.

The inefficiency of using labeled atlases alone stems from passive learning, analogous to learning a language solely from a dictionary or understanding a car only from its manual. This is simply not how we have evolved to learn. Overall, atlases create an illusion of effortless learning.

Other Anatomic Regions

While brain anatomy is unique, similar principles apply to other areas. This includes understanding spatial and functional relationships, clinical significance, and appearance of pathology for many structures. Examples include the purpose and origins/insertions related to bone processes or ridges, the anatomy of fracture patterns or impingement syndromes, learning muscles by groups based on function, compartment, or innervation, and so on.

Furthermore, anatomists have long used the shapes and resemblances of anatomy to remember their names, like sigmoid colon (sigma), the deltoid muscle (delta), nasal concha (seashell), or the hippocampus (seahorse).

Autopsy

Hospital autopsy rates have declined significantly in recent decades.[479] William Osler, for instance, performed nearly 1,000 autopsies prior to joining the *Big Four*.[131] Declining autopsy rates, reduced emphasis on their educational value, and curriculum expansion have limited trainee exposure. Many physicians, particularly pathologists, believe this trend negatively impacts medical care. Understanding autopsies improves communication with families and reinforces their role in quality control. Overall, it is important to recognize this trend as a potential gap in your training and understand the value of autopsy for quality control.

Finally, along with dissection and related activities, our next topics of white coat ceremonies and oaths are time-honored medical school traditions with potential for deeper influence than trainees might predict.

20

White Coat Ceremonies and Oaths

Vance T. Lehman

White Coat Controversies

This chapter explores the deeper cultural influences of white coat ceremonies and oaths. First, physician attire, literally a black-and-white topic, also has figurative gray areas. Before the late 1800s, physicians typically wore black (a professional color) and carried a black handbag.[480] The adoption of the white coat symbolized the growing importance of antiseptic hygiene.[480] This echoes the use of togas by Roman politicians to inspire trust.[480]

The white coat ceremony has become a common early event in many medical school curricula. These ceremonies, typically comprising six key components (Table 20.1), mark entry into the profession and symbolize compassion and healing.[481,482] In addition, the color white represents purity and the rigor of laboratory science.[482] Other community leaders, such as ministers and police officers, also don outfits for honor and identification.

Still, some contend that physicians' white coats and white coat ceremonies signify a hidden curriculum of covert indoctrination. That is, these symbolize caregiving hierarchies, elitism, and social and economic privilege of physicians. Further, these represent medicine's well-established practices of determining membership in the profession.[482]

There are other potential issues, too, such as oaths' content that is not explained to students rendering it meaningless, and a message of tacit separation of students from lay people who will be their patients. Oaths also could turn "trust into entitlement" and send the message that respect comes from a uniform instead of individual behavior.[483,484] This could also contribute to role confusion as a couple years on clinical rotations when students are reminded that they still know very little practical clinical medicine.

However, one study assessing factors of either compassion or elitism in 18 white coat ceremonies found no substantial evidence of elitism.[485] Statements espousing obligations were three times as common as those of privilege and four main themes were identified, including professionalism, morality, humanism, and spirituality.[485]

So, what is the truth and why would it matter to you? The concerns are plausible and perhaps even on some levels true. Certainly, there is symbolism, and the ceremony is meant to be a form of identity transition. Beyond the ceremony itself, debates exist regarding the necessity of white coats, given concerns over hierarchy based on coat length, the widespread use of white coats by other professionals, and the potential for infection.[486]

However, I believe the concerns are more common in journals than in real life and that it is a practice we can continue to endorse and enjoy without concerns of elitist indoctrination.

DOI: 10.1201/9781003633389-23

Table 20.1 Components of White Coat Ceremonies[481]

1. Invitation of family and friends to symbolize support
2. Welcome by the dean and other staff to discuss the school's value system
3. An inspiring address by an attending physician role model
4. The donning of the white coats
5. Swearing of an oath of solemn responsibilities and obligations
6. A celebratory reception

Oaths

Another time-honored ceremony is the swearing of an oath at medical school graduation, such as the Hippocratic Oath. While medical oaths are not highly controversial, and some contend the meaning has eroded over time, they carry significance beyond the immediate messages. For some students, this seems like a simple prerequisite recital to get a diploma. However, these oaths have greater symbolism and influence than is often recognized.

The Hippocratic Oath also symbolizes intergenerational and inter-cultural connections. It transcends human lifespans and continents, serving as a direct bridge between modern and ancient physicians. It encodes central ethical duties that a physician has to both society and her patients such as beneficence and confidentiality.[487]

The oath is also the basis for the Nuremburg Code, guiding human subject research.[487] Though the real origins are a bit convoluted, it has carefully selected words like compassion and joy, both of which have important meaning that continues to be explored in medical practice today.

But both white coat ceremonies and oaths carry a deeper meaning still. Remember that larger human groups are bound and inspired by social narratives rather than simple decree of a local authority or first-hand acquaintances. Ceremonies and oaths are one such conceptual glue that bind physicians together in common mission and service because they are larger than an attending, a dean, or even a hospital president. They cultivate a physician's social identity and initiation into a community. Shared ceremonies and oaths among different schools are effective mechanisms to unite large numbers of people in common cause as a social collective.

Key Takeaways

While white coat ceremonies and oaths are subject to criticism and debate, they remain powerful symbols of the medical profession's values and culture. Through collective public commitments, these help mold trainees' self-image and, by extension, behaviors. Although these activities may seem, in part, a formality, they are likely to have a greater influence on trainees' professional identity formation than many realize. Next, we'll turn to a topic that is central to the mission of medicine but also contains its own surprising controversies—compassion and empathy.

21

Compassion and Empathy

Vance T. Lehman

Compassion and empathy, central to medical practice, directly influence trainees and enable them to positively influence others. These related topics are critical for several reasons: (1) they are core concepts for providing excellent patient care; (2) compassion and empathy can decline during medical training; (3) cognitive empathy lies at the core of understanding how others around you think.

The Difference Between Compassion and Empathy

Still, you may not have a consequential discussion of the difference between *compassion* and *empathy* in your formal curricula. While these two concepts are related, there are crucial differences.

Compassion, a core pillar of medical care, is enshrined in the AMA Code of Ethics.[488] Strauss et al. (Table 21.1) proposed five key components of compassion: recognizing suffering, relating to or feeling it, and retaining objectivity to intervene and alleviate it.[489] This aligns with the expected responsibilities of a physician. In fact, compassion may be viewed as the primary vehicle through which we deliver patient care. Supporting this central role, studies show that decreased physician compassion is associated with decreased quality of care.[407]

Empathy involves sharing the feelings, perceptions, or thoughts of another, not solely in instances of suffering.[490] Unlike compassion, it does not necessarily imply an active response. Empathy comprises cognitive (understanding others' perspectives), affective (feeling others' emotions), and behavioral (communicating with others) components.[491] Later, we'll see that psychopaths are believed to be low on affective empathy but can be cunningly high on cognitive empathy (Chapter 32), for example.

Controversies Over the Virtues of Affective Empathy

The virtues of affective empathy are surprisingly controversial. Psychologist Paul Bloom and others believe that too much affective empathy is overly taxing, appeals to our irrational biases, and leads to poor (and even immoral) choices. In his book *Against Empathy*, Bloom advocates for a more detached, rational approach to compassion.[204] Affective empathy is also mentally taxing and is not automatic.[123] Thus, most people limit the amount of empathy they have for others, especially people they do not know well, and dial empathy way down when they are jealous.[123] fMRI and clinical studies also find that empathy activates different brain regions

Table 21.1 Five Components of Compassion (Strauss)

1. Recognizing suffering
2. Understanding the universality of suffering in the human experience
3. Feeling empathy with suffering and connecting with the distress
4. Tolerating uncomfortable feelings aroused in response to the suffering person (distress, anger, fear) and remaining open to and accepting of the person suffering
5. Finding motivation to act to alleviate the suffering

than compassion and support the notion that empathy is draining whereas compassion is energizing.[122,123]

But surely you should still be an empathic physician, right? Even most critics of affective empathy agree that physicians should listen attentively, demonstrate understanding of patients' perspectives, and communicate with those perspectives in mind. However, if you mirror a patient's fear too much (a display of affective empathy), you could increase their anxiety, and your thoughts may be paralyzed. Therefore, the benefits of empathy in medicine appear most closely linked to cognitive empathy, while excessive affective empathy may prove detrimental.

Many educators recognize the distinct role of cognitive empathy and have emphasized it over affective empathy in recent medical training.[491] Focusing on cognitive empathy makes sense since it is a skill you can both practice and apply to patient care.[491] In addition, improving cognitive empathy may be beneficial for you since it is associated with lower physician burnout, while affective empathy seems to have no substantial association.[491]

Studies indicate that empathy often declines during medical training.[492] While the reasons remain unclear, contributing factors may include a hidden curriculum of role modeling, stressful work environments, managing medical complexity, and prioritizing biomedical knowledge over so-called soft skills.[492] This hidden curriculum may then lead to cynicism, desensitization, distancing from patients, and burnout, with a cumulative effect of lowered empathy.[492] Although diminished empathy is almost always viewed negatively, in certain situations, tempering excessively affective empathy with rational reasoning and cognitive empathy could be adaptive.

Cognitive Empathy and Theory of Mind

Cognitive empathy is closely linked to theory of mind, an understanding of the perspectives, thought processes, and behaviors of others. While most people have acquired a basic theory of mind by kindergarten, there is much more we need to do to understand how people think in the workplace. Optimization of cognitive empathy in training, however, requires integration of many other concepts we have discussed. These include EC, facial expressions, active listening, and understanding personality. These methods help you gain insight into others' thoughts, feelings, beliefs, values, preferences, pet peeves, triggers, motivators, and—importantly—expectations.

Specifically, ways to gain access to others' thoughts hinge on meeting the basic expectations, making a good first impression, looking interested, and asking directly for expectations and feedback. It is also useful to adopt the mindset of "what can I do to help?" If the moment is right, it can be enlightening to ask, "What do you like best about your profession (or working here)?" It is also useful to gain insights from successful predecessors.

Although individual thoughts cannot be definitively ascertained, certain common beliefs and biases should be acknowledged. Most people deploy ego-preserving strategies when their competence could be questioned, tend to be overconfident when they have knowledge but are not yet an expert, and probably even feel superior to you in some way.[176] Thus, most people do not want to be heavily criticized in front of others. Essentially, everybody wants to feel important and respected too.[176]

Key Takeaways

Compassion and empathy are critical for trainees to understand for several reasons, in particular the differences between the two concepts and the importance of both cognitive and affective components. In the next chapter, we'll discuss two topics that are strongly connected to compassion with great potential to impact trainees but that more often remain below the surface in training—religion and spirituality.

22

Religion and Spirituality

Vance T. Lehman

Background

For some trainees, religion is the primary compass for their deepest beliefs, actions, and morality. They may view medicine as a sacred calling, guided by both spiritual principles and science. However, certain scientific teachings may be at odds with their religious teachings. Some prominent scientists (such as Stephen Hawking) reject the role of religion and spirituality in science, because the concept of divine intervention would violate the deterministic laws of nature.[130]

Regardless of where on the spectrum of religiosity different trainees fall, most trainees share these questions or knowledge gaps: What role, if any, should religion play in patient care? What is religion, and how is it different from spirituality? What should I do when religion and science clash? These questions are important to address because, of all influences in medical training, those of religion and spirituality have potential to be the most profound; however, they may be the least discussed. Let's consider the answers to these questions.

First, regardless of your personal beliefs, it is useful to acknowledge that religious and spiritual considerations are central to healing and human experience. Physicians have even been portrayed as an extension of God; in the painting *The Chief of the Medical Staff*, Jesus guides a surgeon's hand during an operation. Early Western hospitals were strongly affiliated with religion.[493,494] Later, during the Dark Ages, Benedictine monasteries became medical centers, serving as both a refuge for the ill and a repository of medical knowledge.[145]

Furthermore, the support of clergy and connection to religion during the 19th century elevated physicians' status and endowed them with moral and spiritual authority.[471] Today, around one-fifth of U.S. hospitals still have religious affiliations.[495] However, official religious ties of medical practice are much less common now than bygone centuries. Physician authority is now more intricately linked to scientific knowledge. To understand the influence on modern medical trainees, we must explore the definitions of religion and spirituality.

What are Religion and Spirituality?

Religion

While there is no single definition of religion, we can conceptualize it in two broad categories: substantive and functional. *Substantive definitions* of religion are anchored in a belief in greater being(s), the supernatural, nonworldly realms; these offer explanations for reality. This definition most closely resembles the common conception of religion and is also most at odds with medical views on pathogenesis, for example.

 DOI: 10.1201/9781003633389-25

Conversely, religious scholars often utilize a broader *functional definition*, originally proposed by Emile Durkheim.[496] As the name implies, a functional religion is characterized by what a religion does rather than what it is. This typically consists of shared beliefs and practices, resulting in social cohesion.

Many concepts fall under the functional religion umbrella, including non-theistic practices like Zen Buddhism, nationalism, sociopolitical ideology, corporate culture, and humanism. Regardless of whether this definition fits your viewpoint, the point is that a profession, an organization, and humanism can have a deeper impact on you than you might realize. In medicine, oaths and the medical culture can be viewed as part of this, or what some refer to as social constructs.[120,471]

Humanism as the Dominant Functional Religion

More broadly, Noah Harari asserts that humanism has now become the dominant religion.[120] In this way, humanism is simultaneously antithetical to traditional religions and a functional religion. That is, humanism implies that humans give meaning to their lives and prioritize earthly needs over reliance on the divine.[1] Humanism can then be seen as a powerful undercurrent that greatly shapes our personal and professional lives.

Spirituality

How is spirituality different from religion? Some consider it a separate topic from religion (Harari says that spirituality is a "journey," while religion is a "deal").[120] However, with an in-depth analysis, theologian Dr. Michael Balboni along with physician Dr. Tracy Balboni contend that spirituality and religion (by the functional definition) necessarily co-exist since they share key characteristics, and one implies the other.[471] Balboni provides a multifaceted discussion on the nuances, differences, and interdependence, but for our purposes, we can consider that religion implies both individual and collective social structures with "beliefs, practices, relationships, and organizations."[471]

Perhaps for practical purposes though, spirituality means different things to different people. It may be an internal experience for some, an ethereal experience for others (or both or neither). Regardless of your individual conceptualization, it can be a pathway to meaning and compassion.[122] Thus, even if you believe physicians should steer clear of their patients' spiritual beliefs, being in tune with your spirituality can guide you as a physician since it fosters compassion, a central role in patient care.

Can Spirituality and Religion Be Disentangled from Medicine?

Balboni argues that separating spirituality and religion from medicine is more challenging than it appears. He contends that, in humanist fashion, we have simply replaced a spirituality of *transcendence* with one of *immanence*, which focuses on physical health and comfort.[471] In turn, medicine has become out of step with the values of many patients and less able to meet the needs of pluralistic beliefs.[471]

Medical care is informed by morals and values, and even if not formally acknowledged, they can fundamentally arise from substantive or functional religious beliefs. Even if we disregard the historical links between traditional religions and medicine, disentangling them

123

remains challenging. One can argue that the void created through de-emphasis of the formal religions effectively becomes filled with a belief in modern medical practice itself, and this belief can be considered a form of religion with a liberal functional definition.[471]

Does Discussion of Religion Belong in Medical Education?

There is a debate over the tacit formal separation of medicine and religion. Regardless of one's viewpoint on this separation, we can make a case for discussing religion and spirituality here on several grounds. Medicine and religion are intertwined both historically and in modern-day practice. They have analogous features like illness/sin, healing/forgiveness, counseling/confession. Compassion, a central pillar of medicine, is advocated by all major world religions. For many, religious beliefs help guide medical decisions, and prayer for the ill is commonplace.

There are many potential reasons why religion has diminished prominence in modern-day medicine. Science, which is at the heart of the biomedical model, may be viewed as replacing and disproving religion rather than coexisting with it. Modern physicians are science-based healers rather than religious figures (or spiritual advisors). The appropriateness of such discussions is open to debate and depends on the context. Truth be told, existing evidence indicates that the discussions are often unwanted by patients (see the following section). But that does not mean that viewpoints on these topics do not factor into patient health and well-being.

It is also important to acknowledge that some interventions promoted by modern medical practitioners have religious origins. While the influence of Western religions in medicine has decreased in recent history, the influence of Eastern religions has grown. For example, some argue that yoga and mindfulness have been largely secularized to gain widespread approval in the West but still represent religious-derived practices.[471] Yoga is most closely associated with Hinduism and mindfulness with Buddhism.[2]

Relevance for Medical Trainees

Although there is more for us to learn on this topic, a survey of religious and nonreligious medical students found that religious students may struggle with identity and self-doubt in training. However, they may be better equipped to deal with some elements of adversity.[471]

According to Balboni, the disconnection of substantive religion and spirituality from medicine may exert a strong socialization effect on trainees.[471] Specifically, we tacitly learn that religion has a limited role in medical care. Additionally, tacit promotion of the spirituality of immanence can undermine the "transcendent calling" of medicine, put physical concerns over the transcendent, promote technical care over personal care, shift our focus to material priorities and efficiency, impede compassion, and increase burnout.[471]

Certain aspects of religious practice that have an acknowledged direct impact on medical care, such as dietary restrictions or beliefs against some conventional medical treatments. Nonetheless, there is value in learning more about common religious and spiritual beliefs. For example, even those who are not Buddhist can gain a useful perspective about mindfulness, suffering, and compassion by studying the *Four Noble Truths* and the *Eightfold Path*. In addition, basic education can improve respect for and understanding of the diverse patient beliefs you are likely to encounter.

Finally, we can debate if, when, and how a physician should address religious and spiritual concerns in clinical practice on multiple grounds.[497] For example, a third or more of patients prefer that their physicians do not broach the topic of religion.[497] It is a complex topic without universal clear-cut answers, but at the very least, you should understand the history, viewpoints, and humanistic assumptions embedded within the system.

Science and Religion

What about the tension between science and religion? Here, there are no universal answers, but keep in mind that you will encounter a variety of viewpoints, even among physicians. If you believe that religion provides comfort for those who do not understand science, as Hawking did, remember that there is a strong human desire to seek spiritual meaning, and for many, physics falls short of offering this meaning.[130]

Additionally, it may be useful to conceptualize different dimensions of medical practice, including a science-backed dimension to guide evidence-based diagnosis, treatment, and prognosis and also a religious-spiritual dimension. Your most appropriate role as a healer will usually be practicing the evidence-based component, but for yourself and perhaps for certain patient situations, the religious-spiritual dimension can be important too.

Notes

1 It is important to acknowledge that the precise definition of humanism is debated.
2 The classification of Buddhism as a religion varies by source.

23

Organization, Productivity, and Habit

Vance T. Lehman

Organizational Skills and Planning

Chapters 24–29 address several challenges in medical training and the skills needed to overcome them. This chapter begins with organizational skills, productivity, and habit formation, which are essential for optimal performance in medical training and can help you stay one step ahead of the hidden curriculum. This topic is crucial because it directly relates to several others in this book, including well-being, effective learning, and efficiency.

To-Do Lists and Alternatives

This often starts with creating a *to-do list* if you have always juggled tasks mentally or have limited attention. Many time-management resources, however, suggest that you replace a to-do-list with other approaches. These approaches include brainstorming and calendar filling, keeping multiple hierarchical to-do lists, electronic methods, or simply choosing one important thing to focus on at a time and bringing it to completion.[498]

You may need to try several methods to see what works best for you. Regardless of method used, relying on your memory to implement the plan is a major potential pitfall. Instead, incorporate it into your routine to make it automatic. In addition, consider creating a "not to-do list" of things that are not worth your time.

The Planning Fallacy

Most people also have a nagging tendency to underestimate task completion time, which is known as the *planning fallacy*. Take one notorious example: the Sydney Opera House. The planning fallacy is why it was nearly $100 million over budget and took a decade longer to build than predicted.[499]

Similarly, attempting to learn a large amount of information in a single cram session is likely to fail. Overall, the best predictor of time needed is comparative historical data from a similar past project. When you must guess, start out by allotting more time than your initial estimate and be sure to budget some time for unexpected events because these often cause delays and rarely speed things up.[500]

DOI: 10.1201/9781003633389-26

Productivity

Basic Challenges and Approaches

Beyond planning pitfalls, challenges to productivity are endemic in our work structures. Interestingly, though perhaps unsurprisingly, workers believe they are more productive than their coworkers, rating their own productivity at 8.2, their coworkers at 7.2, and the company leadership at 6.8 on a 0–10 scale.[501] Even so, a survey of U.S. workers found that they spend only three hours per workday focused on their primary task, with emails and unnecessary meetings identified as the two biggest time drains.[501]

You will find a variety of similar challenges to productivity in medicine, including stringent documentation requirements, EMR inefficiencies, and points of delay among the many intersecting processes needed to deliver patient care.

To help manage these challenges, there are countless guides and resources on productivity. In brief, the common themes include optimization of time, energy, attention, organization, purpose, and priorities.[401,498,502–506] One resource that is relevant to medical training is *Getting Things Done* by productivity expert David Allen. This offers practical methods to manage inbox messages, choose which tasks to prioritize first, determine which tasks to delegate, clear your mind of clutter, and increase focus on important items.[502]

Determine Your Values and General Priorities

Other general steps you can take to optimize productivity start with defining your values and priorities. You must also consider the shared priorities and expectations of your family and significant other. These priorities should guide your time, energy, and attention. You can commit to and clarify these priorities by writing them down and sharing them with your partner.

Optimize Your Environment

Next, set up your environment to support your priorities. First, as a reality check related to your home environment, homeownership often consumes several times as much time and money than expected. More generally, owning things creates clutter and consumes time. During intense medical training, a simpler lifestyle with an easy commute can be beneficial. If you have 16 waking hours in a day, work a 12-hour shift, commute 1 hour each way, and spend an hour on housework, then 75% of your free time is spent on commuting and upkeep.

In addition, choose your friends and manage your conversations intentionally. It is far easier to be productive when we are surrounded by others who value productivity and positivity.

Prioritize Specific Tasks by Asking If, When, and How

With the right environment in place, you can set priorities for individual tasks. There are various recommendations for ranking priorities that consider the amount of time needed, amount of effort required, task urgency, importance to you personally, and/or importance to your career.[502,507,508] The results boil down to answering three questions: if, when, and how you should do a task. The *if* question is answered by considering whether you should do it yourself, delegate it, or forget about it.

If you're lucky, you'll have more opportunities than you can accept. This means you must learn the art of saying "no" to low priority offers. You cannot always say "no" as a trainee, but keep in mind that taking on too many extra projects is counterproductive.

When an unexpected proposal comes your way, it is usually best to say something like, "Thank you for the offer, this sounds interesting. Let me assess my current projects to see if I would have the bandwidth to do a good job and get back to you by tomorrow morning." If you are interested but truly too busy now, you can say "no" but still indicate interest to leave the door open in the future.

To determine *when* to do a task, those that are both urgent and important usually take priority. For example, you might groan over the rigmarole of renewing a state medical license that soon expires, but it is both urgent and important. Things that are neither urgent nor important can wait, and those that are just urgent or just important fall somewhere in the middle.

Many gurus also suggest taking care of the most feared or effortful task early in the day.[507] Save low-effort tasks for the end of the day, when decision fatigue has set in. In addition, it can be useful to factor in your chronotype (basically if you are a morning or night person) as your schedule permits since evidence shows that some of us really do work better at different times of the day.[90]

There are many considerations for *how* to be productive, but a big one is simply paying attention to the task at hand. Despite the many claims some make on the ability to multitask, you are unlikely to do so effectively.[498] In fact, multitasking usually exceeds our cognitive capacity, resulting in a cognitive switch penalty and reducing net productivity.[45,498,509] Further, the commonly held notion that women are better at multitasking than men is not strongly supported in the literature.[510–512] Some evidence, however, suggests women are more likely to prefer multitasking.[513]

Email Management

Moreover, email management is a special consideration for productivity since it consumes considerable time and energy, but there are several steps you can take to mitigate the effects.[508] For example, manage spam emails with filters or by unsubscribing. Drop the auto pop-up notifications for new mail and batch your email review. For quick, routine tasks, open each email just once and then delete or archive it. Many email responses can be completed effectively with just a few short sentences. Store emails that you need to keep in dedicated folders for easy access.

Prioritize Rest and Recovery

While challenging in medical training, sufficient rest is essential. In addition to good sleep and some relaxation on off days, a little rest during a workday is important since medical performance and productivity decline later in a work shift.[514,515] Strategic breaks during the day, even if it is just getting up and taking a two-minute walk to clear your head, are beneficial.

Habits

Case Study: Resident Turn Runner

To help us understand the essentials of habit formation, meet Greg, a second-year resident in a busy pediatric program. His partner works full time as a physical therapist, and they have two children, ages 1 and 3. Until last year, feeling too busy, he had exercised only intermittently during training and found himself caught up in a negative mental feedback loop. Then he made a change.

After self-reflection, he wanted to identify as a physically active, healthy person. He decluttered his house, organized and simplified his chore list, and made a habit of going to sleep early when possible. He started getting up 40 minutes earlier. His alarm was his cue to say something positive about the day's outlook and to put on his exercise gear that he had laid out the evening before. He invested in a solid, residential-grade treadmill and some headphones.

At first, he jogged only a mile and then walked additionally when he was interested. Over time, the mile became easy and automatic, and he gradually increased his distance to two, three, and then four miles. Although he was a bit groggy and sometimes had only mild motivation, he stuck to it because it was easy and enjoyable enough. After all, he could listen to his favorite music and was rewarded afterward with a runner's high and a substantial, but guilt-free, breakfast like high-protein yogurt with fruit and honey. This was also a little time to himself in an otherwise busy personal and professional life.

With time, he started running longer miles on weekends, completed several half-marathons, and identified not only as an exerciser, but as a runner. Now, he could not imagine himself any other way. The habit was set for the foreseeable future.

Overview

Habit formation is important to understand on a personal- and patient-care basis. The topic of habit is as important as ever, with increasing awareness of lifestyle as determinants of personal well-being and the rise of chronic diseases that, in many cases, can be delayed or avoided with lifestyle modifications.

Healthy habits can be particularly useful for you during the time-strapped training years. You can benefit most with a growth mindset and an adaptive response to failure. You may also find habit-forming principles useful for motivational interviewing and counseling.

Greg's story demonstrates many important elements of habit formation: he addressed something that was important to him, so much so that he changed his self-image to match (he became a *runner*). He found a reliable prompt (alarm) and found a reliable reward (runner's high and nice breakfast). He made the habit easy (home treadmill and realistic early self-expectations) and enjoyable (music and time alone). These factors served as provisions for times when his motivation was a bit low due to grogginess. Now, let's explore these factors in more detail.

Layers of Habit

Broadly, habit formation has been divided by various authors into layers, steps, phases, and challenges. With this approach, the layers are[211]

$$\text{Identity}(\text{core}) \rightarrow \text{Processes}(\text{middle layer}) \rightarrow \text{Outcomes}(\text{outer layer})$$

Some sources contend that we must first adopt a new identity, or belief, as a fundamental driver of new habits. If you are going to bike regularly, you can't just be someone who completes a bike race once; you must become a biker. Too often, individuals focus too much on the outcomes (e.g., win a bike race) and then get derailed when the outcome—which may be out of their control—is not as desired.

129

The Basic Formula (Steps): Cue, Response, Reward

There are many resources and models for habit building, but most follow the same basic formula of steps:

$$Cue \rightarrow Response \rightarrow Reward$$

While authors in the literature on habit formation have different perspectives, most ultimately boil things down to this simple operational formula, which is best for general applications. An article on the importance of habit formation in general practice offers a practical view that a habit is formed when we "repeat a chosen behavio[u]r in the same context, until it becomes automatic and effortless."[516] However, as we'll see, effective habit formation also requires optimized cues and rewards.[208]

The cue (sometimes referred to as a prompt) can be an internal thought or external. It can also be modifiable like a strategically placed reminder or nonmodifiable like a certain time in the day. In general, prompts that are part of our current routine are far more effective than relying on internal cues (i.e., remembering).[208]

A *reward* must occur with or immediately after the response to cultivate a habit. Recall that rewards are connected to associative memory, emotions, and expectations. More delayed celebrations are not highly habit-promoting and are better referred to as *incentives*.[208]

Phases of Habit Formation

Finally, habit formation progresses in phases as follows:[516]

$$Initiation \rightarrow Learning \rightarrow Stability$$

That is, an action needs to be repeated regularly many times before it becomes an engrained habit. There is no set number of repetitions or set timeframe required to establish a habit, however. It is usually best to start small so you will succeed even when you lack motivation. The cumulative effect of many small consistent habits can be meaningful.[208,211] We are also more likely to stick to a habit with positive associations and celebration.[208]

Challenges for Habit Formation

The main difficulty with habit formation is the many potential challenges in forming and maintaining them. Changing routines can be hard. These roadblocks could arise from any of the components of the layers, steps, or phases. If you do not alter your core identity (layer), identify an effective cue or reward (step), or aim too high to start, setting yourself up to fail (phase), a habit may not stick.

It is well worth investing time to learn these challenges in more detail with dedicated resources. Here, we'll briefly mention just two related key factors: your environment and mindset. Your environment is key because it contains cues but can also create friction. If your environment is not optimized for a particular habit, it is more likely to fail. Alternatively, an optimized environment decreases the need to rely on willpower and motivation. Mindset is also critical because if a given habit is not truly important to you or if your mindset is fixed, the habit is less likely to hold.

Additional Resources

Three of the excellent many resources about habit you might choose to read are *The Power of Habit* by Charles Duhigg, *Atomic Habits* by James Clear, and *Tiny Habits* by BJ Fogg. While similar, there are some differences in philosophy and scope. For example, the opinions on the importance of willpower and motivation in the equation differ.[208,211] Overall, any one of these books is a great place to start.

24

Failure

Vance T. Lehman

Famous Failures

Born to immigrant parents of modest means, Richard Carmona spent part of his childhood homeless in New York. He faced adversity and setbacks that most never will, and at the age of 17 he dropped out of high school. Still, he changed course, joining the military and eventually special operations. This decision paved the way to serving as medic, then nurse, and later surgeon. In 2002, he was sworn in as the 17th U.S. surgeon general.

There are countless examples of famous people who overcame failure to achieve enormous success—Oprah Winfrey, Dwayne "The Rock" Johnson, or Olympian diver Greg Louganis to name a few. In industry, the introduction of *New Coke* nearly bankrupted Coca Cola in the 1980s. This chapter explores two key questions: what constitutes failure, and does it foster growth?

Types of Failure

There are many types of failure, but here, we'll consider just three broad types of failure relevant to medical training: (1) professional growth-related, (2) sunk cost, and (3) those of medical practice.

Professional Growth-Related Failure

Learning from failure with a growth mindset—and trying again—is key to professional growth. While many, including Pixar founder Ed Catmull, tout this type of failure as a necessary ingredient for success, it turns out that failure does not always make us better. First, negative feedback generally evokes a stronger emotional response than positive feedback.[517] In fact, failure is similarly painful for everyone, from grade-schoolers to CEOs.[179]

One reason for this is that it strikes at the ego and can threaten one's self-esteem.[517] This is especially true when self-esteem relies heavily on external validation. The pain of failure can lead to denial and information aversion, even when it is critical to know, also known as the *ostrich effect*.[518]

Sunk Cost Failure

Conversely, a sunk cost failure occurs when we should abandon a course, regardless of prior effort. In medicine, this could be a research project that, over time, becomes clear that it will not deliver meaningful results (positive or negative). Ed Catmull refers to it when asserting

DOI: 10.1201/9781003633389-27

that failure is one necessary ingredient for success, though he discusses sunk cost in the setting of projects that are abandoned as well.

Medical Practice Failures

In the book *The Checklist Manifesto*, Dr. Atul Gawande, general surgeon and public health researcher, breaks factors contributing to failure of medical care down into two general categories: those of ignorance and those of ineptitude.[519] Ignorance, fueled by common biases, is addressed through improved self-awareness.

Ineptitude—getting something wrong that we ought to get right—is where checklists can come into play, he contends. This is increasingly important given the rising complexity of modern medicine and the potential for failures due to ineptitude.[519] Nevertheless, the scope and heartache of failure is much broader, and checklists are probably only an answer for a narrow set of routine, established activities.

A special type of failure in medicine is a *never event*, or a serious but preventable event that we should always avoid. Examples include leaving a surgical sponge in a patient, giving a patient a medication that they have a severe allergy to, or performing a procedure on the wrong patient. The implications of never events (which we should avoid at all costs) are markedly different from those of professional development (where failure can be a point of growth) or sunk cost (where failure can be an opportunity to redirect resources).

Shame, Guilt, and Perfectionism

Failure of professional development summons one's inner critic, which is always lurking somewhere nearby and secured a foothold in our brain long ago by offering a survival advantage to our ancestors being chased by predators. Though humans have made a quantum leap from hunter-gatherers to city-dwellers in a relatively short 10,000 years, the inner critic persists.

Today, the inner critic casts this ancestral memory onto modern-day setbacks, treating getting a grant rejected as our ancestors might respond to encountering a salivating saber-toothed tiger. When these emotional factors are dominant, we learn less from our own failures than we do from observing those of others.[520] One take-home message is that we should seek out safe ways to share our failures and learn from others, such as with anonymous presentations of medical missteps or with morbidity and mortality conferences.

Everyone's inner critic can show up unannounced. Two gifts it may bring are *guilt* or *shame*. Both involve different aspects of negative self-evaluation, but the distinction between these two concepts is debated. According to author Brené Brown, guilt is the psychological discomfort of failing to live up to our values. The inner critic still has an adaptive role when not running amuck, and appropriately placed, well-managed guilt can steer us back onto a path that makes us proud. Shame, on the other hand, is a deep, intensely painful belief that we are unworthy and intrinsically flawed.

Perfectionists, including many healthcare workers, are particularly vulnerable to this. High standards can be adaptive but also risk increased chance of self-proclaimed failure. Perfectionism mixed with self-criticism can become maladaptive, culminating in frequent failure-criticism cycles and secondary effects like shame. If you are a perfectionist, you should be particularly wary of this inner voice. The inner critic may offer useful insights but often doesn't. After you have considered his points, send him packing…and lock the door with a deadbolt for a time if you must.

Mindset

You should adopt a *growth mindset*, which is described by optimism, positivity, and accepting of the natural need to improve. Essentially, it means embracing failure as an opportunity for growth without excessive self-criticism. It is the view that even if you have not succeeded *yet*, you can, with practice, achieve success. Conversely, a *fixed mindset* can threaten resilience and lead to negative self-evaluation, over-generalization of under-developed skills, and quitting. Your mindset is crucial; it can significantly impact your career and well-being.

A growth mindset can also help cultivate passions. With the right attitude, environment, and success, topics that are interesting to a person can evolve to avid personal pursuits.[521] Conversely, a fixed mindset hinders this transformation. While it is not realistic to develop a deep passion for every area of medicine, a growth mindset can help keep us interested, which in turn spurs social learning and makes conventional learning easier and more enjoyable.

Key Takeaways

There are many types of failure, and each requires different management considerations. The ability to manage failure well is critical for success in training, although often undertaught. Suboptimal responses to failure can result in denial and lack of personal growth. Key ingredients for managing failure well are recognition of its universal nature, a growth mindset, and appropriately high self-expectations. In Chapter 31, we'll see that the ability to guide others through their failures is a crucial skill needed for leadership but again is often not formally taught.

Next, we'll discuss medical writing, another critical skill needed every day in medicine for optimal performance.

25

Medical Writing

Vance T. Lehman

General Considerations

High-quality writing is crucial for success in medicine. This encompasses clinical notes, progress notes, history and physicals, pathology and radiology reports, academic papers, and basic communication. Well-organized writing implies an organized thought process. Poorly constructed notes, however, increase workload for supervising physicians and other clinicians. Medical writing is a skill that few medical trainees master. One reason is that premed English classes often inadequately emphasize the critical analysis and technical communication skills needed for medicine.

Style

This style is closer to that of popular fiction writers than literary authors. Stephen King suggests a simple writing style, emphasizing common words, short sentences, and well-managed paragraph length.[522] This immerses readers without distracting them with complex syntax. Analysis of King's fiction books has found a mean of 4 characters per word and 13 words per sentence.[523]

Popular writers often use similar structures, while literary Pulitzer winners often prioritize complexity.[523] Literary writers may aim for beauty or uniqueness, while professional writing primarily conveys information. However, straightforward writing can also achieve literary merit, as seen in the works of Ernest Hemingway and Toni Morrison.[523] Effective simple writing uses strong verbs and avoids filler words. It conveys its message clearly, avoiding extravagant language.

Despite the need for succinctness, medical writing often includes unnecessary filler words. Overusing phrases like "there is," "is seen," or "unchanged" can quickly add unnecessary length. New trainees often overuse transitional phrases. While some jargon is necessary, overly technical terms are generally unhelpful in clinical notes. Avoid colloquial language; use professional terms instead.

Medical and scientific writing commonly overuses the passive voice. This aims for objectivity but results in weak, wordy sentences. Many authors favor the active voice in popular writing, too, though some are more flexible.[522-524] The passive voice is useful when the action is more important than the agent. For example, it can soften blame by stating "mistakes were made" instead of "he made mistakes."

While sentences affect flow, King emphasizes the paragraph.[522] Paragraph length and structure significantly impact readability. Excessively long or short paragraphs hinder

DOI: 10.1201/9781003633389-28

readability. Trainees often create overly long paragraphs that bury information or use short, choppy paragraphs that are difficult to read.

Finally, use *parallel structure* for consistent grammar and form. For example, use a consistent grammatical pattern (e.g., verb presence and type) for every component for consecutive list items, clauses, or sentences.

Organization

Medical writing often tells a clinical story. The format depends on the context and type of writing. It generally follows a chronological order, as in oncologic histories. Alternatively, some notes start with the most critical information. This usually relates to the main concern or reflects changes since the last follow-up.

Information related to common topics should be grouped for readability. For example, head CT reports often separate brain findings from those of other structures. Mixing anatomical areas muddles the report unless a pathological link exists (e.g., frontal sinusitis with intracranial extension).

For follow-ups, begin with changes since the last encounter. Start with a succinct summary, such as, "Since the last episode, X and Y have changed," or "No significant change since the last encounter."

In sum, clinical writing can be organized chronologically or by importance, topic, or stability.

Editing and Practice

In addition to daily reading and writing, King places strong emphasis on the editing process.[522] He advises against premature submission of manuscript drafts, even to informal reviewers. In medicine, editing is crucial for all forms of writing. Early in training, critical appraisal of clinical notes is a worthwhile investment. This includes *content editing* (ensuring key information is included and extraneous information is omitted) and *line editing* for structure, clarity, and grammar.

Manuscripts always require editing. New trainees often prematurely submit incomplete drafts to staff or other coauthors, perhaps due to insecurity or inexperience. Aim for a complete draft before seeking review, but seek help from your mentor if you are stuck in a specific area. Even good drafts need editing; poor drafts may require rewriting. Clinical notes require careful editing, too, especially initially.

These suggestions—daily practice for writing, editing and organizing composition, carefully reading others' notes—are forms of deliberate practice.

Know Your Audience

Trainees sometimes question the importance of writing quality if the facts are correct, implying that such concerns are overly picky. Before we address this point, consider the audience for medical reports and notes. While the primary audience is usually healthcare providers, it also includes patients, other institutions, billing personnel, and even lawyers.

Remember the first rule of communication—know your audience. The diverse audience requires balancing technical accuracy with readability for non-physicians. In all cases, we are judged by our writing. Others will judge our professionalism, skill, intentions, dedication, and even intelligence based on our writing. Difficult-to-read notes waste time and create frustration.

Confidence

Confidence includes conveying your degree of certainty in your conclusions and inspiring confidence in your abilities. A correct conclusion in a note doesn't inspire confidence in your ability if the reasoning or wording is unclear. Conversely, even if a trainee's conclusion is incorrect, attendings may be impressed by sound reasoning and calibrated (e.g., safe) recommendations.

In radiology reports, for example, stating "there is a possible shadow in the lung that might be an area of nodularity" differs greatly from "there is a spiculated nodule strongly suggestive of malignancy." The first conveys low diagnostic confidence and doesn't inspire confidence in the writer's abilities. The second conveys high diagnostic confidence and inspires confidence in the reader's diagnostic abilities.

Know Who to Imitate

Some experienced staff don't write perfect notes. Even so, they will enjoy being given the benefit of the doubt that trainees and new staff are not. Therefore, create well-structured notes with all critical elements, even if some staff deviate from this practice.

Composing an Original Research Manuscript

First Author Papers Give You More Mileage

While any project participation is useful, aim to be first author on at least a paper or two. This carries more academic weight on early career applications than a middle-author position. The first author typically contributes the most work, writes the first draft, and sees the project through. Completing a project demonstrates commitment and is viewed favorably on applications, especially for academic careers.

Substance and Style

Manuscript writing, a formulaic process, can be unintuitive for trainees. Original research begins with good study design and rationale. You can write the introduction and methods sections early, after finalizing the study design. You can also complete the key references and complete a literature search.

Manuscript writing boils down to substance and style. Prioritize substance over background. The core of the manuscript is the methods and results. The methods section should allow study replication and reveal limitations and biases. Patient selection bias is particularly important in medicine. Each method should have a corresponding result (and vice versa). For example, the Standards for Reporting of Diagnostic Accuracy (STARD) initiative outlines 25 elements for diagnostic accuracy studies, with 23 in the methods and results sections.[525]

The Meat of the Manuscript: Methods and Results

New authors often write lengthy, meandering introductions and discussions, but conciseness is key. A comprehensive overview of the entire relevant body of literature is more appropriate for a review article or book chapter. The introduction should briefly explain the rationale and aims, often identifying a gap in the literature. The discussion should briefly summarize the key results, their importance, and their relation to prior literature. The discussion often concludes by suggesting future directions and acknowledging study limitations.

The Importance of Reasonable Data Interpretation

Misinterpretation of sound methods and results can lead to manuscript rejection. Examples include overinterpreting differences with overlapping confidence intervals, making unsupported assertions, and downplaying limitations. Avoid claiming novelty since it's impossible to know all published and unpublished work. Excessive self-citation can raise eyebrows, though measured self-citation boosts your h-index.

Manuscript hype will be called out by seasoned reviewers and editors. Overselling results in the title is common. The abstract's conclusion is another area prone to hype.[1] This is one reason why abstract perusal does not replace careful reading of the methods and results. Discussion sections can also overstate results with broad, unsubstantiated implications. Avoid self-aggrandizing phrases like *inaugural study* and *pioneering work*.

Peer Reviewers are Infinitely Tougher than Coauthor Reviewers

Writing style improves with practice and accepting (sometimes brutal) critiques. Coauthors are generally kinder than anonymous reviewers. Even when coauthors offer minor comments and praise, reviewers can eviscerate the manuscript. Thus, a careful presubmission critique from a coauthor is invaluable. Further, read peer-reviewed articles from high-quality journals regularly to learn good writing styles.

Case Reports

Case reports require special consideration. Submissions often include irrelevant details, resembling clinical notes. If the case report concerns a cutaneous eruption after exposure to a rare plant, avoid distracting details like the patient's hypertension, social anxiety, or smoking history. Use objective language (e.g., "reported") instead of pejorative language (e.g., "complained"). You should also avoid overemphasizing the number of previously reported cases, as many go unreported.

Finally, include colleagues with relevant expertise and/or who meaningfully participated in patient care when possible. If a case report focuses on a brain tumor with a rare appearance on imaging or pathology, seek expert help. Involve a radiologist or pathologist as a coauthor to select and describe images. Having the relevant expert listed as coauthor can add credibility to the work and ensure that it is accurate.

Book Chapters

One benefit to writing book chapters is that they are generally accepted for publication. However, book chapters generally carry less academic weight than research articles. They are either not peer-reviewed or less rigorously reviewed. This doesn't mean you should avoid writing chapters, but be selective.

Table 25.1 Key Writing Lessons in Medicine

1. Use clear and concise language
2. Avoid redundant or filler words
3. Favor the active voice
4. Favor simple sentence structures
5. Control flow with paragraph formatting/length
6. Use parallelism
7. Edit your work
8. Practice writing and read consistently
9. Use technically correct language but consider avoiding highly specialized jargon for general reports

Submitting a Manuscript and Journal Selection

Use a professionally formatted cover letter and title page (staff often have examples). Careful journal selection is crucial. Submitting to an inappropriate journal wastes time and resources. In addition, there are many other unique features of each journal, including type of access, publication fees, index status, audience, and submission requirements. For more information, see our article "Journal Selection Primer for Neuroradiology Researchers."[526] While focused on one discipline, the principles apply broadly.

Key Takeaways

This chapter introduces key concepts for professional medical writing. Effective writing is a critical skill for patient care and demonstrating competence. Key takeaways are outlined in Table 25.1. Excellent writing skills are crucial for research, the topic of the next chapter.

Note

1   As an important aside, I read the main body of every citation in this book, including full books and articles, not just the abstracts.

26

Research

Vance T. Lehman

Two Trainees with Different Outcomes

Sean and Sara are ophthalmology residents starting an academic program who both desire to enter the same fellowship. Both aspire to enter private practice but must complete a research project as part of their training program. Both opted for retrospective studies, advised as more realistic for trainees. But the similarities end there.

Unsure how to begin, Sean asked his attending about potential research projects. The attending is an excellent clinician and is easy to work with. He tells Sean about an idea he had recently about describing their experience with a rare condition. After a few weeks, Sean asks him how he can start, and he directs him to the research office, which can help him set up an IRB under his name. After stumbling through the IRB process and a month-long approval, he wonders how he will identify patients for the study. He then discovers a clunky, homegrown data retrieval system, requiring a weekend to sort out.

When Sean retrieves the patient data, it is not good news—there were only a few patients in the system. He started trudging through the clinical charts and taking notes about the clinical features, treatment, and outcomes. However, the documentation was inconsistent with substantial missing data. His attempt to categorize the data resulted in a table with numerous gaps, unsuitable for statistical analysis.

To fulfill his requirement, he submits a manuscript to one of the main ophthalmology journals, but after several months of waiting, it is rejected. Upon rejection, Sean and his mentor decide to reformat it and submit it to another journal. On his fellowship application, he lists the research as *in progress* on his CV.

Sara takes a different approach. She reviewed her attendings' research profiles, noting publication topics, mentorship success, and publication rates. She finds a few whose research topics interest her and who publish regularly. She casually asked one attending about suitable projects, demonstrating her preparedness.

The attending offered an interesting, relevant, and practical project. A brief literature search confirmed the project indeed addressed an unanswered clinical question, and she verified sufficient patient data before proceeding. Checking patient numbers was easy, because the attending had already completed an IRB and had a database of basic information ready.

Her attending also developed a straightforward research question and explained how she could collect the data systematically to answer it. The entire process was smooth, culminating in a conference presentation and publication. Her fellowship application included the conference abstract and PubMed citation.

DOI: 10.1201/9781003633389-29

The experiences of new trainees often resemble those of Sean more so than Sara. What makes the difference? Let's explore the importance of background research before starting a research project. We'll then discuss selecting a project, conducting literature searches, and applying the scientific method.

Why Do Research?

Many trainees, focused on patient care, initially show little interest in research. Still, there are reasons that you might want or need to do it. Discovering something new, especially with potential for improved patient care, is exciting. Tangible motivations include CV enhancement and collaboration with a mentor who can provide strong support. Research ultimately connects to education and clinical practice on local and global scales. Further, it can lead to expertise, opening opportunities for speaking engagements, travel, education, and industry collaboration.

While many programs require research, academic programs often expect trainees to pursue additional projects. Staff may view this as essential to your education and a way to contribute to the program and specialty. Some programs allocate research time; in these cases, accountability for progress is expected.

However, the primary focus of training remains clinical care. Thus, avoid overemphasizing research at the expense of clinical competency.

Types of Research

Research endeavors vary in types, goals, and timelines. *Basic science* projects can take months or years, with publication as the tangible outcome. Some basic science projects simply do not work out at all. Most medical trainees pursue clinical research instead.

Clinical research can be broadly classified into *retrospective* and *prospective* studies. Prospective studies are challenging for trainees due to time and resource constraints. Retrospective studies often offer the best return on time investment. In the previous scenarios, both ophthalmology residents wisely chose retrospective, clinically based projects.

Selecting Research Projects and Mentors

Some methods to select research mentors (advisors) and projects are more successful. Consider this common scenario: an interesting case is encountered during patient care, and someone declares, "We should write this up." Despite mutual enthusiasm in the moment, this should be tempered with discipline.

Realize that "we" actually means "you." Spontaneous ideas may yield important contributions, but not always. Such ideas often lack forethought regarding data availability or existing literature. Sean went with an unvetted project, which was not shovel ready.

Do Background Research

In general, like Sara, you should also do some background research on the topic (and mentor) before committing. When considering any prospective mentor, assess their interest, availability, and experience. Determine if they are committed mentors, not just seeking free help.

141

Table 26.1 Traits of an Ideal Research Mentor

Has time and interest to be a research mentor
Tailors a project and degree of responsibility to your level
Has a solid record of publication, including recent years
Has completed numerous first-author publications himself/herself (even if remote)
Is interested in developing your general academic skills, not just pushing through a project
Has no major personality conflicts with the prospective mentee
Has the primary goal of helping you, the academic community, and patient care; not simply to further his/her own career

Review the mentor's PubMed profile to assess their publication experience and journal choices. Proceed cautiously if they have few publications. Ideally, they should have several first- and senior-author publications to demonstrate experience and perspective

First-author publications show understanding of the process; senior-author publications indicate established mentorship. Beware of attendings who haven't published as first authors but enlist trainees for projects as their trainees may not have received experienced guidance needed to be successful. This is not to say that less experienced attendings cannot be great mentors too. Sometimes, they will have fresh perspectives. More experienced attendings may also have competing priorities. So, each opportunity should be evaluated individually, but more experienced attendings will usually have an edge walking you through the process.

Regardless of experience, mentors vary in their level of involvement. Hands-on mentorship is most helpful for inexperienced trainees. Traits to look for in a research mentor are listed in Table 26.1.

Consider the Purpose, Merit, and Feasibility of a Study

You should also evaluate the purpose, merit, and feasibility of a project. Clinical research merit depends on proposal quality and potential impact on patient care. Thus, it is wise to conduct a literature search on the topic before committing to a project. Existing publications aren't a deal-breaker if you can offer new information or resolve a controversy.[1] This might involve addressing limitations of prior work or exploring a new angle, such as a different patient population.

While replication is important, novel information is frequently prioritized for publication. Consider carefully if your study is smaller and similar to previous work. However, some dismissed ideas may have been poorly executed, done in a different context, or require confirmation. Finally, right or wrong, a timely (hot) topic increases publication chances.

Sara's project had a key advantage: feasibility. The feasibility of a project depends on several factors. Retrospective studies are easier; data is readily available, and depending on the design, IRB consent may be waived. Data availability is critical. Some projects offer ready-to-use databases (like Sara's), while others require de novo patient searches (like Sean's).

The study should be large enough for statistical power but avoid impractically large studies. Taking over a partly finished project can be risky; if considering one, assess why the previous lead stopped. Specifically, determine if it was for personal motivational factors or project-related factors. Authorship considerations should also be agreed upon before proceeding. Finally, ensure alignment with your mentor on contributions, timelines, and roles in presentations and publications.

Literature Search Strategies

Literature search competency is crucial given the increasing volume and complexity of medical information. Effective search strategies involve selecting resources, using appropriate search terms, conducting secondary searches, and critically appraising results. Although this is a vast topic, this chapter outlines key strategies that are high-yield and generalizable.

Google and PubMed

You'll encounter many useful search engines and databases. Key resources include Google and PubMed, a widely accessed medical literature database. Google can be a reasonable starting point. It includes articles not indexed in PubMed but has limitations. For example, articles from lower quality or predatory resources may be included. The Google Scholar search engine offers a more refined search. PubMed indexes reputable journals,[2] filtering out irrelevant articles, but is more rigid with search terms.

Consider Google for quick searches, but for substantive research, start with PubMed and then use Google to identify any missed sources. Generative AI tools, such as openevidence. com, can cite peer-reviewed literature and answer questions intuitively (always verify with primary sources).

Search Optimization

Develop skills in optimizing search terms, searching by author, title, or PMID, using overview articles such as guidelines or review articles, and conducting secondary searches of article references. This requires substantial practice. In addition, it is useful to review the *PubMed User Guide*, found on their website.

Evidence for Daily Practice

For quick, real-time answers during busy workdays, you'll need a streamlined approach. With practice, this can be done quickly. Still, you must understand your search limitations and avoid drawing too many conclusions from only a few articles.

Importance and Debates of the Scientific Method

Medical training may not extensively cover the scientific method. It is one of those things in the background that *you should already know*, presumably introduced well before you ever graduated from high school. This is unfortunate, as it's a key foundation of medical knowledge, constantly evolving and debated.

Deductive Reasoning and Falsification

Science is often viewed as an unwavering guide to truth, but its nature is debated. Historically, deductive reasoning dominated knowledge acquisition from Aristotle to the scientific revolution. Francis Bacon, in the 16th century, argued for inductive reasoning—accumulating evidence to reach general conclusions.

The philosopher Karl Popper, in the 20th century, identified a problem leading to a return to deductive reasoning. He noticed a striking difference between the theory of relativity and the prominent psychological and social theories of the day like psychoanalysis and Marxism. He argued that psychoanalysis and Marxism were unfalsifiable, as data could always be manipulated to fit their claims. Thus, Popper asserted that true science uses deductive reasoning and attempts at falsification (to disprove a theory).

This means that a theory can never be *proven*, only supported by withstanding attempts at disproof. Conversely, a single solid (and ideally replicated) failure can invalidate a theory. For example, Einstein's theory of relativity would have been falsified if light hadn't been deflected during the 1919 solar eclipse. Inductively developed, unfalsifiable theories were, in Popper's view, *pseudoscience* (a term considered pejorative today).

Inductive Reasoning and Verification

Given Popper's influence, familiarity with his views and critiques is useful. While Popper's approach remains dominant, critics like Thomas Kuhn have argued against falsification.[527] Kuhn argued that we often must choose the best among competing theories, as none have perfect evidence. Falsification therefore risks rejecting the best available theories.

Kuhn also noted that observations are influenced by preexisting beliefs (*theory-laden*), impacting research objectivity and logical certainty. He advised that we favor a verification approach instead based on the best available probabilities and inductive reasoning.

Other Critiques of Falsification

Popper's approach has also been criticized for being impractical and not reflecting actual scientific practice.[528] It also has limitations for complex fields like medicine (discussed in Chapter 48). Popperian proponents, in turn, critique Kuhn's approach, arguing that falsification deals with more definitive theories than inductive conjectures.[529]

Yet, the notions of falsification and verification do not even enter the minds of many great doctorate level researchers for practical everyday purposes. So, why should you care about the definition of science if even experts still disagree? One reason is that the concept of falsification can help you assess the rigor of a theory.

For example, the popular *central governor theory* in exercise science controversially asserts that performance limits are brain-based protective mechanisms, not physiological limitations. This idea though remains vulnerable to considerable criticism, largely on the grounds that it is not falsifiable.[530,531] Additionally, credible researchers actively seek to disprove their own theories.

Calls for an Updated Scientific Method

Finally, some authorities and even the National Science Foundation advocate modernizing the scientific method.[532] This is due to knowledge derived from non-scientific methods, important findings unrelated to hypotheses, the real world's complexity, and the need for new large data analysis methods.[532] For example, large datasets (e.g., genetic data) may be mined agnostically, rather than hypothesis-driven. Therefore, less rigid, discovery-focused methods may be beneficial.[532]

Notes

1 The value of replication is discussed in Chapter 28, though pure replication studies are often not the best choice for a first project.
2 While reliable, PubMed indexed search results still need critical appraisal and some articles from predatory journals are still included.

27

Statistics

Vance T. Lehman

Introduction

Modern statistical analysis offers excellent tools, but their effectiveness depends on proper application. In medicine, they are too often misapplied or misunderstood. Clinicians often demonstrate low statistical proficiency, coupled with overconfidence.[63] Further, the proliferation of statistical methods highlights the field's complexity. Beyond the pitfalls of statistical application, deeper controversies exist regarding inferential analysis, probability, and null hypothesis significance testing (NHST).

The major problems are that we are not taught enough about statistics and tacitly taught to take the validity of NHST results we encounter for granted. While most of us won't become statisticians, we'll interpret statistically analyzed studies and apply them to patient care. Improved understanding of this topic is crucial. This prevents potentially embarrassing or dangerous misinterpretations. This chapter explores key debates and fundamental concepts often overlooked in training.

Fundamental Concepts and Questions

Descriptive Versus Inferential Analyses

Statistics can be broadly categorized as *descriptive* and *inferential*. Descriptive analyses describe all data points in detail. This is like counting every vote in a general election. Inferential analyses use samples to extrapolate to the larger population, providing predictions with estimates of measurement error and uncertainty. This is like an election poll. Some experts believe that inferential analysis in medicine has substantial limitations, especially when ignoring existing knowledge.[533]

Probability

Probability is another fundamental concept in statistics. It turns out that the definition of probability is debated, impacting the interpretation of statistical results. NHST is rooted in a frequentist interpretation, defining probability strictly as frequency. Some experts argue that this definition is simplistic and undermines result interpretation by ignoring existing knowledge. This viewpoint also reflects the complexity of real-life results.

Is a Coin Toss 50:50?

The coin toss, a seemingly simple 50:50 probability event, illustrates the complexities of probability. Now, if one side were slightly more common, we might assume bias such as

DOI: 10.1201/9781003633389-30

lopsidedness. However, it's more complex. That is, the starting side is slightly, but significantly, more likely to land face up.[534] This likely reflects the complex physics of the toss. Given this complexity for a simple coin toss, consider the impact of frequentist assumptions on more complicated issues.

The Hybrid Origin of Null Hypothesis Significance Testing

In addition to the purely frequentist definition of probability, NHST's controversial nature, in part, stems from its combination of the fundamentally incompatible approaches of Fisher and Neyman-Pearson.[535,536]

These two approaches look similar superficially (like a significant p-value in the Fisher approach and an alpha value in the Neyman-Pearson approach) and use the same tests, which makes it tempting to think we can just combine them seamlessly. This setup can also overstate the definitiveness of single, unreplicated studies.[535,536]

The Normal Curve

Understanding the normal curve's applications, validity, and limitations is also crucial. Many statistical analyses *assume* a normal distribution of data or transform data to approximate it. Normal distributions were initially observed in physical phenomena (e.g., astronomical errors) and later applied to biology and sociology.[533] Then the statistician Karl Pearson coined the term *normal distribution*, implying its widespread occurrence (or the expected, normal, situation). Pearson later realized that many things deviate from it, but despite his attempts to develop a correction, the concept of *normality* stuck.[533]

The normal distribution is useful because many samples approximate it, naturally or after transformation. For example, traits influenced by multiple independent variables (e.g., height) often exhibit normal distributions.[533] [1] However, few, if any, measured things follow it exactly.[537] Since mild deviations from the normal distribution can result in large changes of measured variance, the assumption of normality can be problematic.[537]

Statistical Test Assumptions

You should also remember that conventional statistical tests have assumptions. If the assumptions are wrong, the results can be misleading. One way to classify many statistical tests is as either *parametric* (with parametric assumptions) *or nonparametric*. Parametric methods transform data to fit a known model, often assuming normality.[538] Parametric tests provide exact solutions to a fitted model while *nonparametric tests* provide approximate results without changing the model or assuming a normal distribution.[538] One issue with NHST techniques applied to small samples is *overfitting* of data to a model.

The Perils of P-Values

P-values are among the most misunderstood statistical concepts. In 2016, the American Statistical Association published a firm critique of the overuse and misinterpretation of p-values.[539] Common problems include failing to recognize that a small p-value doesn't indicate effect size or clinical significance.

Uncorrected data can yield spurious (and sometimes outlandish) results, such as correlations between medical conditions and astrology, or brain activity in a dead salmon (fMRI).[540,541] Additional discussion of the numerous other p-values pitfalls such as *p-hacking*, *pHARKing*, arbitrary significance levels, and need for confirmatory studies are beyond the scope of this book but is readily available elsewhere.

Bayesian Analysis

There is a major long-standing debate, under-recognized by medical trainees, over two fundamentally different approaches to statistics: frequentist and Bayesian. The frequentist approach has been dominant since the early 20th century, when NHST was developed.

Key Differences Between NHST and Bayesian Analysis

The fundamental difference between the two statistical approaches is that the frequentist approach treats a difference between two groups as fixed.[542] Thus, probability here is defined strictly, and objectively, by the frequency without factoring in background conditions and biases. Conversely, the Bayesian approach considers the difference to be variable and incorporates a *prior probability* of an outcome.[542] Thus, probability here is defined, in part, subjectively.

With Bayesian analysis, adjusting data with prior distributions yields *posterior distributions* of effect sizes. Thus, posterior distributions provide information on the range of effect sizes. Fundamentally, the Bayesian approach offers a more nuanced view of probability, providing more information about inferences from small samples.

Furthermore, NHST results reject or accept a (null) hypothesis.[533] Bayesian analysis, on the other hand, essentially never rejects or accepts a hypothesis but rather provides an intermediate-level probability that a hypothesis is true, and this probability can be updated with new information.[533] Finally, Bayesian analysis is most associated with verification, while NHST is most associated with falsification, and thus factor into the debates over the best approach to science mentioned in the last chapter.

Potential Benefits of the Bayesian Approach

With a Bayesian approach, an unlikely outcome—like extrasensory perception (ESP) being real—would require *extraordinary evidence*. Amazingly, frequentist analyses have suggested minor ESP effects, but Bayesian reanalyses deem this unlikely.[533] The prior probability of a person possessing ESP ability is exceedingly low. For comparison, hypotheses without prior reason to favor one outcome over another have neutral prior probabilities

In his book *Bernoulli's Fallacy*, Aubrey Clayton argues that many NHST applications are flawed and should be replaced by Bayesian methods. He cites flaws in the frequentist interpretation of probability, overreliance on normality assumptions, underemphasis of effect size, multiple comparisons, and base rate neglect. For example, we may inappropriately extend NHST methods effective in simple cases to complex systems like biological systems that are influenced by unknowable factors.

Bayesians acknowledge NHST's effectiveness in specific circumstances but criticize the need for multiple tests to accommodate various situations. Selection of a statistical test for a given analysis can also introduce operator bias. Further, each test has assumptions and limitations often misunderstood by physicians.

Bayesian methods offer numerous potential benefits, including broad applicability.[533] Bayesian proponents believe that this method works better in many common situations that are problematic with NHST. These situations include hypothesis formulation after data is

Bayes Theorem

$$P(F|H) = \frac{P(H|F) \times P(F)}{P(H)}$$

P(F|H) = Probability of F given that H is true

P(H|A) = Probability of H given that F is true

P(F), P(H) = Independent probabilities

Clinically-Relevant Form

Diagnostic Odds = Disease Prevalence Odds × Diagnostic Test Likelihood Ratio
(Posterior)   (Prior)

Figure 27.1 To illustrate Bayes theorem, let's ask the question: what is the probability there is fog (F) given that there is high humidity (H)? According to Bayes theorem, this will equal the probability that there is high humidity if there is fog adjusted by the independent probabilities of both fog and humidity). There would be a high probability that there is fog when there is high humidity (P(H|F)) when there is a high probability that there is high humidity when there is fog (P(H|F)), when the independent probability of fog (P(F)) is high, and when the independent probability of high humidity (P(H)) is low. Another way to look at this is that Bayes theorem takes the base rate of something into account and updates the likelihood with new information. For diagnostic tests in medicine, we can see the form of where a disease prevalence odds (related to the prior probability) is multiplied by a diagnostic test likelihood ratio to give the diagnostic odds of a test result (related to the posterior probability). In such cases, an initial prior probability is known based on disease prevalence, but this is updated with additional evidence from a diagnostic test. Higher disease prevalence or test likelihood ratios give higher odds of a patient with a positive test having a disease. Note that a likelihood ratio is expressed in terms of odds, which differ from probabilities. For example, 3:1 odds corresponds to a 75% probability expressed as a percentage (3/(3+1)).

collected, small sample sizes, optional stopping of data collection, and multiple comparisons.[533] Modified forms of Bayesian analysis may be used for clinical decision-making as well (Figure 27.1).

Critiques of Bayesian Analysis

However, determining prior probabilities can be contentious, and frequentist methods are entrenched. Frequentists assert that the prior probabilities are susceptible to investigator biases and could rig the results of a study.[543] Bayesians counter that frequentist approaches also involve subjectivity, such as hypothesis formulation and test assumptions.[543]

Many statisticians emphasize proper interpretation over the choice of approach, recognizing roles for both.[543,544]

Statistics, Medicine, and Eugenics

How Statistics and Eugenics Became Intertwined

Formal curricula often overlook the troubling history linking statistics, eugenics, and medicine. Understanding this history reveals how our profession can unintentionally cause harm. This history is relevant because the development of modern statistical methods aimed to create an illusion of objectivity in comparing human populations, making eugenic concepts more acceptable.[533]

149

Key figures in NHST's development—Francis Galton, Karl Pearson, and Rondald Fisher—were influenced by, and espoused, eugenic agendas.[533] Remarkably, Galton coined the term "eugenics."[533] He sought to extend the application of trait distributions (e.g., height) to concepts like intelligence and societal "worth" of populations.[533] The use of objective (frequentist) statistics potentially aimed to deflect accusations of bias.

One viewpoint, however, is that this use of frequentist statistics created an illusion of objectivity and introduced logical errors in interpreting complex data.[533] By this view, this frequentist approach then resulted in the need for an ever-expanding statistical toolkit to try to overcome these shortcomings, which is too complex for most of us to understand.[533]

The remainder of the story of these early statisticians is out of the scope of this book but seems almost beyond belief through the lens of modern times. Here, we'll focus on the impact it has had on medicine and briefly consider the relevance for us today.

Eugenics and Medicine in the United States

Consider that the eugenics movement quickly spread to the United States in the early 1900s, becoming mainstream among scientists and physicians. A prevailing thought was that social class predisposition, morals, and worth were hereditary. Thus, eugenics ideas colored the American view of people with disabilities, minorities, immigrants, and the poor.

Eugenic ideas were prevalent in medicine, promoted by physicians and medical journals. Many states enacted sterilization laws exceeding European precedents.[533] U.S. segregation and eugenicists influenced Nazi ideology, though the extent is debated.[545] However, physicians failed to foresee the ethical implications and devastating consequences that contributed to World War II atrocities.

Downstream Effects of the Intertwined History

Wartime atrocities led to ethically questionable medical experimentation, such as the *Minnesota Starvation Experiment*. The desire to understand wartime behavior also inspired some of the most provocative and (ironically) controversial experiments ever done, including the Stanford Prison Experiment and the Milgram Electric Shock Study (Chapter 8). Moreover, modern research guidelines, including the *Nuremberg Code*, emerged from the atrocities of Nazi experimentation.

This history highlights our susceptibility to conformity and power, medicine's potential for both good and harm, the limitations of real-time moral judgment, and the need for informed consent. Some argue that past eugenic biases persist, raising concerns about birth selection and gene editing potentially leading to a "new eugenics" without adequate safeguards.[546]

Note

1 Another important instance of a normal distribution is found when a population of any distribution with a well-defined mean is sampled many times independently. The distribution of the sample means will approach a normal distribution according to the central limit theorem.

28

Evidence-Based Medicine

Vance T. Lehman, Ajay Madhavan

Overview

This chapter builds on the topics of research and statistics discussion in the last two chapters. Further, it serves as a segue to the next chapter on logical fallacies and cognitive biases, which, along with evidence-based medicine (EBM), are important topics for medical decision-making.

Debates in Evidence-Based Medicine

To start, EBM is a relatively recent development, formalized in 1990s and popularized by a 1996 publication entitled *Evidence-Based Medicine: What It Is and Isn't.*[547] Still, even though formal EBM is decades old, a hidden tension remains between advocates of *traditional medicine*, who think it de-emphasizes the value of clinical experience and has major limitations in complex environments, and those who believe it is a core way physicians can overcome biases and apply best practices to patient care.[111,548] Many physicians fall somewhere in the middle. Thus, you may need to adapt to working with attendings who have a variety of viewpoints on how EBM fits into clinical practice.

One criticism of EBM by the traditionalists is that it promotes an overly dogmatic and algorithmic approach to medicine that discourages thinking and does not fully recognize the uncertainty and complexity of real-life practice.[111] Beyond considering clinical evidence, however, EBM guidelines advocate factoring in patient values, preferences, adherence to treatment, and other factors for individual cases.[549] At the same time, it is true that EBM attempts to mitigate our selection bias for evidence that just confirms our preconceived notions and places the most weight on the highest-level evidence available—which at times seems algorithmic.

Evidence-Based Medicine Is Generally Undertaught

This debate aside, understanding EBM is generally a key part of medical problem-solving and an area where trainees often fall short. Ideally, you would master the basic EBM concepts during medical school. However, you will likely benefit from substantial additional formal training and/or self-education to gain a solid grasp of these concepts. For this, some medical societies provide excellent supplemental EBM courses.

Even though it is unrealistic to expect all physicians to become EBM experts, you should also become familiar with the shortcomings of the current body of medical literature. These include misapplication of statistical methods (as mentioned), variable journal (including predatory) and peer-review quality, hype, and even fraud.

The Scope of Evidence-Based Medicine

We also find that trainees often misunderstand the nature and scope of EBM. For example, at its most basic level, the *evidence* is more than what's found in the medical literature. Evidence can also come from clinical experience, a patient's clinical presentation, and/or test results, though these are usually weaker forms than peer-reviewed literature. A big part of medical problem-solving is tying these different forms of evidence together in the right way.

It is easy for trainees to overlook the scope of EBM, so remember that it can help guide us for all three major components of patient care: diagnosis, treatment, and prognosis. To do this, EBM methods utilize a variety of statistical tools, describe approaches to randomized controlled trials (RCTs) and meta-analyses, describe pitfalls in evidence assessment, and provide ways to assess the quality of evidence and strength of recommendations using the Grading of Recommendations, Assessment, Development, and Evaluations (GRADE) approach.

Dr. Gordon Guyatt, has published an excellent book detailing these concepts, called *Users' Guides to the Medical Literature*.[549] While the book is too long for a most trainees to read straight through, it is worth perusing the major topics and working to understand over time as your career progresses.

The Replication Crisis and Zombie Trials

One important aspect of EBM is determining your degree of confidence in the truth of what you read. This is probably more challenging than most trainees believe, as evidenced by the landmark paper "Why Most Published Research Findings Are False," published in 2005.[550] This paper found a low replication rate in the literature, which has since been demonstrated many times over and is found in medicine and many other relevant fields, leading to concerns that we are amid a *replication crisis*. Most trainees and many staff that we interact with across the world are not highly familiar with this concept. This unfortunately leads to some undesirable clinical decisions based on putting too much faith in a single unreplicated and non-definitive study.

As one famous example in communication, a finding that was completely overturned was the highly publicized finding in one study that people who "*power pose*" increased testosterone and risk tolerance, suggesting that we ought to incorporate this into our body language practices at work.[551] To her credit, the author of the original study has acknowledged that the preponderance of data now shows that power posing effects are not real.[552,553]

Recall, too, that the results of the Stanford Prison Experiment did not bear out in another setting.[162] Thus, we ought to think twice before adopting new practices like power posing based on unreplicated data. We should also recognize that many disproved findings persist in the literature across a wide spectrum on disciplines.

Potential Causes of the Replication Crisis

The replication crisis has multiple potential causes (Table 28.1).[533,550,554–556] Some reasons for low replication rates may depend on the field of study. In behavioral and social sciences, this may partly reflect inherent complexity and difficulty reproducing exact study conditions.[556] In artificial intelligence (AI) research, a mechanism called '*data leakage*' has been implicated as an impediment to replication, which basically means a training data set is somehow connected to the test set in a way that will not occur in real-life applications.[555] According to Aubrey Clayton though (from Chapter 27), a fundamental cause likely lies in the way NHST is applied.[533]

Table 28.1 Potential Causes of the Replication Crisis

Inappropriate use or interpretation of statistics
Low statistical power or other poor study design
Insufficient availability of high-quality reviewers
Failure to consider prior probabilities
Various biases (especially publication bias)
Financial conflicts
Fraudulent publications and data
Emergence of predatory journals
Complexity of behavioral and social sciences
Publish or perish academic environments
Hot topic trends
Data leakage

In a variety of fields, the combination of a hot topic trend and publish or perish environment may promote a race to publish many positive results.[554] Thus, we should be particularly careful in interpreting data from fields outside our area of expertise. On a practical level, the results of any individual study deserve reasonable skepticism and confirmation with replication. Sometimes we have little choice except to make a medical decision with only one study to guide us, but we should do this carefully.

Broader Effects of the Replication Crisis

One broader effect of the replication crisis is that studies with false conclusions or questionable methodology can taint systematic reviews. A 2021 publication assessing available raw data from clinical trials in anesthesiology found that 44% had false data and about a quarter of the trials additionally had such glaring credibility concerns upon reanalysis of individual-level data that these were dubbed "Zombie Trials."[557]

Although impossible to confirm, there is reason to believe that more broadly there are hundreds of thousands of such Zombie Trials.[558] Furthermore, a 2023 publication entitled "Trials We Cannot Trust: Investigating Their Impact on Systematic Reviews and Clinical Guidelines in Spinal Pain" found that studies with "*trust concerns*" impacted the conclusions of systematic reviews and clinical guidelines for various treatments for spinal pain.[559]

Efforts to Mitigate the Replication Crisis

There are recent efforts to curb the replication crisis, sometimes referred to as the *credibility revolution*. Key changes include calls for open data, incorporation of replication projects into graduate-level education, journal-level improvements to manuscript assessment procedures, and calls for changes to academic grant and promotion incentives, among others.

Although it will take time to assess the effectiveness of these measures, it is reasonable to assume for now that this will likely need additional efforts.

Critiques of Replication Crisis Concerns

For a balanced discussion, many experts also believe that concerns about the replication crisis have been overblown.[544,556,560] One paper entitled "Stop Reproducing the Reproducibility Crisis" argues that variable results are expected in fields like biology, given the variability of study conditions, and that the problem lies more in the overinterpretation of conclusions and misinterpretation of statistics than in the data itself.[544] For behavioral and social sciences, some authors argue that research methodology and interpretations should be modified at every step compared to those of the physical sciences and that the low replication rates are less of a problem than often proclaimed.[556]

So, is the replication crisis a real problem for us? There are intelligent arguments and likely validity on both sides, but some of the arguments in favor of a true crisis seem undeniable such as the impact of publication bias and problems with statistical interpretation. The take-home point is that you must learn the basics of EBM and should usually not put too much stock in the conclusions of an isolated publication.

Hype

Even when there are no replication concerns, there may still be many forms of potential hype. Here, we'll explore hype related to individual publications, broader medical topics, new technology, appeal to authority, and the media.

Publication Hype

First, editors may be eager to publish salacious news-worthy papers to increase the journal visibility and impact factor. Second, it can take the form of the exact words used in either the title or the discussion and conclusions sections, which imply a greater impact of the data than the analysis merits. One study found that use of adjectives considered promotional (hype) on successful National Institutes of Health (NIH) grant applications increased 41% between 1992 and 2020; there were 139 such adjectives like "key," "transformative," "scalable," "transdisciplinary," and "unique."[561]

Authors also know that many readers will only view the title and abstract, and sometimes sneak in promotional language that overstates the results. Sometimes a conclusion sentence is an opinion, recommendation, or overgeneralization that is unsupported by the data. Another problem is a *fate (or trajectory) fallacy*, a statement that something is "becoming more recognized" with "increasing evidence." Trajectories can only be determined retrospectively, and we cannot assume, or imply, that future data will continue to support a hypothesis.

The title and abstract are also vulnerable to hype that oversell the results relative to study limitations or small effect sizes. The abstract should be concordant with the main body of the manuscript, which in turn should reflect the data and the limitations. Less experienced authors are particularly prone to producing abstract hype. While this slips through the cracks too often, experienced reviewers will call it out and manuscripts that seem to misrepresent the data with too much hype are at risk of rejection.

Hyped Medical Topics

It is not just individual publications that can be hyped, but sometimes entire topics. There are many examples where conventional knowledge accrued through observational studies has been called into question after the publication of RCTs, which are generally considered a higher level of evidence. A few examples include the impact of hormone replacement therapy on post-menopausal heart disease,[562] the benefit of vitamin D supplementation and perception of widespread vitamin D deficiency, and benefit of vertebroplasty for treatment of painful spinal compression fractures.[563-567] In each instance, RCT results contradicted the prevailing viewpoints.

There are areas of persistent debate and nuance within these topics, however. For example, there may be subgroups who could benefit for each of these examples, methodologies of the RCTs (as any study) could be critiqued, and perhaps we need to be careful not to take overly dogmatic stances after RCTs too. Indeed, there are ongoing debates in all these areas.[563-565,567-569] The full discussion is best left to the experts, the main point is that RCTs can upend previously held dogma, but there may be important nuances too.

In addition, research hype reaches the public directly from the researchers making their rounds on various media outlets. Showcasing impactful, surprising, or sensational studies is a favorite topic. Sometimes the researcher will make rounds promoting his or her research results (and themselves), as a form of careerism. This is not inherently wrong, but there is little time for context or in-depth scientific analysis, and often a news headline is based off a single non-replicated research study. Nonetheless, patients are exposed to this hype even though they may not be equipped to put it into perspective.

New Medical Technology Hype

A special type of hype can come with new medical technology. Both professional and popular optimism fuels a typical natural history of new technology hype with an initial optimism spike, then an overcorrected dip, and finally achievement and acceptance of a true middle ground called the *Gartner Curve*. This parallels to the Dunning–Kruger overconfidence effect that will be discussed in Chapter 29. As an example, some observers in medicine say that the hope and hype of stem cell treatments during the past few decades, especially embryonic stem cells, is a good example, with hopes that we are recently climbing out of the *trough of disillusionment* and on the *slope of enlightenment*.[570,571]

Authoritative Bias/Hype (Appeal to Authority)

We like to read definitive statements. They sound convincing, concise, and authoritative. An article that couches too many things with a "suggests" or probable, or "best current understanding" sounds less authoritative and is harder to read. The problem is that the cited work to support these statements may have flaws. We rarely know something with certainty, and often there is a real reason to question the veracity of statements made in the medical literature—or at least to add caveats to their generalizability.

So, be on the lookout for things that are presented as established fact when the evidence consists of a few case reports or limited retrospective data. This is especially important in new or developing fields, which may still have an underdeveloped body of literature.

Media Hype

Another critical type of hype is found in our media. Every day, the results of the latest medical study make headline news. The lay press presents the information as best they can but are usually not experts on the topic or on statistical analysis. They can inadvertently trick themselves and the public with limited understanding of the term *significance* and with effect size, differences and limitations, biases of studies and importance of a single publication.

Another potential source of misinformation is television shows about medicine, including some that feature physicians. The problem remains that topics extending well beyond the areas of host expertise may be misrepresented. One author (VTL) was once consulted because a group of local citizens became concerned about radiation exposure from a routine imaging examination after hearing misleading information from a celebrity physician. Additionally, even expert guests can hype their own topic as a method of self-promotion and a manifestation of careerism, even if inadvertent.

Academic Dishonesty

Beyond the "zombie trials" and hype, you should be aware of other times when authors intentionally falsify information. There are three major forms: (1) false data reporting, (2) false authorship, and (3) plagiarism. It is important to distinguish these occurrences from inadvertent mistakes which, though unfortunate, are inevitable and forgivable. Further, the retraction of an academic article could be due to either academic dishonesty or to an inadvertent mistake.

The incidence of academic dishonesty was recently heightened due to concerns raised about a series of publications with evidence of fabricated content from, ironically, several high-profile honesty researchers.[572,573] Various types of article fabrication or other misadventures such as random number generator derived data, doctored images, p-hacking, and paid authorship for paper mill prefab articles are now uncovered by watchdogs like *Data Colada* and reported upon by *retractionwatch.com*.

While outright fraud is uncommon (and likely a minor contribution to the replication crisis), you should keep the possibility in mind as you read articles and, of course, never fabricate data. You should also try to work with attendings who will provide an appropriate level of oversight and availability for your projects to help ensure your data integrity.

Unfortunately, there are always gray areas, and it is hard to know where to draw the line. The article "The Dilemma of the Honest Researcher" points out that academics who submit overly optimistic or hyped grant proposals may beat out one that provides a more realistic (honest) proposal. Other examples include carving a project into many smaller *minimal publishable units*, which might be a smart strategy or might be considered dishonest, depending on the circumstance. While there are no universal answers, you should avoid writing with overt hype and use common sense when dividing projects into several minimally publishable units.

Reviewer Considerations

In addition to concerns about quality, hype, and author honesty, the quality of literature depends on manuscript evaluation by an army of volunteer peer-reviewers. While participation is a noble exercise, reviewers receive little formal training, and some have conducted few studies or written few papers themselves. They may also have expertise in only one aspect of the contents of a submission, but lack expertise in statistical analysis, evaluation of AI tools, or other areas. Many journals do not have enough resources to vet all papers with a statistical or AI expert reviewer, even when it could be beneficial.

While tough reviewer comments are expected, sometimes these can be snarky and unprofessional using language that people would never use without the shield of anonymity, which is basically a toxic psychological regression. The number of requests to review manuscripts received by academics can surpass several per day, contributing to an epidemic of *reviewer fatigue*. The bottom line is that tough reviewer comments are expected, and you should not become too discouraged if you receive some questionable reviews.

Finally, articles that have undergone substellar peer review are more common than fraudulent publication. It is important to realize that even publication in a reputable journal does not guarantee a pristine review process, and plenty of questionable quality information slips through the cracks, especially with complex multidisciplinary topics. This is a product of both the reviewers and the investigators.

Scoring Systems and Scales

Explosion in Number

Let's turn to a discussion of scoring systems and scales, a special topic for evaluating and understanding evidence. Validated scoring systems have many uses in medicine such as facilitating management and prognosis. These can also help counter physician biases, but physicians are often (too) reluctant to use them.[574] Reasons include lack of confidence in the scoring systems and belief that they infringe on physician and shared decision-making.[574] The trick in training is figuring out which ones to adopt. This can be a challenge since so many scales exist, scales may have substantial limitations, and implementation varies by practice.

In fact, scoring systems and grading scales are increasing in such epic proportions that even subspecialists cannot keep track of them all.[575] To manage this, we need to figure out which ones are useful.[575] There are different ways scales can be useful such as for assessing disease activity or severity, quality of life measurements, or other outcomes. These may not only inform clinical decision-making but also may have important applications in clinical trials.[575] Useful scales should be clinically relevant, validated, and easy to use.[575]

Other Limitations of Scoring Systems and Scales

Scoring systems and scales, however, may have other limitations. Even if helpful to standardize and guide diagnosis and treatments, they still do not paint a full clinical picture. Later, we'll see that the PCL-R scale for psychopathy gives no direct hint that psychopaths can harm others without showing anxiety (Chapter 32).

Psychological scales have been critiqued on multiple grounds, including that they are overused as an easy and efficient way to generate official-sounding data, contain vague language, oversimplify complex phenomena, achieve numeralization instead of quantification, and other issues.[576] More broadly, the methods of validating scales often fall short such that we are unsure of what a scale is truly measuring, and some authors warn that we should use scales that we do not understand well with caution.[577]

Medical training does not usually explore the nuances of scales in such depth, so remember to be careful when using or citing one. You should understand if it is validated (even if the process is imperfect) and be aware whether others at your institution recognize and use it. You should also understand the limitations, such as overweighting or omission of certain items.

157

Predatory Journals

A final way that the evidence can become complicated or tarnished is through predatory journals, a thorn in the side of the academic world. Hallmarks of predatory journals include exorbitant fees, lack of transparency regarding publication charges or process, insufficient or absent peer review, unduly high acceptance rates, names, logo color schemes, or websites resembling those of legitimate journals, and unethical (but not necessarily illegal) procedures.

They may also have an editorial board full of reputable academics who get lured into the process, often because they recognize other names on the board and trust that it is a legitimate organization. Further, the sophistication of these journals evolves over time to remain under the radar. *Thus, if you submit a manuscript to a journal that you are not familiar with, you must vet the journal's legitimacy.*

Still, vetting journals for legitimacy can be challenging for several reasons. First, truth be told, the definition is not clear-cut, and some features of legitimate and predatory journals can overlap.[578] Signs of a legitimate journal include affiliation with a reputable parent company, indexing in major search engines, and evidence that it follows appropriate peer review and quality assurance.[578]

Red flags include a poor-quality website, poor-quality articles, false claims about indexing, inconsistent information on correspondences, missing information (pub fees, contact information), aggressive article solicitation, and exorbitantly high acceptance rates.[578] Yet no single criterion is foolproof.

Thus, proper journal vetting may require checking multiple criteria and checking that claims of indexing and impact factors are true. In addition, a variety of free or fee-based websites provide lists of predatory journals, but it can be difficult to know if any one of these is complete and up to date.[579] Finally, seeking mentorship at your institution can be a helpful way to recognize and avoid such journals since knowledge about this topic is not heavily publicized.

Landmark Studies

We'll conclude this chapter on a more positive note: the value of understanding landmark studies. In medicine, one encounters a myriad of important clinical trials with creative names that describe what they evaluate like RALES (Randomized Aldactone Evaluation Study) or CLOT (Comparison of Low-molecular-weight heparin versus Oral anticoagulant Therapy for the Prevention of Recurrent Venous Thromboembolism in Patients with Cancer) or imply greatness like COURAGE or IDEAL, or countless others.

This information overload can be simplified by recognizing that there are typically a few landmark trials in an area of medicine that are most important for a newcomer to know. One task when starting a new clinical rotation is figuring out what the landmark studies are and learning the take-home points (though new rotating medical students are often not expected to know too much).

Further, there are usually groups of studies, including sister studies done simultaneously or second-generation studies such as those that followed DASH, assessing the diet with various modifications.[580] In other words, a single study is just a snapshot in time, one piece of a larger story. These stories develop over time as selection criteria are modified, complication rates decrease, diagnostic tests improve, and new technologies are introduced.

Not only does a single study not tell the whole story, but the older results may no longer apply to the current practice environment even if they contain useful information. Unless you plan to specialize in a narrow area though, you will not have enough time to analyze every study for most topics. Therefore, you must rely on review articles, systematic reviews, commentary, lectures, and the insights of your attendings and colleagues.

Review articles may be an update and highlight those in recent years or the past year or may be more comprehensive. Commentary and review articles can offer perspectives and context that reading a single study cannot. Other important encompassing resources are systematic reviews, meta-analyses, and clinical practice guidelines. These too have exploded in number. It is useful to keep a watchful eye on the key publications and clinical guidelines in an area of interest or current clinical rotation. The NEJM publishes *Journal Watch* (www.jwatch.org/guideline-watch), where you can find a curation of impactful articles for a variety of specialties and topics, as well as summaries of key clinical guidelines.

29

Logical Fallacies and Cognitive Biases

Vance T. Lehman

Introduction

When I entered medical training, I knew almost nothing of logical fallacies or cognitive biases. These received little attention in my formal medical curriculum but it turns out that understanding these topics is one of the more useful skills for medical practice. While evidence of impact on patient outcomes is sparse,[581] errors in cognitive reasoning almost certainly have an under-recognized influence on our medical decision-making and recall that we are most susceptible to them when we use System 1 thinking.[582]

Logical Fallacies

In short, logical fallacies arise from over-reliance on heuristics and a lack of awareness.[1] Before I knew what they were, I hardly noticed them. Now, I see that these abound in medicine, both in medical decision-making and in other workplace logistics. I could write an entire book on what I have learned on this topic in medicine alone.

Learning about logical fallacies will help you avoid them, both those you might fall into and those set by others. At first, you may notice only the most overt examples, but with practice, subtler examples emerge too. In fact, the subtle examples are often the trickiest but the most instructive. While we cannot delve into a comprehensive review, here are a few examples of the most common, but under-recognized, ones I have observed.

False Equivalence

One common, but often subtle, logical fallacy found in medicine (as in other work environments) is *false equivalence*. This fallacy typically arises when someone compares the pros and cons of two different things. Since almost any topic is associated with some pros and some cons, the legitimacy or effect of two different things can often be portrayed (intentionally or inadvertently) as being overly similar, while the true balance of the pros and cons is ignored.

A blatant example is a statement that routine childhood vaccines all have some pros and some cons in a way than implies that both pro-vaccine and anti-vaccine stances are equally valid when, in fact, vaccine benefits are great, and adverse effects are rare. Thus, it is important to watch out for this fallacy when someone appraises medical evidence.

DOI: 10.1201/9781003633389-32

Another instance of false equivalence occurs when a leader implies that the situations of two different groups of subordinates are similar (perhaps to keep the peace), when the degree of sacrifice or reward is objectively inequitable. For example, consider two residents who are each assigned four new patients on a shift, but one resident gets straightforward single-problem admissions, and the other gets complex multi-problem admissions. Both have the same number of new patients, but the work distribution is not equitable.

Or, if two sets of residents are each assigned ten hours shifts, but the shift for one set is overnight and understaffed and for the other set is during normal working hours and is fully supported and staffed, the two assignments are not *equal*, even though they may be sold as such.

Be cautious, as a future leader, against falling into the trap of claiming false equivalence (even if more subtle than these examples) since some of your followers can easily notice the logical error and become insulted or upset.

Politician's Fallacy

Yet another elusive logical fallacy is the *politician's fallacy*: there is a problem, so we must do something. This fallacy arises from attempts to fix a suboptimal situation, such as a medical treatment regimen that does not seem to be working, with some action—ANY action—without consideration that the status quo may be preferable to poorly conceived solutions. I've seen very intelligent people seduced by this line of thinking over the years. This is not to say that we should not try to change course when something is not working but that we should do so with intentionality, because sometimes the proposed change is worse than the original situation.

Proof by Lack of Evidence

One logical fallacy that can easily evade detection is *proof by lack of evidence*. This fallacy assumes that something is true because it has not been refuted. For example, a new faster or cheaper, but untested and potentially problematic, diagnostic protocol of any sort (MRI, pathology, clinical algorithm) might be implemented clinically after only a brief period of beta testing with the rationale that it has not been proven inferior. While this might be acceptable with ongoing monitoring, the flaw in logic should be recognized to ensure appropriate data collection continues.

Quantitative Fallacy

The final under-recognized logical fallacy in medicine we'll consider here is the *quantitative fallacy*. This is a tendency to place too much weight on the significance of quantitative, compared to qualitative information. For example, white blood cell counts may be given greater weight in clinical decision-making than qualitative information such as a patient's subjective report of her symptoms and clinical findings on examination.[583]

Learning Other Logical Fallacies

These examples do not include many of the best-known logical fallacies since you may have already heard of these such as *ad hominem* arguments, circular reasoning, false choice fallacy, hasty generalization, red herring, slippery slope argument, strawman argument, and sunk cost fallacy. Still, it is worth reviewing these common fallacies in relevant resources. You will find that there are many other fallacies too. While the names can quickly become overwhelming, there are various ways to group them into broader categories, which can be enormously helpful.

One approach is to divide this broadly into groups of erroneous and misleading use of language or errors of relevance.[584] Further, there are three major types of errors of relevance: (1) fallacies of premise and conclusion, (2) fallacies of appeal (to emotions or qualifications), and (3) fallacies of inductive reasoning.[584] There are also other, less technical, ways to categorize logical fallacies that some trainees might find more intuitive such as ones that avoid the question, make assumptions, use invalid statistics, or employ propaganda.[585] In addition, you can practice identifying logical fallacies by watching the news, analyzing politicians' speeches, or reading books about mystical types of healing.

Cognitive Biases

Even though the impact of cognitive biases on medical decision-making is better known now than in the past, I think most trainees still underestimate their effect. Recall the case of the brain metastasis that masqueraded as a benign vascular mass from Chapter 5. This case introduced several cognitive biases including anchor bias, availability bias, confirmation bias, and prior report bias. We have also seen examples of base rate neglect, health optimism bias, and the halo effect. These cognitive biases and many more are prevalent every day in any medical practice.

This is a broad topic and the point here is not to illustrate every bias, but to encourage you to use dedicated resources to learn more about them. Once you know them, you will see them arise daily both from within and from those around you. As an introduction, we'll review a few more examples that are particularly useful in medicine and then look at three special cases that have a substantial impact on the hidden curriculum: overconfidence bias, in-group bias, and disadvantageous inequity aversion.

Recency Bias

Consider a hypothetical ED physician deciding whether to order a chest CT angiogram for a patient with chest pain. She decides to order it and the CT reveals a pulmonary embolism. Over the next month, several more patients arrive at the ED with chest pain and now she is now much more likely to order chest CT examinations with the recent pulmonary embolism diagnosis in mind. She has seen countless patients with chest pain over the years but is letting her most recent experience have a disproportionate impact on her judgment.

As a companion example, after a proceduralist experiences a complication, he may become more risk averse for time. In my experience, even the most seasoned physicians can be susceptible to this error in reasoning called *recency bias*. So, even when it seems obvious to an external observer, it can easily elude us from within.

Therapeutic Illusion

Now, here is a lesser known and perhaps more subtle cognitive bias that has specific relevance for medicine: the *therapeutic illusion*. This occurs when physicians or patients believe that medical interventions are more effective than they really are.[586] This arises when a physician attributes random success to their actions and selectively notices positive outcomes as a confirmation bias.

This, in turn, can lead to inappropriate recommendations and treatments. Another example in medicine occurs when patients do not follow up in clinic and their physician assumes the treatment worked. This example also reminds us that cognitive biases can co-occur and that variants of similar biases are described with different names (another more general name for therapeutic illusion is the *illusion of control*).

Overconfidence Bias

Overconfidence is common and one of the biggest potential pitfalls for anyone at any stage, but especially novice trainees.[14,587] This is probably why it is one of the best studied biases. Consider that around 90% of people consider themselves to be above average drivers.[110] In medicine, one study found that 40% of ICU physicians who were "completely certain" of their patients' diagnoses were deemed wrong at autopsy.[110] Overconfidence can arise consciencely or unconsciously[588] and can be conveyed by either verbal or non-verbal communication.[589] The point is that you may be completely unaware of your own overconfidence even when you project it to others.

In fact, overconfidence is a prototypical *stealthy bias*—that is, a bias that hinders its own detection.[588] Further, there is objective evidence that American students are objectively overconfident, at least when it comes to standardized tests. Specifically, it has been shown that American students who score in the middle of the pack on standardized tests show confidence levels higher than top-performing students from other countries, and this tendency likely applies to medical training too.[349,590] In fact, residents tend to rate their performance higher than their attendings do.[590]

To understand why novice trainees are often overconfident, consider the *Dunning–Kruger effect* (Figure 29.1), which describes how people (like trainees) who know just a little bit about a

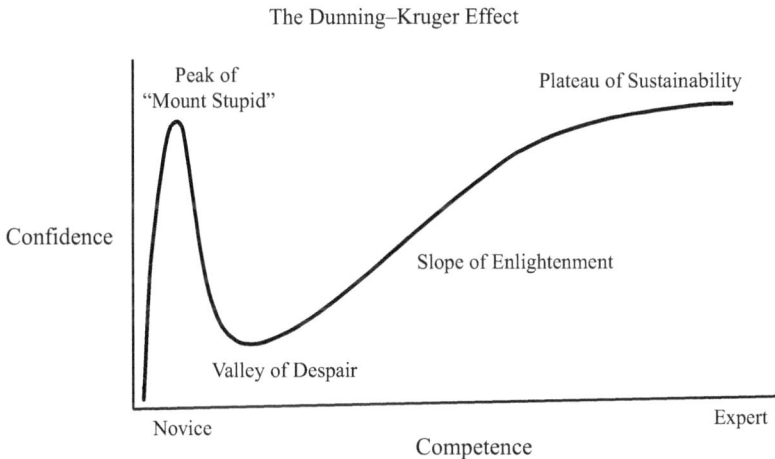

Figure 29.1 The Dunning–Kruger Effect. An individual's confidence in their ability to execute a skill rises quickly with just a small to moderate amount of knowledge, outpacing their true competence level. The summit of overconfidence has been referred to as the peak of "mount stupid." As competence increases with learning, so does the awareness of how much more there is to know. This awareness leads to decreased confidence; the nadir called the valley of despair. Continued learning and skill development lead to the slope of enlightenment and eventually the plateau of sustainability. Only after this cycle and considerable purposeful practice does one reach a concordant high level of confidence and competence. This is a common trend, though there is certainly interindividual variability, and awareness has potential to mitigate the overconfidence. While some recent evidence suggests that the Dunning–Kruger effect may be overstated and may be due in part to statistical noise, overconfidence bias is real and the perception of being overconfident can backfire for early trainees.

topic tend to have disproportionally high confidence levels.[110] This overconfidence varies by person but is already present in first semester medical students.[591] This effect is particularly problematic if a trainee (inappropriately) disregards a staff order or is overly skeptical of staff who take a clinical approach that the trainee does not understand. While some recent evidence suggests that the Dunning–Kruger effect may be overstated and may be due in part to statistical noise, overconfidence bias is real and the perception of being overconfident can backfire for early trainees.

While the focus of the Dunning–Kruger effect is the evolution of confidence in novices, experts are often overconfident in certain situations as well.[592] For example, a subspecialist (say neuro or cardiac radiology) radiologist with extensive expertise in CT physics still can overestimate his own ability in this specialized arena. Further, he might generalize this confidence to believe that he knows best how to set CT protocols and interpret CT examinations for *every* organ system head-to-toe and could even naively dismiss input from radiologists with substantially more clinical (but less physics) experience evaluating other body systems.

The Right Confidence Level Depends on the Subject and Situation

How can trainees understand and regulate their confidence levels? First, consider that conventional wisdom has long suggested that an outstanding trainee acts with confidence. The idea is that confidence makes you look competent and trustworthy, and humans tend to favor confident people—recall, this is common business school advice too. Showing confidence requires walking a fine line though, since overconfidence can be a source of negative evaluations and/or perceived as arrogance.

In addition, there are many plausible mechanisms by which overconfidence could lead to medical error including resistance to opposing opinions, failure to follow appropriate guidelines, or skipping use of practice guidelines altogether.[588] In the worst-case scenario, overconfidence could lead to adverse patient outcomes if the trainee makes decisions without proper oversight.

The ideal confidence thermostat setting probably differs by rotation and attending. Remember too that confidence in yourself is different than confidence in your ability for a particular task.[177] If you have never done a task, you have little basis for confidence in your ability. This is particularly true during the third year of medical school. Premature confidence can leave you looking naïve or arrogant. But this does not mean you cannot have, and cannot show, confidence in yourself as a person (i.e. confidence that you will try, learn, and eventually succeed).

You should also have confidence in your ability to collect and present basic information. When presenting on rounds, your team needs to trust that your report is accurate. Stating that a chest radiograph was "read as normal" (a fact) is different than saying "the chest radiograph *is* normal, so there's no chance there's a lung cancer" (an appraisal that is not entirely true). When you are asked a question, it is usually best to answer it directly. Provide just the facts and don't confabulate by answering questions you weren't asked directly. Most importantly, if you don't know something, don't guess!

Overall, the trick is to consciously balance the polar forces pushing you to either overconfidence or to impostor syndrome and strike a balance with appropriate confidence and humility. When others offer viewpoints that differ from your own or offer critical feedback, do not dismiss it immediately, even if you feel certain your approach is better.

Table 29.1 Key Areas of Impact of Overconfidence Bias in Medical Training

Trainee overconfidence is a common topic for feedback in some specialties/rotations
Some rotations might reinforce overconfidence
Learners remember less from didactics than they think they will
Physicians may think they are more immune to the effects of sleep deprivation than they really are
Promotion of other biases such as planning fallacy or illusion or skill
Misdiagnosis can result from overuse of heuristics
Schema maintenance (see Chapter 3)

Recognize that everyone is better at you than something, and every viewpoint has something to offer. Look to your objective experience to guide your actions. Do not take on something that you are not objectively ready to attempt based on self-belief alone, as this could be dangerous. The major areas where overconfidence is relevant to training are shown in Table 29.1.

In-Group Bias

Understanding in-group biases helps us understand the medical world on multiple fronts. While in Western cultures, we tend to think about ourselves as individuals, we also have a *social identity*.[593] According to the book *Wrong* by Dannagal Goldthwaite Young, this social identity has a large impact on our behaviors and perceptions by fulfilling basic needs called the 3Cs: Community, Comprehension, and Control.[43]

There is compelling evidence to support this assertion in multiple arenas, including sports fandom, political beliefs, and overestimation of the accomplishments of one's country.[263,594-596] The effects become hardwired in our brains; when our deeply entrenched group-based beliefs are challenged with counterevidence, fMRI studies show that we activate our limbic (emotional) brain regions more than our rational prefrontal cortex.[597]

Why are in-group effects so powerful? During human evolution, groups had a survival advantage over a lone wolf, with key advantages of acquiring scarce resources, status, protection, and power.[43] For these and other reasons, humans evolved to have a comparatively low rate of intra-group aggression (reactive aggression) and violence, certainly much lower than that of chimpanzees who (along with bonobos) are the closest primate relatives.[121]

In stark distinction though, humans exert extreme violence (proactive aggression) against out-groups, which may reflect an evolutionary fight for scarce resources. These traits have been observed in various hunter-gatherer tribes throughout the world and in are reflected in war.[121] Anthropologist Richard Wrangham has called the juxtaposition of these two types of aggression the *goodness paradox* that we alluded to in Chapter 6.[121] We also have a distorted perception of out-groups, including exaggerated differences from the in-group and homogenization of out-group members.[43]

These concepts materially impact our experience in the medical system through in-group/out-group effects and *social comparisons*. In medicine, we could identify with multiple groups such as those pertaining to job role, areas of specialty, stage-of career, being a parent-physician, being male/female/nonbinary, being first-generation, and so on (Table 29.2).

Table 29.2 Key Types of In-Groups Encountered in Medical Practice

Generational (e.g., millennial)
Hierarchical status (e.g., trainee or attending)
Professional type (e.g., physician or nurse)
Specialty-based
Gender-based
Clinical physician (versus administrative, research, etc.)
Medical society member
Multigenerational physician status (or first-generation physician)

There is a complex web of such in-groups in a typical medical practice, especially in larger departments where in-group status shifts depending on context and could be the division, department, or the institution. We have a natural tendency to size up our situation with that of other groups through social comparisons, subconsciously interpreting what we see through the biased lens of our identities and our previously held beliefs.[43]

Through in-group effects, we tend to attribute in-group member errors to situational factors and out-group member errors to malintent.[43] In-group effects can amplify turf battles or other complaints among different departments, specialties, or professional status (like physician, nurse, administrator, etc.). In the worst case, we even dehumanize out-group members.[598]

In-group bias has also been found to have effects on patient care based on race, gender, and LGBTQ status.[599] On a broader scale, this cultivates distorted perceptions, as in-group members are viewed as more pleasant and successful than out-group members.[596,599]

Disadvantageous Inequity Aversion

Another concept that has substantial impact on our workplace experiences is *disadvantageous inequity aversion*. This one is really a constellation of biases (and a mouthful!) but basically says that we have evolved to care far more about fairness than about objective rationality. Human decisions factor in emotions and other psychological human factors beyond pure calculations. Cold objective calculations conclude that something is better than nothing, but most people would rather get nothing at all than a raw deal.[120]

For example, if you receive a 5% pay raise (by itself, a cause for celebration) but your peers all get twice that, you will be upset. This concept explains a great deal of workplace behavior and can be related to in-group bias, when one group (usually, the other one) is perceived as getting a *better deal* than another (usually, one's own).

Managing Cognitive Biases

Beyond what we discussed already with overconfidence bias, the first step to mitigating your cognitive biases is to acknowledge that you have them. However, this is challenging (and often impossible) since biases are often unconscious and sometimes stealthy (or self-amplifying).[588] Examples of stealthy traits include overconfidence, close-mindedness, and complacency.[588]

The next steps of cognitive bias mitigation include learning what they are and how to pivot from System 1 to System 2 decision-making when faced with diagnostic uncertainty.[582] Beyond formal training, some specific methods you can use to mitigate cognitive biases include reflection, seeking feedback, instituting standardized decision-making approaches, and bias control measures like self-blinding to prior diagnoses when formulating an opinion.[588] Additionally, it is useful to factor in evidence-based knowledge into clinical decisions and consider alternative explanations (including chance) for positive tests or outcomes.[586]

Finally, once you learn about logical fallacies and cognitive biases, you will frequently find someone else falling into the traps, but often the best course of action is to do nothing unless the consequences of the erroneous reasoning are high. If you must call them out, be sure to do so with humility and tact. Sometimes, this is best in the form of a question such as "I see your viewpoint. I'm wondering if you also thought of the possibility that…"

Note

1 There are two broad categories of logical fallacy: formal and informal. Formal logical fallacies arise from errors in deductive reasoning and invalid inference. This type is less common and is not discussed here. In distinction, informal logical fallacies are formed in natural language and can arise from erroneous or misleading content and invalid induction.

30

Social Media

Vance T. Lehman

Overview

Part III concludes with four important chapters related to professional development, starting with the power and pitfalls of social media. Social media can have substantial positive or negative effects for trainees. We'll discuss these effects in the context of several major social media considerations: (1) education, (2) networking, (3) personal branding, (4) health, and (5) problematic posts.

Social Media and Education

Social media has become a powerful educational tool. Various platforms like X (formerly Twitter) can be used to disseminate information directly or to call attention to resources like excellent review articles or original research. Social media also has potential to improve the treatment of patients around the world through increased accessibility of information in low to middle income countries.[600]

Numerous learning formats (e.g., webinars, podcasts, tweetorials, blogs, one-off tips, surgical videos) and resources are readily available. There are also many different content creators, including institutions, departments, training programs, journals, societies, and individuals. So many, in fact, that sifting through the content to discover the gems is challenging, time-consuming, and even overwhelming. Just navigating the sea of social media information is becoming a specialized skill.

The ease of creating low-to-medium quality content contributes to this deluge. On the other hand, it is difficult to create high-quality content. Additionally, influencer-mediated popularity of a post or topic can be conflated with merit.[601] There are numerous other limitations to relying too heavily on social media for learning material. These include superficial content, potential misinformation, variable content creator credentials, and protean platforms.[601]

There are also many advantages of learning with social media including interactive and bidirectional capabilities, image-rich electronic environments, individual or group options, diverse perspectives, and pre-filtered content. Videos, as mentioned, can be advantageous for dynamic processes like procedures. Learning with social media can mirror our natural ability to learn well in collective, social environments through stories, shared experiences, and shared viewpoints.

Overall, social media is poised to have a large and increasing role in medical education, but it is a moving target and far from optimized. Currently, it is probably best viewed as a supplement. Choose your sources wisely, favoring those from reputable sources such as highly

DOI: 10.1201/9781003633389-33

rated institutions or journals without getting caught up in unproductive chat areas. Occasionally, trainees try to learn primarily by using a hodgepodge of semi-randomly picked videos or other content, which usually leaves noticeable knowledge gaps. Instead, select one or two key resources that fit your specific learning needs and review these systematically along with the formal curriculum.

And if social media is not for you, remember that many physicians have achieved greatness without using social media at all.

Social Media and Networking

Social media can be an effective way to find and build community among individuals with similar interests or goals. This comes in a variety of formats (e.g., physician-restricted access, trainee-focused, physician-parent focused, general purpose, etc.) and serves a variety of purposes (e.g., general networking, select topics like finance, institutional or program advertising, medical topics, and nonmedical life topics). Popular physician-restricted forums include Sermo and Doximity.

Overall, these platforms offer valuable resources for a variety of medical and nonmedical questions, including discussions on managing a family, personal finances, or other personal or professional situations. These groups can also be a source of humor and online camaraderie. Like other forums, the groups migrate, evolve, and sub-groups may evolve over time. Also, many of your patients will find online support communities related to their condition. One important benefit is that some physician platforms will let you seek advice on difficult medical cases.

You may find information about certain schools or training programs online. For example, in radiology, this has been available since around the year 2000, soon after auntminnie.com was established.[602] While online discussion of this topic has since largely migrated to other platforms, some of the principles remain the same. That is, the information varies greatly in quality. Much true insider information never makes it onto these platforms, for example. Misinformation or exaggerated negatives about a program can result from troll activity or (anonymous) disgruntled individuals. Additionally, junior residents or even medical students can post with impunity and masquerade as experts.

Social media can also be a rich source of other insider tips for surviving and thriving in training. The *#hiddencurriculum* tag (among others) has been used to garner online advice for a variety of practical topics like sleep schedule optimization ahead of call.[601] This offers another avenue for exploring the topics discussed in this book

Social media has also become a source of information and moral support for patients, with both good and bad effects. The bad effects relate largely to misinformation. For this reason, it is useful to have reputable suggestions for your patients who might benefit from it, directing them to groups such as those found on https://connect.mayoclinic.org/.

Personal Branding[1]

Some trainees leverage social media for personal branding, such as during residency interview season. You might create a professional profile with your professional interests and experiences, for example. That said, it is difficult to say much that cannot already be gleaned from your application. Further, profile claims that are not substantiated by evidence, like a stated interest in a topic, are not compelling. It is far better if you have done research, volunteerism, or some other tangible activity for any professional interest you highlight. Through posts and comments, you can also promote yourself and your cause, but keep in mind that your professionalism and the quality of your posts and content will reflect on your reputation.

Social Media Impact on Health

As a physician in training, familiarity with the views of Congress and the surgeon general on social media is important. In 2021, the U.S. Congress held a session called "Disinformation Nation: Social Media's Role in Promoting Extremism and Misinformation" with social media CEOs.[603] During the hearing, the CEOs asserted that they are taking strong measures to counter misinformation and denied that their products are addictive.

A follow-up congressional hearing in 2024 grilled social media executives on the potential for negative effects on the mental health and safety of our youth.[604] U.S. Surgeon General Vivek Murthy also weighed in, issuing an advisory on the potential negative effects of social media on youth in 2023 and calling on Congress to enact a formal Surgeon General Warning in 2024.[605]

There are potential problems, but is social media use something we need to advise against (and avoid ourselves) as physicians? Some of your patients will read books like *The Anxious Generation* that make the case that social media use is increasing youth anxiety.[352] Other experts, though, refute this idea and believe the negative effects are smaller than often claimed.[606–609]

It seems that the major problems usually arise with what some have called "problematic social media use," or continued use despite psychological distress or impaired functioning; this type of use can have negative effects such as increased risk for depression through social comparisons to the status of others.[610–616] This is particularly true for upward social comparisons to someone perceived as higher status (e.g., popularity, fitness, success, attractiveness).[613] Other factors include amount of time, content (which may be violent, sexual, or harassing), and degree of disruption of activities, socialization, and sleep.[605,609]

Even the surgeon general's office has also acknowledged that the topic is incompletely understood, and that social media can offer many benefits for youth as well, including community for members of marginalized or minority groups, can be a source of general social support, facilitate expression of creativity, facilitate connection with friends, and can provide link to mental health support.[605] Still, we should remember that the long-term risks and benefits of social media on mental health and education remain undetermined.

Problematic Posts

The main ways one can land in trouble professionally on social media are posts that are unprofessional or offensive, breach patient privacy, or unduly criticize your workplace or employer. Such posts can have serious professional consequences.

While we enjoy a constitutional right to freedom of speech in the United States, statements that might be perceived as deeply offensive by certain groups can have important employment implications. Social media posts are public, easily accessible, amenable to propagation, and permanent. Approximately 40% of patients consult social media content when selecting a physician.[617] Remember that potential PDs, employers, colleagues, and patients can view your public-facing online posts.

There can be repercussions from posts considered unprofessional, whether related to the workplace or other topics. For example, one physician was fired for making anti-Semitic posts on social media.[618] Next, we examine a controversial study on residents' social media use.

A Controversial Study

In 2020, an article entitled "Prevalence of Unprofessional Social Media Content among Young Vascular Surgeons" published in the *Journal of Vascular Surgery* sparked a firestorm of backlash and debate and was ultimately retracted.[620,621] The study surveyed 480 vascular surgeon trainees and concluded that 26% of those with social media accounts posted unprofessional content. The response raised questions about professionalism, personal versus public life, and the appropriateness of research methods that could be interpreted as an intrusion into our personal lives by members of the medical establishment.

While some reported professionalism violations were clearly unacceptable like Health Insurance Portability and Accountability Act (HIPAA) violations, many categories assessed were more debatable. Examples include swimming attire, holding/consuming alcohol, profanity, controversial political topics, and controversial religious topics.[621] Still, even if you think that your institution has no business probing into many of these topics, it is in your best interest to use reasonable discretion with your public posts.

Violations of Patient Confidentiality

Other serious violations that you must always avoid are breaches of patient confidentiality. Blatant HIPAA violations with clear patient identifiers are clear-cut transgressions, but in other cases like posting a clinical scenario for educational purposes the lines can get blurry. For example, in 2023 a plastic surgeon was stripped of her state medical license after she live-streamed operations to a large following on TikTok for "educational purposes" over multiple concerns.[622]

Other examples may be appropriate, but considerations include the specificity of clinical features, uniqueness and recency of a case, presentation format (like description, photograph, and/or medical imaging), the precise platform (physician only versus fully public platform), manner of presentation, informed consent status, and purpose (patient care, education, humor, or shock-value). For example, in 2021, a group of medical residents made national headlines after they posted a "Price is Right" game to guess the weight of pictures of human organs at surgery.[619]

General complaints about patients or a patient encounter, even if not identifiable, can also be viewed as unprofessional. Overall, you should use extreme discretion and, if there is any question, do not make the post.

Criticism of Your Employer

As another caution, public criticism specifically targeting your employer on topics like quality of patient care or treatment of patients and employees on social media is typically inadvisable. For example, one physician was fired for what she says was speaking out about equipment shortages at her hospital.[623] You should address concerns through official internal channels rather than public criticism.

Know the Guidelines

Given the numerous landmines, you should review your institution's social media policy before posting anything that might fall into any of the categories discussed. The perspectives here are purely for educational purposes, and one's hospital policy trumps these opinions.

The AMA has also published recommendations regarding social media ethics, including the need to maintain patient privacy, a suggestion to separate personal and professional accounts, and the responsibility to address unprofessional posts by colleagues, among other items.[604] Other resources are available as well.[624-626] And remember that PDs, employers, colleagues, and patients might view your public-facing online posts.

Note

1 The value of personal branding has been questioned by some experts, arguing it is usually best not to turn ourselves into a brand that is depersonalized and impossible to perpetually live up to.

31

Leadership and Management

Vance T. Lehman, John C. Benson

Overview

Key principles of leadership and management, as well as politics as we'll see later, have transcended cultures and historical eras. Leaders who are poorly equipped for the job and lack integrity can bring down even the world's greatest empires. For example, the failings of the Roman Emperor Commodus, who was sometimes lazy, subcontracted out too much work without oversight, and unjustifiably killed gladiators to enhance his personal image, are seen as key reasons for the fall of the Roman Empire. Nearly 2,000 years later, these lessons for leadership still resonate in medicine, as well as in other workplaces and in politics.

Why should this topic matter to you? Even as a resident, you will be positioned to weigh in on some decisions such as medical student match rankings to residency selections. You will also be seen as a team leader at various ranks (intern, junior resident, senior resident, etc.) as you climb the clinical hierarchy. Ultimately, having a firm grasp on leadership and management principles is an essential skill for a successful physician.

Titles, Leaders, and Managers

You should know the differences between a person with a title, a leader, and a manager. A title usually carries the expectation that the designee will be a leader and/or manager. Some with titles, however, are not leaders or managers, but rather people who accept a role without taking effective action—or any action at all. Warren Bennis, in his 1989 book *On Becoming a Leader*, contrasts leadership and management with illustrative examples.[152,627] In brief, Bennis says that a manager focuses on the technicalities, practicalities, logistics, and execution. In contrast, a leader focuses on vision, innovation, inspiration, and purpose.

Much has changed since the late 1980s, however, and middle management roles in organizations, including medicine, have taken on more of a leadership nature.[152] Most roles blend leadership and management, with one often emphasized more than the other. At the same time, pure management roles, especially related to business considerations, are now filled by administrative partners.

Management in Medicine

Furthermore, management in medicine has some specific organization-level and individual-level considerations. The book *Lessons in Management from Mayo Clinic* describes organization-level management in terms of a strong culture derived from philosophy and

DOI: 10.1201/9781003633389-34

lived example of the Clinic's founding Brothers Mayo. This philosophy centered on three main ideas: (1) putting the needs of the patient above all else, (2) pooling talent and working as a team, and (3) delivering care efficiently as a destination medical center.[628]

Resources also exist to guide individual-level management, particularly for medical trainees. For this, *The One-Minute Manager* is an excellent resource on the topics of goal setting, praises, and reprimands that can be read in full during a short flight or a few lunch breaks.[629]

Definitions and Types of Leadership

There is no universal definition of leadership. One reason is that there are different types of leaders for different roles. In his landmark 1978 book *Leadership*, James MacGregor Burns categorized leadership as either *transactional* or *transformative*, although his concept of transactional leadership is arguably better described as management.[152,630] Harold Leavitt offers a more comprehensive definition encompassing three main traits: persuasion, competence, and the ability to inspire transformation.[152]

These definitions, though, may be more applicable to formal roles in a transformative environment and large-scale projects than for medical trainees, though they still bring some valuable lessons. Leaders of large groups of people like a hospital CEO, remember, must rely on shared narratives. Experience shows that they also need the right environment.

For example, Ed Catmull's ideas on animation did not gain traction when he worked at George Lucas Studios.[157] His ideas were ultimately successful, but he had to implement them by first separating from Lucas Studios (amicably), joining forces with Steve Jobs, and ultimately forming Pixar.[157] So, if you have a transformative idea but are running into friction, remember that you might need to find the right environment to make it happen.

In clinical practice, most routine leadership roles are more organic and personalized. For these roles you truly can, and should, know the people on your team well. Despite the differences, many of the same principles of effective leadership apply to transformational leaders and frontline leaders alike.

Effective Leadership

Effective leaders of any type need baseline competency for the task at hand complemented by a skillset of basic leadership traits. For example, as former U.S. Special Operations Commander and University of Texas System Chancellor William McRaven points out in his book *Make Your Bed*, a good leader works alongside his people but puts them ahead of himself, leads by example, persists after failure, and stays positive when things are unfair.[631] He also points out that heartfelt commitment trumps innate talent.[631]

Beyond that, there are many tactics that you can use while working in small groups to increase effectiveness, largely related to organization, communication, and example setting. Here are five of the most important tasks:

- **Know your team members well**. This means knowing their personality types, strengths, areas for growth, values, motivators, and goals. Recall that this differs from being a leader of a group over 150 people (or so) where it is impossible to know everyone well and one must rely on shared organizational beliefs.

- **Set clear values locally**, even for small care teams or committees, and to align the layers of culture-shared assumptions (beliefs), values, and artifacts (actions) as close as possible. For example, you believe, say, and show that the needs of the patients come first on a clinical service.
- **Set clear expectations**, tailored to individuals' abilities, that challenge them safely and constructively. This is an evolving process with adjustments made as skills progress.
- **Learn to manage failure, both yours and those you lead**. This means supporting your team members, both privately and publicly, when they've made a good-faith effort but have fallen short. Provide constructive feedback in private. Failure to help guide others through their failures can lead to a maladaptive response and long-term consequences. You acknowledge your own failures and devise a plan to improve. When there is a team failure, the leader assumes ultimate responsibility.
- **Lead by example**. When the workload or complexity increases, they should take the extra hospital admission or sickest patient first. Always maintain the highest level of professionalism, tell the truth, and avoid the biggest team-related mistakes (taking undue credit and gossip), we'll discuss later.

There are a couple of other aspects of leadership worth mentioning. We must strike a balance between being a pushover and being a bully. Both extremes are bad, but being a bully is usually worse. The epitome is probably *The Prince* by Machiavelli, which embodies the sentiment that it is *better to be feared than loved* and that *the ends justify the means*.[632] Unfortunately, some modern leadership books follow suit and recommend Machiavellian leadership strategies that encourage leaders to act in psychopathic ways.[633] This approach will not work well for a young (or really, any) physician.

Micromanaging

One common criticism of suboptimal leadership centers around micromanaging. At times, you will be micromanaged. When you are just getting up to speed on a task for example, this does not necessarily indicate lack of trust or desire for control, but rather a commitment to your success. At other times, though, excessive micromanaging is usually frowned upon and can, in truth, be frustrating for both sides of the equation. You may find yourself micromanaging others too, even if you have sworn off the practice.

Beyond proper staffing, the best way to avoid micromanaging is to set clear expectations, establish methods for assessing results, and then largely leave the details to the team. Notice that the opposite extreme, *absentee leadership*, is not the solution to micromanaging and is in fact another suboptimal leadership style. If you are being micromanaged, you can also try to proactively set the expectations with your boss and share your plan for execution and follow-up with her.

Although you want to avoid excessive micromanaging, you should also realize that just asking someone to do something does not ensure it will get done. Ensuring follow-through is an art. How can you increase the odds? Taking a few moments to explain the reasons and importance of an ask in person, as opposed to an email that sounds like an afterthought, can help. If there is any chance there is any confusion, tactfully check for confirmation that your request is understood. It also helps to have clear deliverables, a completion date, and an exact plan for touching base to ensure follow-through.

Other Leadership Pitfalls

There are worse mistakes than micromanaging though, including undermining your followers. A trap that is easy to fall into is criticizing, in front of others, a subordinate who made a good-faith effort to do something you requested because you did not like the approach or outcome. This is a serious leadership error that can quickly alienate your team.

Finally, the leadership approach must be adjusted when outside of clinical care settings. For example, brainstorming or creative endeavors require risk of failure, lateral thinking, heightened team member independence, and the right environment.[157] As we saw with Commodus, succession planning for key roles like the next chief resident is critical, but the crowned prince/princess approach is not advised.[152] It is better to cultivate a talent pool to choose from.[152]

Leadership Aspirations

Some Aspire to be Leaders

As you progress through training, you will increasingly notice that many physicians aspire to be leaders. Some will state an ambition to become *a leader* outright. This ambition may stem from a desire for advancement, a wish to make a broader impact, emulation of role models, or a response to encouragement. Some have specific goals, which might reflect a sense of a *calling* to medicine and to their community, while others seem to have a vision of themselves as a leader of people in a general sense with any specific goals or positions being secondary factors. Surely every situation is unique, but this prospect is now enabled by workplace cultures with more leadership opportunities than in the past.[152]

You should also be aware that some colleagues with this leadership (or other advancement like fellowship procurement) ambition are working aggressively behind the scenes to tilt odds of advancement in their favor. Coaches might advise them to employ strategies such as associating with influential people, even if this means deciding "if you can't beat them, join them." These hustlers will actively seek out leadership roles for important projects such as a practice improvement initiative and will be sure that the decision-makers recognize their involvement.

They also express interest in roles and offer their services for opportunities before they are officially available, which sends the message that they are go-getters and want to help. Even if some of these strategies seem inorganic, this is reality, and even if these are not for you, it is useful to know what your *competition* is up to.

Leadership Training in Medicine Is Often Inadequate

Nonetheless, many physician leaders have had little formal training in leadership and management. In medicine, this can affect you from both sides. You have physician supervisors doing their best, but without formal training and mentorship, so there can naturally be some unforced errors. You may also be asked to fill a role but remember that many young physicians underestimate the need to work on the skills needed to be an effective leader and manager, believing they can surely get by with their natural intelligence. Thus, if you seek out mentorship, coaching, education, and other resources, you will be ahead of the curve.

Ask Yourself Why or Why Not?

But if you aspire to be a leader, it might be worth asking yourself why? Is there something specific you would hope to accomplish? Are you motivated by having an increased voice when advocating for a group of colleagues? Are you caught up in the culture of chasing titles? Perhaps a better goal than seeking a specific leadership title is to ask, "How can I use my skills, interests, and talents to make a difference?" This route is more likely to bring meaningful work and possibly organic leadership opportunities down the road.

The inverse scenario also occurs. Perhaps you would rather avoid leadership roles, but you still may be compelled to take them. Adopting some leadership positions, like being a senior resident on service, may come naturally. As a physician, you might find it difficult to avoid leadership roles altogether. If you find yourself avoiding leadership opportunities, consider whether *impostor syndrome*, burnout, or a lack of interest is at play.

With this background in mind, in the next chapter, we'll examine a couple of related topics, including what you need to know about meetings and working with others.

32

Meetings, Workplace Politics, and Difficult People

Vance T. Lehman

Meetings

The infamous Wannsee Conference of 1942 serves as a stark example of meeting dynamics and tactics. Reinhard Heydrich convenes a group of Nazi officials around a table to determine the fate of Jewish people. At first, the officials seem to have a chance to offer input and raise concerns. During breaks, Heydrich corners dissenters individually to persuade them to support the plan. As the meeting unfolds, the real ploy is gradually revealed, and it becomes clear that the plan was predetermined. The deck was stacked.

Why Trainees Need to Learn About Meetings

Fortunately, trainees are spared from most administrative meetings. However, as you transition to a staff role, you should start to gain some meeting competence and might even be invited to participate in some, like education committee meetings. Like other topics in the hidden curriculum, knowledge surrounding how to best navigate professional meetings is neither typically taught nor intuitive. In addition, it is useful to start to learn about effective and ineffective or counterproductive meetings before leaving training.

Ineffective or Counterproductive Meetings

While an extreme example, the Wannsee Conference illustrates tactics commonly employed in business meetings. First, formal meetings often do not represent the primary decision-making forum. Rather, decisions are often made during unofficial dialogue, including pre-meetings where a select subgroup of key people set the real agenda.

Sometimes key people meet with dissenters in private to try to understand their point of view and/or to try to convert them to the prevailing thinking. Some meetings conclude with an abrupt, predetermined decision, such as a surprise vote. The net effect is the illusion of decision-making and of achieving a group consensus, while the unsuspecting meeting attendees leave the meeting feeling disoriented or blindsided.

Meetings get a bad rap, mostly with good reason. They consume our limited time and energy. Many meetings are held too often, too large, too long, and poorly run. These gatherings may veer off-topic, turn into complaint sessions, waste time on supplying routine information that could be disseminated by email, or may be recurring without any specific agenda at all.

 DOI: 10.1201/9781003633389-35

A few strong personalities can drown others out or lead to groupthink, which can result in suboptimal or even devastating business decisions.[634,635]

Even when decisions are made, follow-through and action plans can be absent. As the Wannsee Conference illustrates, some meetings serve hidden agendas or deflect responsibility from the true decision-maker. The potential shortcomings of meetings are well-recognized by people who prioritize productivity. Jeff Bezos, Mark Cuban, and Elon Musk all minimize meeting time.[636]

A *Harvard Business Review* article entitled "Stop the Meeting Madness" points out that meetings incur a high cost in terms of time—a zero-sum resource—and of money since the opportunity cost of having paid employees to spend time in meetings can be considerable and is usually under-recognized.[637] They are also unpopular, with one survey of over 2,000 corporate workers in the United States finding that two in five people would rather sit at the DMV than in a pointless meeting.[501]

Meeting Etiquette and Pitfalls

Effective meeting participation requires careful consideration of your role and contribution. It's important to gauge what is expected of you, based on the nature of the meeting, its participants, and the subject. When it is the right time to speak up, be sure to do so with relevance and tact. Avoid dragging the conversation down a rabbit hole. While tangential conversations may have a place at times, they can also cause frustration among leaders trying to achieve a goal or among time-strapped colleagues who can see the meeting may need to run late.

Also, be sure that you are not talking through a half-formed, off-the-cuff idea unless it is clear you are in a brainstorming session. Further, public disagreements should be handled respectfully, thoughtfully, and with acknowledgment of common ground.

Finally, avoid agreeing to a surprise vote that you have not had time to mull over or that might require additional information before being finalized, when possible. For instance, in resident meetings, insider senior residents might hastily vote on call schedule changes, leaving junior residents shortchanged. Even in smaller groups, hasty decisions on significant matters should be avoided whenever possible. Instead, respectfully explain that you take the decision seriously and that the group may benefit from having more time to gather background information and to discuss the advantages, disadvantages, and alternatives.

Workplace Politics

Workplace politics are not limited to traditional office settings. Unfortunately, workplace politics can be found in any place of work, including all types of medical practice. Broadly speaking, political tactics are one of the most enduringly stable features of society, similar today to those of ancient Rome and Greece.[172,437] Workplace politics originate from forces like ambition, personality differences, professional jealousy, ulterior motives, favoritism, and special interests.

These forces may be concealed but are nearly ubiquitous and thus can start to affect you (overtly or covertly), even in training. Actions that seem to stem from in-group special interests, such as turf battles, contribute to politics in medicine. Some political tactics are relatively benign (or even advisable, as in the case of networking) while others are destructive to overall dynamics and cohesiveness.

Though you shouldn't be thrown full-force into the throes of workplace politics and political agendas during training, you will likely feel spillover effects. For many of us, this is disheartening, since politics can serve as an unwelcomed distraction from the overarching desire to take care of patients. Many physicians may be poorly equipped to deal with office politics, but in the worst cases, the effects can be detrimental to careers. So, it is worth taking a few moments to learn a few key points.

Overall, workplace politics help explain why many outcomes in training and beyond are unrelated to ability, dedication, or fairness. We'll categorize these into four main areas: (1) turf battles; (2) promotions, resources, and opportunities; (3) political tactics; and (4) difficult people. Of these, the need to work with difficult people is especially important, and we'll delve into specific types of difficult coworkers such as those with psychopathic tendencies in more detail.

Turf Battles

In medicine, *turf battles* refer to conflicts between providers or departments over patient management, hospital admissions, procedures, and other responsibilities. Turf battles occur on both national and local levels. Trainees usually have virtually no control over these matters but do need to know which providers or specialties are responsible for various tasks. Also realize that local turf battles or simple turf division of labor differ by institution. Thus, turf boundaries may be blurrier than predicted. It is usually best to refrain from any political comment on turf divisions.

Promotions, Resources, and Opportunities

Competition arises when demand for opportunities and resources exceeds supply. This becomes political when the allotment of promotions, resources, or other opportunities are based on subjective factors, interpersonal relationships, or other peripheral factors. It turns out that these other factors are considerations to some degree or another in almost all such decisions. Whether it is selecting chief residents, candidates for a fellowship spot, recipients of research opportunities, staff positions, committee appointments on a national society, or anything else, political factors play a role.

Political Tactics

Political tactics can be constructive (e.g., discussing a topic with individual key stakeholders before a meeting to allow time for reflection and to improve the quality and depth of group conversation) but may also be destructive (Table 32.1).

For example, someone might try to *bait* you into providing a response or action that is detrimental to your best interest. The instigator may use of your known triggers against you to get you to overreact or may casually ask you a benign-sounding question to see if you respond *correctly*. For example, an interviewer may test you to see if you are willing to badmouth another specialty or institution (possibly one he has a hidden affiliation with) by asking a subtly probing question. Since you cannot always know if this is occurring, the best offense is to understand your own triggers and to keep your conversations reasonably positive and professional.

Another political tactic that can affect trainees is alliance forging. Some trainees forge alliances and secure strong advocates, helping them to secure future fellowship or staff positions. In contrast, less proactive trainees may find themselves at a disadvantage.

Table 32.1 Examples of Political Tactics at Work

Tactic	Brief Description
Campaigns	Various campaigns for various positions continue in medical training and beyond (e.g., for a chief resident or PD position)
Alliances	Groups to further a common interest
Quid Quo Pro	There are many potential quid pro quo situations in medicine and academics
Backdoor Deals	Important decisions are often made behind closed doors
Insider Trading	People who are positioned to have knowledge or access to resources that others do not have can use this advantage to their benefit
Baiting	This is a test where someone with an ulterior motive asks a question or brings up a topic to see if you answer correctly
Divide and Conquer	This classic strategy persists since it is an effective means to exert group control. Essentially, a group divided into factions that are pitted against each other, which converts a larger in-group into opposing out-groups[643]
Pawns	A leader makes a self-serving decision that helps them even though it may be disadvantageous to others below them
Fall Guys	In the medical-administrative hierarchy as elsewhere in business and politics, the top dog can get off scot-free while someone lower in the chain takes the heat for something they were directed to do
Hidden Agendas	The stated reason for decisions or policy changes (usually one that cannot be argued with, such as the need to take care of patients or fend off financial disaster), is different from a true underlying motivation[644]
Gaslighting	Overt gaslighting is uncommon, but subtle forms can occur such as attempts to make workers question the validity of their own complaints[645]

There are also ways in which alliance forging can help trainees get the experiences they desire. For example, trainees on loosely structured surgical rotations can also forge alliances with other trainees to strategically divvy up available OR cases to gain a preferable selection of experiences or exposure to different attendings.

Since we work in an inherently political environment, some of your attendings and colleagues will be expert politicians. Understanding this fact can help you make sense of some of the decisions and actions around you. A politician's decisions consider the preservation and expenditure of their political capital. They may respond to your concerns with a shoulder shrug or with a sugar-coated response to keep the peace (or just to make it go away). This response may feel to the trainee like they are minimizing a real issue; it is necessary for the trainee to convey how important the topic is and why.

In addition, a politician might rationalize actions with logical fallacies. Remember though that some actions that seem political might have other explanations that are not immediately apparent. Thus, avoid making too many assumptions.

Difficult People

The prevalence of difficult individuals in the workplace underscores the prominence of this topic in resources on workplace politics.[172] The book *Working with Difficult People* defines ten categories, each of these is divided into three sections from the viewpoint of a boss, colleague, or subordinate, and these are each, in turn, divided into several subcategories.[638]

The myriad ways individuals can exhibit difficult behaviors necessitates a more practical approach to categorization. While the book is a useful reference, a more practical approach is to group the types of people into three broad categories: (1) inconsiderate coworkers, (2) incompetent coworkers, and (3) snakes (people who show psychopathic or Machiavellian spectrum behaviors). It is also useful to recognize that some types of difficult coworkers are very serious (like saboteurs) while others (like overly talkative ones) are more of a time drain.

Finally, the term *difficult people* implies they have a long-term fixed pattern or trait. In addition, in medicine, we all encounter people who are being difficult in the moment. This often occurs after hours when people are taxed, and the full contingent of daytime services are unavailable. Sometimes this comes from residents who are stretched thin. There can also be a fine line passionately between advocating for a patient when you disagree with other practitioners and being disrespectful. In general, it is never OK to be unduly disrespectful to anyone at work regardless of your position.

Psychopathic Behavior

Perhaps the most difficult type of colleague in medicine is a psychopath. We should acknowledge that the term engenders controversy from both diagnostic and stigmatizing standpoints and is not included in the *DSM-5*. In practical terms, it is more important to focus on the type of behavior than the label. That said, psychopaths constitute about one percent of the population (though estimates vary) but wreak disproportionate havoc in the public and at work.* The effects arise from the potentially callous nature of their actions and their proclivity to seek positions of power.

Though psychopaths date to prehistoric times, the modern work environment has become more susceptible to psychopathic infiltration. Now, they can use impression management to influence subjective evaluations, take advantage of being judged only by short-term results, manipulate others below them in the hierarchy to do their work for them, ingratiate themselves with those above them (but discard them later), show outside-the-box thinking (which has become valued), jump around among work areas and positions before being outed, and leverage nebulous job descriptions found in many leadership positions.[633] Many of these factors are probably at work in many medical practices.

Diagnosis of Psychopathy

Psychopathy is formally diagnosed using the Psychopathy Checklist-Revised (PCL-R) but is not formally included in the *DSM-5*. The main features include lack of guilt/remorse, a shallow emotional experience, low to absent affective empathy, and antisocial behavior. However, some experts suggest that the PCL-R may lead to overdiagnosis of psychopathy, is incomplete (such as not factoring low anxiety), and is too heavily weighted toward traits associated with bad behaviors (which can be seen in people with any empathic status).[204,639] The diagnosis holds other apparent paradoxes such as reported low empathy but also high cognitive (manipulative) empathy.[204]

Psychopathic Charm

In addition, psychopaths are often superficially charming, quickly befriending you or anyone around them who might be of use. They may tell you secrets (selectively) and try to pry secrets out of you too. They are also insincere shapeshifters, finding ways to show you that they are *just like you* and are expert pity-petitioners. In doing so, they form an illusion of trust and camaraderie to create a *psychopathic bond*.[633] After cultivating a strategic relationship, psychopaths will use their insider knowledge and kinship to their advantage at your expense. Behind the scenes, they gaslight, lie, and sabotage.

Clues to Psychopathic Behavior

Informal diagnosis of psychopathy is unreliable and inadvisable. One reason you should not try to label coworkers as psychopaths is that people are capable of this type of behavior for a variety of factors. In fact, around 10% of coworkers could be classified as some sort of *snake*, with psychopathic or antisocial behaviors.[633] These factors include other diagnoses like antisocial personality disorder, professional envy (which lowers empathy), personality traits like plain meanness, anger management problems, or Machiavellianism.

In fact, one emerging viewpoint is that Machiavellian behavior[1] (using duplicitous, self-serving, and ruthless tactics) is a more destructive force at work than psychopathy since it is less impulsive, more strategic, and more common.[640]

Still, several indicators may suggest interaction with an individual with psychopathic tendencies. For example, if you find yourself constantly feeling sorry for someone, it could be the effect of a pity petitioner.[641] Another clue is too many *slips* of responsibility with untoward effects on others even if shrouded in excuses.[641] More generally, finding that you are getting to like someone much faster and more than usual—a clue that you might be associated with a manipulator even though it could just be a friendly, relatable person.[160]

Managing Psychopathic Behavior

Many trainees are unaware of the impact of these behaviors, rendering them perfect prey, but there are other actions you can take to protect yourself. Importantly, always optimize the impressions you give to offset any false rumors about you, try not to engage in altercations, document unusual interactions, and avoid psychopathic bonds. Always be very careful revealing anything personal that could be used against you.

It is also useful to learn more about the topic and consider reading at least one of several manageable books about it, including *Snakes in Suits*, *The Sociopath Next Door*, and *Without Conscience*.[633,641,642] [2] Additionally, the book *The 48 Laws of Power* primarily details Machiavellian behaviors to avoid, while offering insights into behaviors warranting caution.[205] [3]

Notes

1 Like psychopathy, Machiavellianism is not a formal diagnosis in the *DSM-5*.
2 These books have nuanced usage of the terms *sociopath* and *psychopath*. *Without Conscience* uses the term *psychopath*.
3 One thing this book warns of is the risk of mixing friends and work, claiming we may not know them as well as we think, and that there are many other potential problems with the setup. In any case, it is important to choose to divulge at work wisely.

33

Mentors, Sponsors, and Role Models

Vance T. Lehman, Amy L. Kotsenas, Kendal Weger

In this chapter, we'll turn from difficult people and focus on those who help us achieve our professional potential. First, mentorship's origins can be traced back to a wise goddess guiding a young man in Homer's account of Greek mythology. When Odysseus sets sail for Troy, he leaves his son Telemachus in the hands of a man named Mentor. When Telemachus needs guidance, encouragement, and optimism to keep his birthright to the throne and maintain hope his father was alive, the goddess of wisdom, Athena, takes the form of Mentor and saves him from disaster.[646] The recognition of the importance of mentorship holds true today as much as ever given the complexities and competition in the modern medical workplace.

Mentors and Sponsors Are Underutilized

Although the virtues of mentorship have been recognized since ancient times, it remains a glaringly underutilized opportunity in medicine. Several factors may contribute to this underutilization, including a lack of awareness of its importance and the prior success of many trainees without mentorship. That is, trainees may not recognize the value of these relationships. Additionally, hesitancy to approach potential mentors could be addressed by programs formally encouraging mentorship.

Mentorship and sponsorship address critical aspects of the hidden curriculum, encompassing knowledge and skills not readily acquired through formal training. In fact, it is *necessary* to seek and foster these relationships to optimally navigate both the hidden curriculum at large and institution-specific challenges. Mentors can direct you to useful information, introduce you to people and opportunities, alert you to pitfalls, help you through difficult situations, assist with development of specific professional skills, and provide perspective and feedback.[143,647]

Mentorship is important at every stage while sponsorship is most important at points of career advancement such as securing a fellowship or job, academic promotion, or a professional leadership position.

Types of Mentors

There are different types of mentors who may be formally assigned through a mentorship program or informal. You can have multiple mentors, some with different areas of focus such as providing career direction versus interpersonal skills support. Close mentoring relationships

DOI: 10.1201/9781003633389-36

require nurturing, prioritizing quality over quantity. Many different traits of an effective mentor have been described. In general, you will want someone who is available, interested, insightful, and trustworthy. One article described a mentor as "someone who has more imagination about you than you have about yourself."[647]

Formal and Informal Mentors

The necessity of these relationships for success is why formal mentorship programs are critical; if an organization relies only on informal mentorship programs, many people will be left behind. Even with formal programs in place though, it is still beneficial to seek out additional informal mentors with complementary perspectives. However, informal mentors generally don't come to you; rather, you must actively seek them out.

Finding a Mentor

This could be fostering a relationship with someone you already know or reaching out to someone you do not know with a specific purpose. Ideally, this will be someone you resonate with and look up to as a positive role model. Basically, this is someone who does something you want to do and/or someone you aspire to emulate in some way.

A brief, respectful inquiry expressing admiration for their accomplishments and requesting a brief meeting to discuss their experience is usually sufficient. If they agree and your first meetup proves to be a good fit, additional meetups can come organically with just a little proactive push. While great mentors can be found at all career stages, it's generally beneficial to seek established mentors who are not in competition with their mentees.

Supportive and Challenge Mentors

Mentors can be categorized as supportive, challenging, or a combination of both.[648,649] Supportive mentors are unconditionally encouraging, while challenge mentors push you to be your best, even if this means giving you brutally honest feedback. It is probably best to have a mix of both types, but too much support has downsides like dependency on the mentor and most trainees (or people in general) could benefit from more challenging mentorship.[648,649]

In fact, the original Mentor of Greek mythology was a challenge mentor. However, this is one area where lots of us (trainees included) go wrong; we misinterpret well-intended challenge mentorship as an ego-threat or something more malignant. A growth mindset is beneficial when interpreting well-intended challenges from a mentor.

Mentorship Is a Two-Way Street

Successful mentoring relationships are reciprocal, requiring active participation from both mentor and mentee. Outside of medicine, such as real estate, mentees may help with basic tasks (for free) or pay for the mentorship opportunity. In medicine though, as in many pursuits, this can be just the joy that they are passing on a legacy or your expressions of gratitude.

Mentors will also have greater joy if you are open to their suggestions. You should also try your best to accommodate their schedule (instead of vice versa) and proactively schedule regular meetups. Finally, the mentor-mentee relationship works best when expectations are known upfront, and it may be up to you to be sure these are set.

Sponsors Help Most When They Know Your Goals

Sponsorship differs from mentorship in its focus on active advocacy, often for specific career advancements such as job offers. Mentors provide guidance while sponsors provide advocacy. Trainees may mistakenly assume mentors are actively advocating for them when this is not the case.

For instance, a trainee may take on a research project with an individual in hopes they will advocate for a position in a fellowship or staff, but this might not even be on the research mentor's radar. This possibility underscores the need to convey your goals to your mentors and to ask them if they can provide strong support for you when needed. Since a strong sponsor can be very impactful, it is important to seek them out as well. This may be a mentor-turned-sponsor or another key player at work who you meet up with and make your case to.

Mentorship for Women and Underrepresented Minorities

Specific considerations exist for mentorship and sponsorship of women and underrepresented minorities. Currently, these groups often receive ample advice but limited opportunities.[650,651] In other words, they are more likely to be given advice than given opportunities.

As their careers advance however, informal mentors and sponsors can become sparse for women and underrepresented minorities in medicine.[652] This results from our tendency to gravitate toward, and promote, others who are like us. But both groups are underrepresented in leadership positions and those who are there may need to expend political capital to keep their own careers afloat. One way to address this challenge is seeking mentors and sponsors from other institutions.

Ineffective Mentorship Situations

Truth be told though, there are several ways a mentoring relationship can lose effectiveness or go sour, including both mentee- and mentor-driven factors. The mentee must maintain their authentic enthusiasm, openness, availability, and so forth as mentioned. The mentor may lack time or requisite experience. A junior mentor who is not yet established in their career may seek to glean academic productivity from the mentee, which can conflict with a mentee's best interest. There might also be issues with boundaries, bias, or managing the transitions of the relationship to a post-mentorship phase.

Breaches of confidentiality pose a serious risk. A mentor might find herself with a conflict of interest such as being a mentor but also a member of a selection committee for a position in which the mentee is applying. While this may be unavoidable, this does need appropriate management and disclosure. Finally, there may also just be an irreconcilable mismatch of personalities or perspectives.

Other Supportive Relationships

There are many other important types of professional relationships, as summarized in Table 33.1. In particular, it is critical to identify positive role models since they play a particularly prominent role in influencing the development of your professional persona.

Table 33.1 Types of Relationships That Support Career and Personal Development (Hill)

Relationship	Description
Mentor	Serves as a subject matter expert and confidant(e) who listens, supports, guides, and provides perspective
Sponsor	Advocates for a specific position
Role Model	Is one you seek to emulate
Ally	Is a colleague with a connection
On-Boarder	Orients newcomers
Supervisor/Preceptor	Oversees clinical duties or a rotation
Research Advisor	Assists with research execution
Consultant/Coach	Assists with development of a specific skill or sets a strategic goal and plan

Key Takeaways

Actively seeking mentorship and sponsorship is crucial yet underutilized during training. These relationships offer many benefits, including opening doors and helping you navigate the hidden curriculum. The topic is so important, in fact, that it serves as an excellent segue to Part IV, where we'll focus specifically on topics that are directly related to clinical practice.

Part IV

Part IV will apply many of the main points we have discussed already to clinical rotations, beginning with the transition from classroom to clinical settings. The general topics from Part I remain critically relevant, with some topics that we'll discuss in more detail, such as effective learning methods.

DOI: 10.1201/9781003633389-37

34

Introduction to Clinical Rotations

Vance T. Lehman

The importance of each theme of the hidden curriculum comes into full force once you step foot on the wards or in the clinic. This period is marked by significant change, cultural immersion, increased hierarchy, new challenges, and rising expectations. A new level of professionalism becomes necessary. Well-being faces greater challenges. Mastery of interpersonal psychology and communication skills becomes critical. Gender considerations become increasingly salient. It is very important to review the suggestions for managing major transitions we discussed in Chapter 10. Consider the relevance of these themes as you explore the following topics.

The additional themes and topics from Part III are all relevant too. During clinical clerkships, it is essential that you prioritize honing cognitive empathy, maintaining personal organizational skills, managing failure effectively, optimizing your medical writing, and seeking mentorship. To navigate all this complexity, it is more important than ever before to use our six central strategies: (1) get the easy things right, (2) use effective learning methods, (3) be proactive, (4) understand how others think, (5) identify influences, and (6) embrace challenges.

Detailed advice for each rotation is beyond this book's scope. That said, the general principles given here apply well to most rotations when tweaked for the specific situation. For example, there is one fundamental factor that disproportionately impacts how your attendings/evaluators are influenced to rate your performance: *Did the attending's day improve because of the trainee's presence?* Most doctors in academic practice choose that career path because they love teaching motivated trainees, even though it requires extra energy and effort. Nothing is more discouraging, though, than if a learner does not arrive with a good attitude toward their own learning or substantially impedes the flow of the day by not being prepared.

If you're a newer trainee, the answer to the question may rest on your level of interest, preparation, and positivity. If the answer is yes that the attending's day did improve because of your presence, she is more likely to offer more favorable feedback. If you're an experienced trainee, this determination may rest on whether you made the day easier for the attending by functioning at or above the expected level, going above and beyond to help the care team, offering helpful intellectual contributions at appropriate times, and so forth.

Above all, continuously strive to emulate the thought processes and actions of an attending physician while also being mindful of your own inexperience and other limitations.

DOI: 10.1201/9781003633389-38

Context Matters

While previous discussions about clinical rotations have offered a general overview, the specific expectations, challenges, and influences in clinical settings vary significantly by context. Your training program location (e.g., urban versus rural) and model (e.g., university vs. community) matter. The roles of PAs or NPs (if present) on teaching services should be known. Expectations vary by specialty (and even among services within specialties), by your training level, and by the type of problems your patients have (e.g., straightforward versus complex).

This requires careful consideration. A common error is applying assumptions from one context to another without verification, which occurs as trainees jump from service to service. Thus, it is essential to be nimble and uncover tacit expectations for every new context.

Things That Don't Necessarily Predict Success

Let's briefly examine factors unrelated to success as a competent physician. Though widely used for hiring and promotions, interviews and letters of evaluation actually have limited ability to predict performance. Most other factors used to select students or residents (such as pre-entry test scores, age, gender, or study of physical sciences) have limited ability to predict performance too.[653]

In fact, most objective measures on residency applications are poorly correlated with clinical performance during residency.[654–658] Successful physicians come from diverse backgrounds. Thus, do not develop impostor syndrome if you have followed a "nontraditional" pathway.

Joe's Story

Now, it is time to revisit your classmate Joe from Chapter 2. Recall that he was able to access the hidden curriculum in ways that you (the former you) were not. But how did he do it?

It boiled down to a combination of not only preparation but also a decent amount of luck. It turns out he has an older sister who recently completed a chief resident year at a large internal medicine training program. Without insider guidance, Joe's sister had made many avoidable missteps along her training journey.

Fortunately, she was able to recover (though not without unnecessary stress, energy, and effort) and grow from her experiences, and by the end was even selected for the chief resident position. Attending a lecture at a national conference during her chief year, she learned about the hidden curriculum. The talk resonated with her personal experience and that of the residents she now managed. "*Why hadn't I been told of this earlier?*" she thought.

Managing a large group of trainees as chief resident, Joe's sister's perspective shifted. She encountered many resident issues ranging from professionalism to conflict resolution to clinical competency concerns. By the year's end, she noticed many patterns and gained insight into differentiators of performance. These all seemed so obvious to her now, and she wondered why no one had been there to clue her into them when she was in training earlier. She also reflected on choices in her personal life that she would have handled differently in retrospect. Looking out for her younger brother, she called him up one day: "*Joe, there are a few things you should know about medical training…*".

That was it—one fortunate circumstance that set the stage for Joe. And now, we'll cover some of the advice Joe's sister might have given him by building on the topics of Parts I–III and incorporating the six central strategies for success.

Road Map

Beginning by building on the foundational topic of effective learning from Part I, Part IV now turns to one of the most mentioned themes of the hidden curriculum: professionalism during clinical rotations. This section emphasizes the importance of collegiality, teamwork, and interprofessional competence and offers specific advice for outpatient rotations, inpatient rotations, procedures, and learning the roles of pathology and radiology.

Finally, we'll cover some important general topics, including social determinants of health; evaluations and feedback; conferences, medical societies, and industry; and the application process for residency and other positions.

35

Learning Strategies on Clinical Rotations

Vance T. Lehman

In addition to the fundamental effective learning methods from Chapter 3, several higher-level concepts are incredibly useful for understanding and organizing a large volume of information in the clinical setting. These include (1) hierarchy of knowledge, (2) collective knowledge, (3) experiential learning, (4) time-strapped strategies, and (5) content creation. There are also other approaches, such as mastery learning, which are detailed elsewhere.[659,660]

We'll explore each of these ideas and then briefly touch upon test preparation. We'll also apply basic concepts from *Revised Bloom's Taxonomy* of cognitive skills, which includes (in order of increasing complexity): remembering, understanding, applying, analyzing, evaluating, and creating.

The Hierarchy of Knowledge

Throughout your medical education, you'll be inundated with a vast amount of information. Often, the sheer quantity of information can feel overwhelming, and it can be difficult to organize. This section introduces a *hierarchy of knowledge*—a framework I use for prioritizing and retaining information based on its importance in clinical practice (Table 35.1). This framework can help prevent you from feeling overwhelmed.

The truth is that not all information is created equal. Some facts and concepts are more critical to master than others. When we treat everything as being equally important, we risk diluting the key takeaways and ultimately forgetting what matters most. This hierarchy acknowledges that strategically managing what you retain and what you *file away* can be a practical and powerful learning strategy.

Unlike *Bloom's Taxonomy*, which emphasizes depth of understanding, the hierarchy of knowledge system prioritizes the relevance of a given piece of information in clinical medicine. Thus, the hierarchy of knowledge and *Bloom's Taxonomy* are complementary.

For the hierarchy of knowledge, information can be sorted into one of the following three buckets: (1) knowledge requiring effortless recall and application, (2) knowledge that should go in your back pocket, and (3) information that should be tucked away in your mental file cabinet.

Now, let's look at each bucket in more detail.

DOI: 10.1201/9781003633389-39

Table 35.1 Hierarchy of Knowledge

Category	Knowledge that Requires Effortless Recall and Application	Knowledge that Should Go in Your Back Pocket	Information for the File Drawer
Brief Description	Essential knowledge that every trainee is expected to know, particularly information critical for your current rotation or class. Think of it as the information that should roll off the tip of your tongue	Knowledge that you should be able to recall with a bit of effort. These are concepts and facts that are important enough to revisit occasionally	Everything else that is not entirely discarded – information that you can recall with considerable effort or after a review and that isn't essential for day-to-day practice
KeyFeatures	– Very common – High clinical importance – Clinically relevant level of detail – Applies strongly to current situation (e.g., rotation or class)	– Common – Moderate clinical importance – Mildly exceeds a clinically relevant level of detail – Applies moderately to current situation	– Uncommon – Lower clinical importance – Level of detail exceeds clinical relevance – Low applicability to current situation
Examples	– Treatments for common emergencies – First-line treatments for common conditions – Basic common knowledge such as common routine screening or vaccination recommendations – Basic procedural skills (e.g., suturing) – Heavily tested material	– Important enough to be represented as headings or figures in major textbooks – Relatively common conditions or treatments, but not the most common – Simplified sketches of clinically relevant aspects of basic science processes	– Most mathematical formulas that are not used routinely in clinical practice – Basic science details like enzyme kinetics or intermediate molecules – Experimental information outside your area of subspecialty – Uncommon things that are easily found in reference material

195

Knowledge Requiring Effortless Recall and Application

This bucket contains the essential, foundational knowledge that every physician trainee should know cold. This includes information critical for your current rotation or class—the things you need to recall instantly without hesitation—as well as for any emergencies you may encounter unexpectedly in any setting.

However, remember that this effortless recall bucket is prone to spillage; if you don't actively practice retrieving this information, it will gradually migrate to the back pocket or file cabinet buckets. Realize that much of what you need for one rotation may be less critical on the next. It's also important to note that pure recall is just the first step. According to *Bloom's Taxonomy*, remembering information is the lowest level of cognitive ability. To truly master something, you must strive for higher levels of understanding, application, and analysis.

Knowledge That Should Go in Your Back Pocket

In contrast to the information you need to know instantly, your back pocket holds clinically useful, but less critical or less urgent, information. These are the concepts and facts that are important enough to revisit occasionally but that you can take a few seconds to recall.

While it's tempting to try to cram everything into your back pocket, remember that space is limited. You can amass a large knowledge base, but you can only actively practice so much. Prioritize the information that is most relevant to your current learning goals and clinical experiences.

Information That Should Go in Your Mental File Cabinet

Everything else—information that isn't essential for immediate recall or regular use—goes into your mental file cabinet. This doesn't mean you should ignore these topics entirely. What seems irrelevant today might become crucial with medical advances during your career.

A broad knowledge base, even of *filed away* information, can also help you make connections in research and clinical care. This category includes information you can recognize and recall with either more considerable effort or substantial review. Think of it as knowing enough to know what to search for when the need arises. For example, you might not remember the specific details of a rare genetic disorder, but you know enough to search a medical database for more information if a patient presents with relevant symptoms.

How to Determine Which Category Is Best

It's understandable that determining which information belongs in each category can be challenging, especially for trainees. This skill develops with experience, but a few clues include (1) frequency with which the topics are encountered, (2) clinical importance, (3) level of detail (reductionism), and (4) rotation-specific relevance.

Here are some specific examples for each bucket category:

- **Knowledge Requiring Effortless Recall and Application**. To determine what knowledge belongs in this category, think of the general knowledge expected of all physicians, such as common vaccine recommendations and screening guidelines. For specific rotations, consider the following:
  - Open-source questions from prior exams (approved for dissemination).
  - Routine medical situations (e.g., first-line treatments for hypertension while on an internal medicine rotation).

- Emergencies you're expected to address.
- Insider information gathered from prior trainees.
- Information actionable in everyday practice. For instance, knowing that sickle cell anemia arises from a GAG to GTG mutation is less clinically relevant for most physicians than knowing that its inheritance is autosomal recessive.

- **Knowledge for Your Back Pocket**. To determine what knowledge belongs in your back pocket, focus on the key take-home points that form the framework of knowledge. These may appear in

  - textbook headings and subheadings,
  - textbook illustration content,
  - textbook summaries, or
  - simplified sketches of basic science processes.

  For example, venous collaterals that underlie varices secondary to portal hypertension are clinically important, while uncommon variants of jejunal veins are best left to subspecialists. For a process such as a biochemical pathway, sketch it out. The summary sketch with only the key inputs, outputs, and potentially critical regulators are back pocket information. Without emphasizing the big picture, we risk putting everything into the file cabinet, even the information we really should keep closer at hand.

- **Information for the File Cabinet**. To determine what goes in your file cabinet, think of things that are not used during routine clinical or that can be readily looked up, such as the following:

  - **Many Mathematical Formulas**.
  - **Enzyme Reactions**. Detailed biochemical pathways that aren't directly relevant to clinical decision-making.
  - **Niche, Unsubstantiated, or Experimental Content**. Information that is highly specialized, lacks strong evidence, or is still under investigation.
  - **Lookup-able Lists**. Information that can be easily accessed when needed.

Exceptions depend on circumstance; for example, radiology residents should keep the NASCET equation, a simple accepted equation to calculate the degree of internal carotid artery stenosis, in their back pocket rather than in the file cabinet.

Collective Knowledge

One of the greatest benefits of medical training is access to the collective knowledge of physicians. Remember that humans have learned through social learning, sharing, and passing down knowledge for millennia. This collective knowledge—encompassing perspective, historical context of medical treatments, experience-based heuristics, and effective clinical reasoning strategies—is invaluable for real-world practice. Through this shared wisdom, you're connected to generations of medical professionals, even legends like the Big Four at Hopkins. It's crucial to tap into this resource.

How to Access Collective Knowledge

Access is often as simple as cultivating interest, enthusiasm, inquisitiveness, and proactivity. Don't let a reliance on textbook knowledge hinder your clinical learning. Remember, you must *do* things, not just *know* things. Engage actively in the clinic to understand how attendings and senior trainees think. Ask well-timed questions that are relevant, thoughtful, and directed at your attendings' areas of greatest experience. Attendings find it rewarding to teach engaged and interested learners, but disinterest or arrogance can be detrimental to your learning experience.

Experiential Learning

Let's expand on the central role of experiential learning, especially in the context of clinical decision-making and social learning. It's crucial to emphasize this, because many trainees overemphasize websites and flashcards when higher-yield clinical experiences are available.

Experiential learning connects to learning priorities and collective knowledge. It is specific to medical practice and acknowledges complexity, further discussed in Chapter 48. When done well, experiential learning becomes the cornerstone for applying knowledge using deliberate practice and mastery learning techniques. Chapters 3 and 6 also highlighted the historical and evolutionary basis of social and experiential learning.

Why Experiential Learning Matters

Nothing shatters the illusion of knowledge faster than trying to apply it in a real-world setting. The gap between textbook knowledge and clinical readiness is typically vast. Studying for trainees is like learning music theory and practicing warm-up exercises for new musicians wishing to learn to play an instrument—necessary but insufficient. Real-life experience, even when it pushes you into your discomfort zone (with proper oversight and patient safety measures), is essential.

Maximizing Experiential Learning

- **Know Your Patients**. Relate patient care experiences to your knowledge base and connect seemingly disparate topics.
- **Explore the Differential Diagnosis**. During admissions, investigate all realistic possibilities, not just the primary consideration.
- **Craft Excellent Notes**. Take pride in creating well-reasoned (but appropriately concise) admission and consult notes that organize your thoughts and demonstrate critical thinking.
- **Be Curious**. Look up background information on your patients' conditions to learn volumes.
- **Recognize Exponential Benefits**. Notice that clinical experience yields increasing returns in both knowledge and efficiency.

Time-Strapped Strategies

Clinical rotations differ significantly from classroom learning by offering far less dedicated study time, including preparation for exams. To succeed, you'll need to develop efficient learning strategies. These will help you balance clinical responsibilities with studying for test preparation. Some trainees excel at using time-strapped methods, while others take a more casual (and often less effective) approach. The first principle is simply to start early, or even ahead, of a rotation. In addition, here are some steps to boost your efficiency:

- **Personalized Flashcards**. Create electronic flashcards (keeping in mind the previously mentioned caveats) that connect topics and synthesize information in a meaningful way, rather than simply regurgitating facts. Make it a habit to use these cards during short periods of downtime.

- **High-Quality Resources**. Seek level-appropriate, high-quality resources that are reasonable in length and number. One excellent resource is better than two mediocre ones. A resource you actually read is far more valuable than a dozen that sit on your bookshelf (or desktop). A first-rate question bank that promotes problem-solving, develops topic synthesis, and provides well-thought-out explanations is invaluable. Consider high-quality podcasts from reputable medical journals for commutes.
- **Strategic Downtime Planning**. Plan how to use short periods of downtime effectively. Five or ten minutes here and there can add up quickly. Brief review sessions can strengthen partially learned concepts and leverage the advantages of spaced repetition. However, the best use of downtime depends on the rotation. Some surgical services may expect trainees to use it for clinical errands, research, studying, or assisting in the OR. Factor in specific rotation expectations when planning your study strategy.

Content Creation

Content creation, the highest level of *Bloom's Taxonomy*, is a powerful tool for learning medicine.[442] This can take many forms:

- **Personalized Learning Tools**. Designing your own flashcards or practice tests that synthesize information.
- **Educational Writing**. Writing a review article for a medical journal.
- **Conference Presentations**. Creating didactic or case-based conferences.

Content creation is closely linked to teaching. By teaching with created content, you organize your thoughts, identify knowledge gaps, practice active recall, motivate yourself to research, and ensure you can confidently explain concepts.

While content creation may seem time-consuming, it offers a high long-term return on investment. Creating high-quality conferences, whether didactic or case-based, is one such method. Focus on formulating images and patterns for your audience, finding connections, and discussing problem-solving and differentiating features of conditions, rather than simply regurgitating facts.

Studying for Shelf Examinations

Core clinical rotations often conclude with shelf examinations—standardized tests based on previously used (or *shelved*) USMLE questions. Just as studying alone isn't enough for clinical excellence, clinical practice alone isn't enough to ace shelf exams. While there is no single formula for success, the following guidelines can help:

Key Study Strategies:

- **Plan Ahead**. Create a detailed study plan that distributes study sessions throughout the rotation, starting early. Cramming is never optimal and is virtually impossible during clinical rotations. Incorporate the effective learning techniques discussed in Chapter 3.
- **Prioritize Knowledge Gaps**. Fill in major knowledge gaps first, and then focus on the details. Some details matter more than others. Details with little direct applicability to patient care (e.g., the specific chromosome where a gene resides, except perhaps for X-linked diseases) are typically lower yield.
- **Form Connections**. Connect study material to your clinical experiences, even if indirectly. As you progress through rotations, think about how common topics

interconnect. For example, many internal medicine concepts apply to surgical patient care and vice versa.

- **Utilize High-Quality Resources**. Use a level-appropriate, high-yield book (or equivalent) designed for clerkships. High-yield bullet point resources are useful for downtime review, but don't forget that comprehensive content is crucial for building your knowledge base. Rehearsing buzzwords is a low-effort activity, best reserved for only limited times when you're tired. Focus on connecting topics, learning clinically relevant pathophysiology, and distinguishing between similar conditions.
- **Emphasize Question Banks**. Use a high-quality question bank with explanations.[661] Many students find that focusing on one question bank is more effective than rushing through multiple banks. The National Board of Medical Examiners (NBME) website also provides practice questions.[662] Question banks encourage active learning, identify knowledge gaps, and incorporate information into clinical context. It is useful to use question banks for both learning and testing. Be wary of questions found on unverified sites on the internet, as some of these are inaccurate or not level appropriate.

36

Clinical Professionalism

Vance T. Lehman

Back to the Basics

This chapter builds on the basic expectations outlined in Chapter 2, with a focus on respecting colleagues, patients, and confidentiality. Key aspects of professionalism include maintaining a professional appearance, being punctual, demonstrating preparedness, and exhibiting politeness.

Professional Attire

Considering professional appearance, there are practical reasons for a dress code. The first reason relates to patient preferences. As mentioned in Chapter 14, most patients prefer a formal, professionally dressed physician in clinic (or scrubs) and prefer white coats.[370] This aligns with research suggesting that professionals in higher-quality business attire are often perceived as more competent.[160] The second reason is safety, including prevention of injuries and hospital acquired infections.[663] For example, closed-toed shoes may protect healthcare workers. It is not acceptable to wear the same scrubs from home to the OR. These standards are expected of attendings too.

Arrival and Departure

While punctuality may have seemed less critical during preclinical years, it is now of paramount importance. Of course, any reasonable person will honor exceptions for an emergency or other one-off situations. Otherwise, it is never wise to ask to leave before duties are done, even if it is late and rounding is being very inefficient or if you want to get to Pilates class or tend to personal errands.

One special case is the desire to leave town for personal or other reasons. This is a time you need to plan and be sure your transportation is amenable with your schedule. For example, avoid scheduling flights that necessitate leaving work early without prior approval from your program. For situations like this, an attending may feel his hands are tied and let you go, but at the expense of a mark on your reputation.

In addition to arriving and departing at appropriate times, it is to your benefit to show up to required trainee-focused conferences and other educational activities. You should not aim to barely clear the bar. If the required conference attendance rate is set at 80%, you should still aim for 100%. Emergencies, of course, take priority. But these are exceptions. Aim for 100% attendance, even if the minimum requirement is lower.

DOI: 10.1201/9781003633389-40

A particularly unprofessional example is requesting to leave duties for a conference but then going home or to the resident lounge. While staff may not track your every move, attendance patterns and frequent trips to the parking lot or break room are noticeable.

Even scheduling too many optional work-related meetings during the day such as research project meetings can create problems. When you must have a research meeting during normal working hours, be sure to check with your staff ahead of time. Also, make sure it is not a disruptive online meeting or loud phone call in a shared workspace.

Preparedness

Considering your preparedness, you should always arrive ready for a workday. If unsure about preparation requirements, ask a senior resident or attending promptly to ensure you meet or exceed expectations. Expectations vary by service and staff. When in doubt, err on the side of thorough preparation; this will maximize your learning. Remember that preparation should not be pure busy work. Seek to understand the patients' conditions, imaging, and prior treatments, as well as the problem-solving methods employed during prior visits.

Finally, always be courteous and professional, in person, on the phone, in the hallway, and even in your clinical notes. Strive to present your best, most professional self.

Be Available When Others Are

Another important consideration of professionalism pertains to respect for others' availability. If anyone, especially an attending, agrees to meet to help you on any account (mentorship, research discussion, education topic, remediation, etc.), do your best to accommodate their schedule. Avoid inconveniencing them to meet yours. Do not say you are unavailable during a research day because it is mildly inconvenient for you to come in for a meeting. This is surprisingly common behavior and can be perceived as entitlement. It is generally viewed negatively when one expects others to invest more in their career development than they are willing to invest themselves.

Similarly, while it is important to set boundaries on personal time, you should not defer reasonable requests just because they are inconvenient for you. For example, if an attending wants to set a meeting up or asks you to give a presentation on your academic day, it is usually poor form to outright refuse.

Further, there is a legitimate debate over how to calibrate our boundaries for off-hours emails. However, ignoring an email from an attending or taking more than one workday (when you are not away) to answer is generally seen as a mark against your professionalism and/or respect toward the sender.

Disagreements over Patient Care

In addition, it is helpful to learn productive ways to handle disagreements over patient care. When these arise, do not pollute the EMR with squabbles, and never throw another colleague under the bus. You will inevitably disagree with the approach of other physicians and might feel frustrated or even cornered. Perhaps you think a consulting service should take immediate action, but their assessment is that treatment can wait a couple of hours.

Even if you feel you need to document your service's viewpoint to cover yourself, be very careful how this is documented in the EMR. Anything documented that could be perceived as exaggeration or unfair blame-shifting is inadvisable. Instead, seek respectful, direct dialogue and, when needed, advice from your senior trainees or attendings.

Judging Other's Competence

You should never prejudge anyone's ability and never make a public statement about another's competence. You will hear whispers of reputations of various attendings or other professionals. It is critical to understand that these perceptions are often incorrect. Even if you think you are making a positive statement, it is a risk, as it can easily be interpreted to (inadvertently) imply comparison among the staff.

For example, do not inadvertently insinuate that certain attendings are *the good ones*. In addition to being poor form, you as a trainee are in a poor position to judge the competence of attendings. Some of the most astute attendings are unsung heroes who stay out of the limelight.

The reputation of physicians among their peers is an imperfect measure of their skill. Some reputations are built entirely from research or presentations at national conferences, which may or may not reflect excellent patient care. As an example, in *How Doctors Think*, Jerome Groopman recalls a personal story where he flew far and wide to find the most renowned hand surgeon for his own condition, but in the end, it was the hand surgeon who took the time to carefully and thoughtfully evaluate his situation who found the answer.[111]

Avoid Unwarranted Absences

There are many stories of trainees (or others) who are not fully forthcoming about their absences. This can take many forms: moonlighting when your training program is paying for you to go to a national conference, going to a national conference but attending very little or none of it, implying you are too unwell to do a task but are seen out on the town doing fun things that are more strenuous, and so on. Unwarranted absences can severely damage your reputation and sometimes are grounds for formal disciplinary action.

The Worst Mistake

There are endless mistakes one can make, but one stands out as the worst: taking credit for the accomplishments of others. One survey of bad boss behaviors found that people rate this number one.[664] It has been referred to as the worst "trait," but here we say "mistake" since the word trait implies a fixed intrinsic personality flaw, whereas "mistake" recognizes that anyone could potentially falter, and offenders can change.

Murky Areas of Credit Attribution

But this topic can be murky. In some corporate cultures, it is customary for a project team leader to claim credit. Giving a lab leader the last authorship position on a paper for which he did little direct work is a common example in medicine. Further, colleagues can forget where an idea originated or may make a presentation that inadvertently leaves out recognition.

For example, patients with unusual diagnoses may be presented at conferences or in the literature without acknowledging the individual who first recognized the diagnosis. While frustrating, these situations are inevitable. Overall, there is a difference between customary or inadvertent credit transfer and unscrupulous credit snatching. Avoid claiming credit for the work of others and realize that others will probably (and often inadvertently) take some credit for your ideas.

Perceived Versus Real Efforts in Group Projects

A related phenomenon is the degree of credit taken for a group project. The *Harvard Business Review* article "How (Un)ethical Are You" reminds us that we tend to overrate our own abilities and contributions.[203] This is also true among highly successful professionals like physicians. A Harvard experiment found that the sum of perceived effort on group projects was an average of 139%.[203] This creates a mismatch between perceived credit and perceived contribution. Everyone on a team can feel like they are doing more than their share and can ironically react by doing *less* in response.[203]

In medicine, we must sometimes diplomatically manage perceived effort and ensure we (and others) are recognized for legitimate efforts while still being a team player. While this is challenging, an approach that uses indisputable objective data and examples can help. This topic is further complicated by the medical hierarchy.

That is, you want to make your superiors and mentors look good without the extremes of outshining them too much or conversely getting fully excluded from recognition. Be gracious with your credit and try to make others around you look good. It is possible for an entire team to succeed and feel good about themselves.

This does not mean you should downplay your accomplishments. Be sure to shine, but just make sure you aren't stealing someone else's reflected light. Make it your own.

Avoiding Gossip and Rumor

While taking credit for other people's work is the worst mistake, workplace gossip is a close second. But gossip is more insidious, nuanced, and common. It is an interplay between two or more people rather than a solitary offense. A harmless much needed *vent* can drift to it. It may seem like no active harm is being done. If someone is willing to gossip about others, why would they not do the same about you?

Too often, strategic sabotage, one-sided or false information, can unfairly taint someone's reputation. It can become an attempt to discredit or dehumanize someone. It is a subtle odorless poison that infiltrates the air and slowly and stealthily wreaks havoc on a workplace. People will not respect you more if you gossip. And recall that gossip is a time drain that hinders productivity.

Nuances of Gossip

This topic is nuanced though. Gossip can be functional and is impossible to eradicate. Remember that human language evolved for gossip within bands so everyone in a group could know who to trust. We should also not fear discussing real problems simply because it might be construed as gossip. If there is a problem at work, how else are people to find solace from others who understand?

Ideally, though, such discourse minimizes speculation and is geared at finding a solution. But it should not become a perpetual tribal habit, which can devolve into poisoning the well, labeling, *ad hominem* attacks, out-group battles, and group-level bullying. In sum, there are many reasons why it is in your best interest to avoid being pulled into too much gossip.

Never Disparage Anybody or Anything

Not only should you avoid gossip and rumor, but you should never badmouth any other specialty, clinical team member with different credentials, or other colleagues. Many physicians are partnered with other clinic or hospital employees, and you might be unaware of it, especially if they keep different last names. They also have close friends or children with these positions. Others have close friends or relatives in the rival hospital across town. Assume that everyone in healthcare knows everyone else outside of work, especially within an institution.

Banishing Your Inner Napoleon

Once residents start taking call, they are typically granted much more responsibility and authority. This is a time of stress, results-based evaluations, and an apparent shift in the hierarchical position. Unfortunately, it is also a time when a trainee's inner tyrant, even one they did not know exists, can emerge.

This is quickly noticed, however, and one misstep can make its way up the chain of command quickly. Letting loose your inner tyrant damages your reputation and does not help patient care. It is also time for an ego check, especially since we all need each other more than ever in this world of increasing medical complexity and subspecialization.

There will be times when you must take a firm stance for patient care, even if it is unpopular. However, these times are rare and essentially never require a tyrant. But this task is harder than it sounds, especially when you are tired, irritable, and at your wits end; by analogy, the first time Napoleon was banished to an island, he came storming back and attempted (unsuccessfully) to reclaim his throne.

Accepting Responsibility

According to *self-affirmation theory*, we are driven to protect our self-image of competence. Sometimes blame will fall unfairly on you (and everyone else) via multiple mechanisms like retrospective bias, but other times, we find a situation where we really should accept responsibility. However, resistance to taking responsibility can become problematic.

If you find yourself thinking or saying, "The staff made me feel this way" when they were "too hard on me"; "the staff blamed me for something that was really his fault"; "the staffs' standards are unrealistic"; "I did it just perfectly; it is not my fault," it is possible you are not accepting responsibility.

Special Considerations for Interactions with Attendings

Everyone has insecurities. Even after years of coiling cerebral aneurysms, administering anesthesia in the OR, or managing women in labor, your attendings will have moments of self-doubt. Understanding this is crucial for a couple of reasons.

First, realize that this is normal and, while more prevalent in training and early in a career, that feeling never goes away completely. That is, an intermittent impostor syndrome can persist long after training is done. Second, you will witness attendings deal with difficult situations.

These are key learning opportunities, but when your attending needs to focus, it is not a good time to ask nonurgent questions.

Attendings will not know every answer, and don't press them too hard if they are not sure about something (instead find another resource). Always stay tactful to avoid being labeled (unfairly) as an overly skeptical trainee. The issue is that well-intended questions could be misinterpreted as questioning an attending's ability. Never hold back a question, though, if you truly believe patient safety is at risk.

Respect Others' Time

While some people are busier than others, everyone thinks they are busy. Always be careful when suggesting that someone else should assume a responsibility instead of you because you are too busy. This implies you believe the other person is less busy.

Work Environment

There are some differences in professional norms among rotations. Inpatient, outpatient, pathology, radiology, psychiatry, pediatrics, and others can have different expectations for dress and/or behavior. While you can possibly show up to inpatient or surgical rotations in a T-shirt and change into scrubs, clinic may require proper business attire.

This does not mean rigid conformity, loss of all individuality, or Rolex watches, but there may be basic dress codes to follow. To instill the highest degree of confidence in your patients and team, it is advisable to make sure your hair and clothes are not disheveled or unclean.

Making a Positive First Impression

As we have already seen, we are heavily influenced by first impressions.[665] These are best delivered with a genuine smile, focused interest, and appropriate eye contact. In medicine, this also means timing an introduction with tact. If an attending is clearly in deep thought or focused on a task, it is usually best to not interrupt.

You should also know who your attending is from day one. This means their name, what they look like, and the basics of their areas of clinical expertise. Finally, while you should never be late to a clinical rotation, an on-time arrival is ten minutes late if it is your first day.

After the introduction, it is usually an opportune time to show that you are eager to do well and to seek performance feedback. It is also an opportune time to have an initial discussion about rotation expectations. Taking this initiative can help fend off a cycle of attendings' confirmation bias of any of their own intergenerational biases.

First Impressions and Labels

At the introductory stage, the labeling effect is powerful. First impressions create labels that trigger feedback loops with long-term consequences. In addition, your reputation can be propagated by second-hand labels passed on attending-to-attending. Once this occurs, your subsequent first impressions start with a baked-in positive or negative bias. Such reputations may have a disproportionate effect on your evaluations early on since you do not have substantial clinical skill to be judged by. A positive first impression confers a *halo effect* that colors future evaluations.

Though impactful, first impressions are often misleading. Recall that some of the best ones are made by psychopaths.[633] Or sometimes a new acquaintance has just had a bad day. It is best to base your interpersonal assessments of others from a series of observations, ideally based on objective criteria. Making a good first impression is not foolproof though and, over time, it is possible to fall from grace. Still, it is easier to maintain a good reputation than recover from a bad one.

Know Your First-Name Culture

You should also know the first-name culture of your institution. In some institutions resident physicians are on a first-name basis with attendings, and in others, they are not. In general, if you are not sure, it is best to use formal names first unless asked to do otherwise. Sometimes residents are used to being on a first-name basis but must adapt to a new culture when going elsewhere for a fellowship.

There may still be gray areas for using first names when there is an established relationship and one person transitions to a new status like resident or attending. First names are common practice in these situations, but when unsure, it is best to assume formality. Finally, when addressing another physician of any status in front of a patient, it is best to use their formal title instead of their first name.

Key Takeaways

The main points of professionalism during clinical rotations still revolve around the basic expectations and include punctuality, respect, and avoiding the worst mistakes. The professionalism principles apply in all settings but are particularly relevant to the topic of teamwork, which we'll discuss in the next chapter.

37

Teamwork

Vance T. Lehman

Effective teamwork across professional settings shares key features: decisive leadership, clearly defined roles, closed-loop communication, adaptability, and psychological safety. These principles generally apply to diverse teams, including clinical services, OR teams, and research groups. However, each situation presents unique considerations. Interactions with team members also depend on their professional roles (e.g., senior physician, junior trainee, nurse, administrator).

Group IQ

Team success depends not only on individual members but also on group dynamics. Collective intelligence (group IQ) depends on emotional intelligence (EQ), not just IQ.[47] For example, teams must foster inclusivity, preventing vocal members from dominating discussions. This is why a team leader must set a safe tone, encourage diverse viewpoints, and maintain momentum.

Setting the Stage for Effective Teamwork

Building on the concept of collective intelligence, it turns out that the initial moments of team formation are crucial for establishing a productive work environment.[178] Thus, you should project a team-oriented approach from the start. In medical teams, orientations offer leaders (typically attendings or senior residents) a chance to set expectations and tone. For instance, this is an opportunity to dispel myths about zero-sum performance evaluations among medical students, fostering collaboration over unhealthy competition.

Teams with strong psychological safety and positive rapport can express differing viewpoints and tolerate constructive conflict.[178] However, recall that excessive group harmony can lead to ineffective groupthink, stifling creativity and hindering clinical decision-making.[178] So, be on alert for groupthink as it can impede effective clinical decision-making.

For example, a team member might assume an epidural abscess in a low-income patient is due to intravenous drug use. However, this overlooks other potential causes, leading to an inadequate workup. If another team member, especially a senior one, agrees, others may follow suit instead of identifying a potentially devastating error.

DOI: 10.1201/9781003633389-41

Being a Team Player

While setting the stage for team dynamics is important, effective teamwork also requires that the individuals act as true team players, even though individual and group success can sometimes conflict. In sports, this might mean passing the ball instead of taking the shot; in medicine, it might involve sharing opportunities or credit. How can we resolve this apparent conflict?

Remember that it's not a zero-sum game. In medicine, strive for excellence while supporting your team, but not at the expense of others. Giving credit generously benefits everyone and enhances team function. It also increases the likelihood of reciprocal support. Conversely, withholding information from others so you can later *save the day* degrades team morale.

Maintain flexibility because team disruptions are inevitable. Colleagues get sidetracked, become ill, or tasks fall through the cracks. If a teammate is unavailable but you're free, help if appropriate and communicate this to the team. A team-oriented approach benefits patients, your team, and yourself.

Unmotivated Team Members

Despite the need for team players, not every colleague will be collaborative. A subset only participates in tasks that garner credit or help when superiors are nearby. It's tempting to reciprocate this behavior, but this harms the team and patients, perpetuating dysfunction. You should also resist such reciprocation from a selfish perspective because the resultant internal conflict or negative perceptions from others can negatively impact you.

When selecting teammates, remember that past performance is the best predictor of future performance. A person's track record is more important than their promises. Also, recognize that people are generally either *talkers* or *doers*. These are self-reinforcing traits: doers don't need to boast, and talkers talk because that's how they contribute. If possible, work with doers.

When Individuals Outperform Teams

It is also important to be aware of some pitfalls of team decision-making. Effective groups usually outperform individuals in cognitive reasoning tasks. However, the outcome sometimes relies on a single member with a well-reasoned counterargument.[112] Furthermore, teams can underperform due to groupthink or a lack of decisive leadership, allowing dominant individuals to silence less aggressive individuals or introverts.[198]

Brainstorming also requires a different approach than other forms of teamwork because group efforts and stifle creativity.[112] For example, groupthink eliminates bold ideas, leaving only conventional ones. If a clear expert is present, their opinion might justly outweigh others.[112] Group work is also costly in terms of physician hours, and the benefits may not always justify the cost. Therefore, carefully weigh the pros and cons of a team approach for each task.

Team Member Roles on Clinical Rotations

Most work in medicine, however, remains teamwork oriented, and for these situations, understanding each team member's role is crucial. In emergencies like resuscitations, roles may be assigned on the spot, but usually, they are predetermined. The most obvious stratification is by training level (medical student, intern, senior resident, etc.). Each level has specific expected roles, varying by institutional culture and clinical service.

Clarifying Roles and Closing Loops

Roles become more nuanced with nontrainee staff (physician assistants (PAs), nurses). Be sure to clarify expectations for each member early on. For example, clerical tasks might fall to an intern on some teams and a PA on others. During team discussions, ensure task responsibility is clear. If unsure, ask. After completing a task, close the communication loop so everyone knows it's done, preventing redundant effort.

As a senior resident or chief resident, ensure task delegations are clear, assigning each task to a specific person with a clear follow-up method. When assigning multiple tasks, it can be useful to review the list during rounds to ensure shared understanding.

Interprofessional Competency

Since effective teamwork requires understanding the roles of all team members, it is useful to work on interprofessional competency to better understand the expertise of all the various professionals in medicine. Interprofessional competency and collaboration can improve teamwork, patient care, and morale.[666] Medical education, however, often silos professional programs, limiting interaction between trainees (MD, RN, pharmacy, PT, OT, social workers, NP/PA, etc.).

Therefore, interprofessional education remains inadequate, with no consensus on implementation or effectiveness.[667,668] Interprofessional education approaches can paradoxically heighten division and hierarchical relationships, for example if allied health staff are promoted as "independent experts" who can substitute for physicians in certain situations.[669] More generally, such efforts can paradoxically increase division if done competitively rather than collaboratively.[160] Thus, if you participate in interprofessional training, view it as a team-building opportunity.

Until interprofessional training improves, you should proactively learn the roles and responsibilities of various team members. A fully integrated approach is necessary for optimal patient care in various settings (outpatient clinics, inpatient wards, multidisciplinary conferences).

You should also know everyone's appropriate titles. For example, do not call a *technologist* a *technician*. This is easier said than done, however. The number of titles, degrees, and roles in medicine are overwhelming. While we cannot cover all these here, the next section introduces some of the most common roles.

Allied Health Professionals: Physical Therapists, Occupational Therapists, Social Workers

- **Physical Therapists**: Specialize in human movement, working in various settings (outpatient clinics, hospitals, schools). They focus on prevention, rehabilitation, and conditioning, often using guided movements or exercise. PTs may be involved in inpatient or outpatient treatment plans and assess mobility needs before discharge.
- **Occupational Therapists**: Work in schools and healthcare settings, helping people perform daily activities. They assist with adaptive equipment, fall prevention, and daily routine planning.

- **Social Workers**: Work in diverse settings (schools, hospitals, clinics), helping people integrate into social settings. In medicine, they are instrumental in inpatient discharge planning and may provide mental health counseling. Various degrees exist (LCSW, LMSW, MSW, DSW).

Physician Extenders and Related Providers

Advanced practice registered nurses (APRNs) and PAs have different educational paths (at least a master's degree) and roles, varying by background and state laws. Duties can include running clinics, managing pre- and post-procedural care, performing clerical work, or providing consults. Different types of APRNs exist (e.g., nurse practitioners). Roles vary across practices and departments.

CRNAs, Psychologists, and Physicians

- **Certified Registered Nurse Anesthetists (CRNAs)**: Sedation and anesthesia delivery depends on the practice, case needs, and medical complexity. Simple cases might involve a nurse trained in sedation, with the physician managing medication and complications. Complex cases require a CRNA working under an anesthesiologist or an attending anesthesiologist.
- **Psychology**: Various professionals provide psychological counseling, diagnosis, and treatment. Social workers provide some counseling. Doctorate-level psychologists have either a PsyD (clinically focused) or PhD (research focused). Neuropsychologists focus on brain function testing. Psychiatrists are medical doctors who may focus on complex situations and medication management.
- **Physicians**: In the United States, MDs and DOs have merged accreditation and matching processes, though some differences remain in educational philosophy. Both lead to similar careers. MBBS and MBBCh are medical degrees from UK schools. Additional fellowship titles (e.g., FAAD, FACR) are bestowed by societies with variable requirements. Research the training and roles of other professionals you encounter.

Working with Allied Health Professionals

You must always maintain professionalism when working with allied health professionals, especially ones you do not know well. Established relationships offer more leeway; a misinterpreted mood with someone you don't know well can lead to complaints.

If someone becomes upset with you and makes a complaint, it won't contain just the dry facts but will be colored with perceptions and feelings. Remember too that permanently hired nonphysician staff often hold higher positions in the job stability hierarchy than trainees. They may be union members or friends with attendings, increasing the stakes of a complaint.

Anatomy of a Complaint

A typical complaint might be, "I asked Dr. X for help, but they got angry and were short with me. They didn't want to help and made me feel unappreciated. I love my job, but I don't know if I can continue feeling this way." This reflects negatively on you. Nonphysician staff are often above trainees in the job stability hierarchy, potentially union members, and friends with attendings. As a trainee, you are accountable.

However, allied health professionals can be among your best allies. They will often know the system better than you do and value positive relationships with physicians. Allied health professionals can get you out of a bind and take pride in their important roles for patient care. It is to your benefit to foster positive relationships with them.

Personality Types of Nonphysician Staff

Nurses, technologists, and other hospital staff are essential and deserve respect. However, some may present personality challenges (overconfidence, underconfidence, undermotivation, resistance to physician trainees, taking advantage of allyship with superiors, low threshold for complaints, snarky comments, passive-aggressive behavior).

Remember, though, that people who can seem like the most difficult to work with are often the most committed to their work and patient advocacy. In the end, these often become your best team members. Rarely do people intentionally make life difficult out of spite.

38

Outpatient, Observational, and Visiting Rotations

Vance T. Lehman, Julia S. Lehman

Now that we've reviewed the basics of learning, professionalism, and teamwork in the clinical setting, let's discuss the practicalities of daily clinical work. Medical training often focuses heavily on inpatient rotations, which differ in tempo, objectives, and expectations compared to outpatient rotations. Thus, though medical acuity is generally lower in outpatient settings, the change of pace of clinic can be a challenge. There are, however, several ways you can prepare to enhance your outpatient clinic experiences. Here, there are special considerations for preparation, patient evaluation, efficiency, and professionalism.

Preparation for a Rotation

Review Common Conditions and Management

Ahead of the rotation, you should review relevant common and critical conditions, medications, specialty-specific clinical examination maneuvers, and frequently ordered laboratory tests, and do your best to determine the true learning objectives and expectations.

For patient management, start by learning the first-line treatments and high yield guidelines for frequently encountered diagnoses. When multiple management avenues are available, learn the major reasons for selecting each one. For instance, know when and why you might move beyond a statin for treatment of hypercholesterolemia. Review the most common medications, including indications, side effects, interactions, pregnancy/lactation categories, and contraindications.

Later, you can fine-tune your knowledge base details of the doses, course duration, and administration frequency or of second-line treatments. Finally, start to familiarize yourself with the main points of relevant sentinel papers or guidelines.

Consider Heuristics and Differential Diagnoses

When first learning how to approach management of common scenarios, focus on those where you can develop System 1 heuristics, such as managing common complaints like low back pain, headaches, or dizziness. This does not mean, though, that you can ignore the differential diagnoses or replace all contemplation with an algorithm.

Furthermore, instead of learning about diseases one-by-one, think about differential diagnoses for a given clinical presentation and how the possibilities are distinguished. Consider what specialty-specific topics come up frequently. In dermatology, asking about whether

DOI: 10.1201/9781003633389-42

sunlight ameliorates or worsens a skin rash may be high yield, while in infectious disease, travel history can be particularly important, etc.

Practice Your Presentation Skills

It is also useful to practice a few patient presentations ahead of clinic. Find a practice "patient," perhaps a clinical scenario provided in a textbook, and rehearse your presentation delivery out loud. Remember to include pertinent positives and negatives from the history and physical examination, to provide a short differential diagnosis (in order of probability), and to offer a suggestion on additional required testing and/or management. Also, learn or review common specialty-specific vocabulary. The chief complaint and essential related information should roll off the tongue using standard terminology.

Preparation for the Day

One of the biggest mistakes medical trainees make is arriving at clinic underprepared. For many outpatient practice settings, it is critical to look up the patients beforehand, noting the type of visit, main concerns, prior test results, and anything else that would be useful to know upfront. There is too much information to memorize, so write it down using shorthand for common items. The notes should be readily accessible in clinic, and it should be clear to your attending that you have done your *clinic homework*. Read about your patients' conditions, including all common conditions and those uncommon ones that are being considered in the differential diagnosis for your patients.

Every attending has his own expectations, biases, and assumptions. When working with an attending for the first time, you should solicit their expectations. Briefly review your attending's main areas of interest. If you have time, it can be useful to read any articles your attending has published, as these can reveal their areas of interest and viewpoints.

Finally, it is beneficial to touch base with the nurses and other clinic staff at the start of the day to foster a strong working relationship and to learn about the operations of the clinic, how you can best help them, and how they can help you in turn.

Patient Evaluation

You will see patients for a variety of visit types including problem-focused visits, referrals, follow-up visits, routine check-ups, and care establishment. In medical school, the history and physical examination may be each taught as one comprehensive construct, but these need to be tailored to the clinical question. Thus, you must learn and apply the specialty-specific, topic-specific expectations for targeted history and physical examinations. For example, the comprehensive neurology examination you mastered during a neurology rotation is almost never needed in dermatology clinic.

Avoid Assumptions

There are many tasks that trainees must master, but here are a few areas where trainees seem to get derailed. First, it is often appropriate to question if a presumed diagnosis is correct, particularly when a patient is not responding to appropriate treatments. This questioning may occur by revisiting the grounds upon which the diagnosis was based (e.g., previously documented physical findings, biopsy results, laboratory test results). This practice is important to avoid diagnostic momentum, compounded by labels and assumptions. These approaches acknowledge that diagnoses made with inductive reasoning are provisional. Further, trainees often forget to consider the important question, "What is the most important thing I could be missing?"

You should confirm what treatments the patient has tried and what their impression of their response was. A common mistake is assuming patients complied with prescribed treatments without asking them what they have actually taken. There are many reasons why patients may not adhere to a proposed treatment regimen, such as expense, intolerability of adverse effects, fear over the list of possible side effects, difficulty with the medication modality (e.g., difficulty swallowing pills, intolerance of the greasiness of ointments).

In addition, patients may weigh the risks and costs of treatments and judge them to be not worth it in relation to the degree of their symptoms or the seriousness of their condition. It is also important to consider these factors when offering medical recommendations, as shared decision-making improves patient adherence.

Complete Examinations

Initially, trainees may feel uncomfortable asking patients to remove (or to lift up) an article of clothing for the physical examination section of the patient encounter. However, this request may be necessary to perform a high-quality physical examination (e.g., auscultation of the chest by inserting the stethoscope underneath someone's shirt), and it is often helpful to share this with the patient too. For example, it can be useful to normalize this ask with verbiage such as, "In order to perform a thorough skin examination, I ask all my patients to remove their clothing and put on this clinic gown. Is that ok with you? If so, I'll step out for a few moments for you to undress."

Providers must always ask patient consent before lifting or lowering clothing, and it may be prudent to have a chaperone present where feasible, depending on the nature of the encounter.

Staying on Schedule

One skill that requires practice is keeping the visit on task while still completing an unhurried examination. Asking open-ended questions and engaging in active listening do not mean you can veer too far off course. When a conversation goes astray, gently bring it back into focus, or try out wording such as, "Thank you for sharing that. With the time we have, it's important that I understand [xyz]… Can we talk more about that?" New trainees often find this challenging due to lack of experience with steering conversations and due to concern over being impolite to the patient.

Patient presentations to the attending staff should be focused and pertinent. Be ready to briefly summarize the reason for the visit, the relevant points of the visit, and your impression and plan without prompting. Trainees sometimes relay information but freeze at the impression/plan phase. While you might not have enough information to arrive at a diagnosis, it's ok to state that and share your thought process on what would be required to do so.

The plan of a problem-focused visit could consist of suggested additional tests, a treatment trial, an intervention, patient counseling, or a consultation with other colleagues. Additionally, define the format (phone call, electronic communication, in-person visit) and timing of follow-up. If you don't have any idea, at least make it clear you were thinking about it in context of the patient goals.

Regardless of your stage of training, try to help in clinic as much as you can. Early on, there may be very little you can do. However, if a patient needs someone to help them maneuver their wheelchair or needs a glass of water, or if the attending needs to convey a message to the front desk, for example, be willing to jump in and help. Once you have more experience, you can create clinic notes, enter test orders, write out care plans for patients, etc.

If shadowing, you do not have to be silent but be sure not to talk over the attending or ask unnecessary questions that distract the patient or staff from the issues at hand. Finally, be warned that some patients will have new or different information for your staff once they walk in the room. In fact, patients may tell them something entirely opposite of what they told you. Probably everyone has experienced this phenomenon, and generally, staff understand, particularly if you have otherwise been accurate and reliable.

General Efficiency During Outpatient Rotations

Efficiency is the product of preparation, clinical skills, presentations, and teamwork. Remember that clinic days can be fast paced. For the trainee, staying on schedule is a balancing act. Too much focus on moving quickly can lead to patients or staff perceiving that you are rushing, while being overly inefficient can delay care for other patients in the day and add stress to others on the care team. Avoid asking excessive questions of the attending that are not directly related to patient care during busy times. If you have questions you would like to ask but don't have time, schedule a time that works for the attending to sit down and get them answered.

Observational Rotations

An Unexpected Challenge

Observational rotations paradoxically can be among the trickiest to navigate as a trainee. You must be seen to be interested but are necessarily less involved, and you must also be proactive about learning but not be in the way. With some rotations or staff, the expectations are nil, but with others, these are hidden. Some rotations may be graded while some have little formal evaluation.

Without the appropriate approach, these can set the trainee up for relative failure, such as receiving a default Pass or lukewarm (or negative) comments (such as "he looked tired" or "she did not seem interested")—results that often are more reflective of the passive environment than of your own potential as a future physician. So, what can you do?

Prepare for the Day

When working with an attending for the first time, do not assume that you can simply show up and shadow. For clinic, look up the appointments the night before and take notes. Have the notes ready so you can answer questions and provide visual evidence you are taking interest. As with any rotation, do not bury your head in a smartphone, which gives the impression of being distracted or disinterested (even if you are actually reading about the patients or their conditions).

Additionally, do not work on other projects (including academic ones, which are usually best-done during off-hours or clearly established downtime) when you should be focusing on clinical duties.

Be Present, Helpful, and Unobtrusive

Ask the attending what her expectations are upfront and what you can do to be helpful. For example, on radiology rotations, there is little visiting students can do to facilitate image interpretation, but they can help dig up clinical information for complex cases, for example. If you have any (realistic) goals of things to learn or see on the rotation, tactfully make those known as well. Always remain respectful of the value and expertise of the specialty.

Avoid making the day more difficult for the attending. If they are in an active decision-making mode, consider saving questions for later. No gum-smacking, whistling, excessively loud talking, or strong scents. Be aware that when you are looking at your phone, this can be interpreted (accurately or otherwise) as you being disinterested. Respect personal space. Do not assume that unapproved absenteeism will go unnoticed, and do not hint you want to leave when you do not need to. It is easy to look bored or tired even if you are not, and so you should make a conscious effort to appear authentically engaged.

Take Advantage of Extra Time

Finally, when done for the day, read about topics related to the types of cases you're seeing and that align with your goals. Get enough sleep, make sure to exercise and eat healthy food, and take advantage of the *off-season* to get ahead for your next rotation.

Key Takeaways

Observational rotations require proactive (but not intrusive) engagement. By preparing in advance, being present, self-aware, and helpful, and respecting the attendings' time and expertise, you can gain the most benefit from these rotations.

Visiting Rotations

Planning Considerations

You might pursue a visiting rotation in medical school for various reasons like auditioning for a residency application, learning about a program or region, gaining access to research or case report opportunities, or seeking out letters of recommendation. As medical school grades and now the USMLE Step 1 exam have transitioned to P/F scoring, it is possible that visiting rotations could be weighed even more heavily than in the past.

Each program is different. Some residencies have formal programs and frequent visitors. For those that do not, it is probably more important to have some sponsors or assurances there is truly a valuable experience to be had. Formal programs may require an application. You might also need to find your own housing. You might want to consider whether the programs you are targeting tend to take internal candidates (i.e., those they know). If a program fills entirely with internal candidates, you are shut out.

Advantages and Pitfalls

A visiting experience can help you match into that specialty or even that particular program, as your taking the time to prioritize their program shows interest and willingness to live in a region and gives you an opportunity to meet individuals who might influence candidate ranking (like the PD). But these rotations are like prolonged interviews; you must be on best professional behavior and find ways to go above and beyond—staying late, being helpful where you can, showing gratitude and interest, etc.

You might also want to take on a realistic research project (small, retrospective, but high quality) or an excellent case report. These may earn you a letter writer or even a sponsor, though you should never assume that such a relationship will result.

There is also no guarantee you will match at the programs through which you rotated, and the experience even has potential to be a liability if you inadvertently annoy the wrong person. You might merely receive a courtesy interview or none at all. Further, being held at an institution other than your own, the experiences are typically observational (since short-term visitors usually do not gain personal access to the EMR, for example).

Therefore, you will not get the full experience of what it is like to be a resident in the program, and you likely still will not ascertain all the insider information. To be considered at most programs, a visiting rotation is by no means necessary. Overall, these can be useful, but the circumstances vary, and you must perform well for it to help you.

For more information, consider talking to the PD at your home institution, who might know about other programs and will know specialty-specific nuances. Also, seek out online resources like the following AMA's informational web page: https://www.ama-assn.org/medical-students/clinical-rotations/residents-answer-top-student-questions-about-away-rotations.

39

Inpatient Rotations

Vance T. Lehman, Michael W. Cullen

Overview

In this chapter, we'll turn from outpatient to inpatient considerations. The key to stellar performance and an enjoyable inpatient rotation is preparation. When you are new to an institution, this includes identifying the customs, quirks, and physical layout of the local system as soon as possible, potentially before the rotation starts. For each rotation, prioritize knowing which patients you are responsible for before it begins. Also, clarify rotation expectations with your supervisor and senior trainees early on. Speaking to colleagues who are rotating off service as you begin the rotation can significantly facilitate this process.

New trainees should seek to quickly grasp basic workflows and clinical topics. Specifically, you should understand the admission, rounding, and discharge processes. Reviewing prior patient notes (when available) helps you familiarize yourself with common terminology and approaches for a given rotation.

For medical students, studying for a test such as a shelf examination ideally starts before the rotation too. This provides more learning time and allows immediate application to patient care. Attendings won't expect in-depth knowledge of scoring systems and landmark clinical trials initially, but absorbing this information over time is beneficial.

Institutional Jargon (Slang)

Familiarizing yourself with institution-specific vocabulary minimizes early confusion, especially during your first rotation. While most medical terms are standardized, there are often some institution-specific preferred terms (sometimes, but not always in the category of jargon or slang). This includes the titles used for professionals, work areas, medical conditions, abbreviations, and types of codes. For example, staff physicians are usually called attendings in the United States but are called consultants in some institutions. Still, it is usually best to avoid abbreviations to prevent confusion. Consider that "p.o." usually means taken by mouth, but in rare settings "PO" is used to indicate "postoperative."

Additionally, there is no universal standard for hospital code designation. These are usually designated as colors, such as a Code Blue indicating the need for acute cardiorespiratory support. However, designations vary across countries and regions. There are certainly countless other examples of institution-specific terms. The take-home point is to learn these and, if a term is confusing, ask what it means early in your rotation.

DOI: 10.1201/9781003633389-43

Physical Layout of Clinic/Hospital

The physical layout is different at every hospital and clinic, such as parking, lounges, work rooms, wards, ICUs, OR location, radiology reading rooms, lockers, cafeterias, laundered scrubs areas, on-call rooms, and so on. While sometimes easy to determine, this can be time-consuming and create unnecessary hassle in larger institutions. When you arrive at a new institution, take time to learn where places are. If not covered in orientation, find these key locations yourself.

Functional Layout

Every institution has a unique functional layout. An early major obstacle will likely be learning the EMR. While some EMRs are used at multiple institutions, there may be local modifications or even some home-grown programs. Expect to encounter several different EMRs throughout your training and practice.

You should learn how to use the paging system, who to page for specific questions, and *pager etiquette* (i.e. typical customs and practices surrounding appropriate pager use for a given institution, department, or specialty) as soon as possible. For example, most institutions utilize service pagers for general communication about patients under a team's care. It is usually more appropriate to call a service pager before paging a senior resident, fellow, or staff directly. It is always important to page the appropriate person and number, especially for communication after standard business hours.

Discharge Planning

The primary goal of hospitalization is generally outpatient recovery. The axiom *discharge planning begins on admission* applies to nearly all hospitalized patients. One of the first things you should learn on a new rotation is the discharge process. Consider the steps needed for discharge every day during rounding. This is one area where you can stand out as a medical student or junior resident since you will often have more time than other team members to become well-acquainted with patients and their social support, living situation, goals, and concerns that can facilitate safe and timely discharge.

Discharge planning is a complex process requiring a team effort involving the patient and their family, primary medical team, nurses, social worker, OT/PT, and occasionally consulting medical services. Discharge processes vary across institutions and services; this chapter cannot cover every detail. The primary point is that you should do everything you can to understand the discharge process at your institution and for your assigned service as early as possible in your rotation. For this, it is useful to identify a mentor such as a resident to show you the process. Often, hospitals employ specialists such as social workers who can be great sources of information.

Consider a typical day in the patient's home life. How will they accomplish their activities of daily living? What support do they have from family and friends? Are there other considerations for their life goals or occupational demands? Can ongoing treatment be adapted to the outpatient setting? It is useful to track recommendations from consulting services or on radiology reports such as follow-up of an unexpected imaging finding. Discharge requires timely organization and advance planning. Some examples are included in Table 39.1, but it is useful to create discharge checklists for your specific hospital and rotation.

Table 39.1 Example Discharge Considerations[a]

Ambulation, Fall Prevention, PT/OT Needs
Nutrition
Restroom Use
Drains, Lines, Wound Management
Medication Reconciliation and Preauthorization
Pain Management
Patient Education
Primary Care and Subspecialty Follow-Up Appointments
Follow-Up Tests
Destination (i.e., home versus skilled facility)
Long-Term Intravenous Access

[a] Items may or may not be needed depending on patient requirements.

Rounding

Prerounding

Trainees spend a reasonable percentage of time in the hospital rounding. Some programs or rotations will expect medical students to *preround* ahead of the formal rounds, but the usefulness is currently debated. However, most agree there are both pros and cons and that efficiency could be improved.[670] Regardless of your situation, leverage the advantages of either approach.

If not required to preround, proactively check in with your patients during the day to establish yourself as their primary point of contact. You should still prepare for rounds by reviewing lab and morning test results, identifying any overnight events that necessitate attention from the team, and checking with nursing. From this, you might start formulating a provisional care plan.

If you are required to preround, take advantage of the opportunity to construct assessments and plans. To optimize your efficiency, identify in advance the information you will gather and how you will present it. Regardless of the rounding format, help the team by creating concise well-organized notes. Have an organized system to ensure you follow-up on all tests and interventions during the day. Check the status of your patients at the end of the day before signing out to the overnight team.

Rounding Customs

The rounding customs will vary by reason for admission and clinical service. Some common items you will assess include vital signs, ins/outs, flatus, ambulation, targeted physical exam, wound/dressing status, telemetry tracings, and thromboembolism prophylaxis. You should also note any interval events, test results, or consult recommendations and keep the discharge criteria in mind. When possible, communicate directly with the nurses. Always pay attention to every patient your team visits since you can learn from each. Even when the focus is not on one of your patients, do not bury your face in a device or appear otherwise distracted or disinterested.

Presenting on rounds is part gamesmanship. While flawless presentations aren't necessary, a well-rehearsed, organized, and succinct format is desirable. The words matter too. It is important to use precise, professional, technically correct terms. As we saw in Chapter 4, colloquial, highly informal, and/or degrading terms and phrases such as "sprinkle in a little Lasix," neologisms like "surgerizing," reference to a patient as a "COPDer," and many other examples are sometimes used, but are not advised.[671]

For each patient, have a concise summary of admission date, reason, and current status. You do not need every detail at your fingertips, but if you are only following a couple of patients, you will be expected to know them well and have all material details readily available.

Staff Interactions

When interacting with staff, always use your professionalism skills, maintain a respectful tone, and be considerate of their other demands. You want to make others look good and feel good. As a bonus, strive to do so while still decreasing their effort. They will appreciate it, give you higher marks, and have more time for teaching.

Addressing attending errors requires careful consideration. This will happen since everyone makes mistakes, and attendings make countless decisions every day. How should you handle this? It depends on the importance of the mistake and the potential to cause patient harm. First, recognize that a perceived error might not be one. Perhaps the attending is simply using an alternative, but equally valid, approach or line of reasoning that you have not encountered.

Assuming there is a mistake, first consider its gravity. Minor verbal blunders usually require no action. Potential sentinel events or patient harm (e.g., incorrect site information during a time-out) require respectful intervention.

Trainee Teaching and Hierarchy

Interns and residents provide much of the teaching and oversight of early trainees on inpatient rotations. This has pros and cons. On the upside, it can be easier for early trainees to ask basic questions to other trainees. Trainees at both levels learn something by teaching or being taught. Disadvantages include lack of formal teaching instruction, varying interest in teaching, time constraints, limited teaching incentives, and ongoing self-learning. Junior trainees should ask how they can assist the team. Making the job easier for the senior trainee will be appreciated and can free more time for teaching.

Overall, an ideal situation might encourage more direct attention and teaching from attendings and better instruction of teaching methods to trainees. In the short term though, there is probably little you can do to substantially change the situation of their current training program. Instead, leverage the pros and manage the cons at every stage as best you can.

Many principles of interacting with attendings also apply to senior trainees (though less formally). These include always using your best self-presentation, remembering the basics of professionalism, looking interested, asking questions but not when others are busy and concentrating, and clarifying expectations.

Interactions Between Services

It is important to understand the different roles of primary versus consulting services and the related etiquette. Occasionally, a well-intended trainee on a consulting service will make recommendations that step beyond the scope of the consultation. Further, a consulting service may be charged with making recommendations while the primary service needs to approve the recommendation and place the order. Understanding service boundaries is also helpful, but trainees should avoid turf debates or critiques.

Patient care requires teamwork among clinical services. Avoid blocking reasonable requests for consults or admissions, or transfers from other services. This causes frustration, harms your reputation, and hinders patient care. Conversely, avoid exaggerating the urgency of a request to secure a consult, procedure, imaging examination, or other test done for convenience or so you can *look good* on rounds. This undermines your credibility and collegiality.

Finally, when answering a page or calling someone else, identify your role on the phone. Callers should immediately know if they're speaking with a nurse, NP, PA, physician, medical student, lab technician, or desk staff.

Efficiency on Inpatient Rotations

The clunky inefficiency of inpatient rotations stands in stark contrast to assembly-line regularity of outpatient clinics. It's a different machine, not just a lower gear, and can sometimes seem inefficient. This inefficiency is amplified for you, the trainee, as nearly nothing clinical is designed around your schedule. Inpatient care also requires coordination of many people and events that do not always align in availability, leading to unpredictable delays, human inefficiencies, and imperfect communication.

One of the main challenges in training is time management; systemic inefficiency in the inpatient setting confounds it. Inefficiency also hinders job satisfaction, limits teaching time, and reduces educational opportunities.[672] Resultant frustration and lack of control can erode morale.

However, counterproductive reactions like acting out or emotional suppression must be managed, for example with peer-support and well-being measures. Suppression erodes joy and can lead to sorrow, anxiety, or disillusionment. These untenable mental states can lead to learned helplessness, burnout, or clinical mental health disorders.

You will have limited ability to improve the efficiency of the system as a trainee. Realistically, manage inefficiency by focusing on controllable factors like organization and preparedness. You can also seek to leverage intermittent downtime of inpatient rotations for your own learning, completion of administrative tasks, and pursuit of scholarly endeavors.

Now that we have explored considerations for outpatient and inpatient rotations, we'll discuss how to excel at learning procedures.

40

Procedures

Vance T. Lehman, Kai Miller

Introduction

A strong performance on procedural rotations include preparation, purposeful practice, humility to accept feedback, being a good team player, maintaining a positive attitude, and effective communication. To illustrate these, let's first consider a counterexample:

Years ago, I (VTL) assisted a senior radiology resident struggling with a lumbar puncture (LP).[1] The resident repeatedly encountered bone, the patient was anxious, and the needle angle was clearly incorrect. I patiently explained how adjusting the fluoroscopy alignment could improve access and shared techniques for patient reassurance. I expected this real-time feedback to be welcomed, but the resident responded defensively, insisting on their own approach.

Honestly, I was a bit taken aback. Having performed thousands of LPs, more than most neuroradiologists, I had learned from excellent mentors. At the time, I didn't address the defensiveness directly, attributing it to the pressure of the moment. Now, I would handle it differently. But I know a lot of attendings would give that kind of feedback indirectly—through evaluations or even behind the scenes.

This incident highlighted a lack of a growth mindset. Novice trainees often exhibit overconfidence or under confidence in their procedural skills, stemming from the same unavoidable root cause: insufficient experience. Underconfident trainees become discouraged by their limitations, while overconfident trainees underestimate the time required to achieve proficiency.

It's important to remember that LPs are just one type of procedure. They involve awake patients, local anesthetic, relatively low risks, quick planning, minimal recovery, and are commonly performed. Understanding these factors is crucial when learning any procedure, as we'll explore further.

Procedure Preparation

Thorough preparation is key to maximizing your learning and participation in any procedure. A helpful framework for preparation involves asking, "Who, what, where, when, how, and why?" Let's break it down:

Know Your Patient (Who?)

Beyond the basics (name, procedure, indication), familiarize yourself with relevant medical and social factors, especially those impacting anesthesia and coagulation. Also, identify the

DOI: 10.1201/9781003633389-44

attending physician and, if possible, learn about their expertise and approach—through discussions with your colleagues and/or by reviewing the attending's publications. Get to know the rest of the team too: other physicians, anesthesia staff, nurses, techs, and even industry reps. As you progress, think about how you can proactively prepare the team for a smooth procedure day.

Know the Procedure (What?)

Understand the procedure itself, the clinical indication, and the potential risks, benefits, and alternatives. This often requires background reading on the disease, its progression, the workup, and the procedure. Master the consent process, understanding the rationale and likelihood of each risk. Ensure the consent form is filed. Finally, be aware of any complicating factors like prior interventions or anatomical variations.

Know the Location (Where?)

Confirm the location of the patient before, during, and after the procedure. This usually means knowing the specific OR or procedural suite.

Know the Timing (When?)

Be aware of the patient's arrival time (if outpatient) and the scheduled procedure time. If you're involved in the patient's care, try to speak with them before the attending, unless you're rounding as a team. Remember that schedules can shift, so check in and arrive early. As a trainee, the schedule won't revolve around you. And if you get a moment for a break, take it!

Know the Rationale (Why?)

Understand why this procedure was chosen over other options, considering factors like evidence, local expertise, and patient preference. Also, know the procedure's purpose: screening, palliation, diagnosis, treatment, or research (often combined with another goal).

Know the Steps (How?)

This involves the technical and logistical aspects. While more relevant for senior trainees, it's helpful to start thinking about these early. Begin by studying relevant anatomy on imaging, focusing on structures in the planned path. Consider which vessels or critical structures to avoid and the size of anatomy you'll be traversing.

Plan the necessary instruments and implants (if any), sometimes requiring anatomical measurements. Consider patient positioning and the type of incision or access. Understand the type of anesthesia and its rationale. Ensure all equipment, medications, and resources are available before the procedure begins. Advanced trainees will also develop contingency plans for potential complications.

Other Considerations

Beyond the specific questions for each case, keep these general points in mind. Answering those pre-procedure questions requires tapping into various resources. Start by asking senior trainees— they often know practical details like which instruments are typically used. Also, consult with other team members, review clinical notes and imaging, and do some background reading. If you weren't involved in the initial consult, be sure to carefully review the notes.

Don't worry if many of these considerations seem overwhelming at first. If you're stuck, make a note and ask someone to explain the step when you have a chance. Similarly, don't get bogged down in the specifics of implant models or technology, as these can change rapidly and are sometimes influenced by nonmedical factors. Instead, focus on understanding the underlying principles behind the choices.

In addition, prioritize acquiring fundamental skills early on, such as suturing, scrubbing, and mastering sterile techniques like donning gloves and gowns. Always offer to assist the surgical nurses and assistants—you'll learn invaluable practical knowledge from them that you can't get from books or videos.

Finally, remember that complex procedures can feel like a blur at first. It's easy to get lost if you haven't prepared adequately. Trainees often underestimate how much preparation attendings do, which is one reason why they make it look so effortless. So, make sure you do your homework!

Intra-Procedural Considerations

During the procedure, remember to make a good impression, understand expectations, be prepared, and show genuine interest. When working with an attending for the first time, clarify their expectations and communicate your experience level—don't assume they know. If you're inexperienced, be honest but emphasize your eagerness to learn and participate. Ideally, attendings would proactively assess your experience, but often, it's up to you. Be sure to clarify your role (observing or participating).

If you're new to a procedure, you might only have a basic understanding. Creating a mental outline (or physical sketch) of the key steps can be helpful, filling in the details as you gain experience. You can learn these steps from your initial experiences, procedure reports, discussions with attendings, and videos. Remember, understanding *why* is often more important than *how* at first, although learning basic procedural steps is always useful.

Your experience will vary depending on the attending's philosophy and experience. Newer attendings may perform most of the procedure themselves, as they are still gaining confidence and may be more cautious about complications. However, they can be excellent instructors because they still remember the training experience well. Working with attendings of varying experience levels is ideal, as they each offer unique insights.

Regardless of the attending, be helpful and engaged, but avoid being a distraction. If you have questions, wait for a less intense moment or save them for after the procedure. Always ask if it's okay to ask a question first. Make sure your questions are thoughtful, well-prepared, and genuine. Beyond that, the attending is likely not interested in you trying to show off your knowledge during the procedure.

Post-Procedure Considerations

Your role in post-procedure patient care will vary, so always clarify expectations. For inpatients, if you're responsible for ordering overnight tests or other necessary items, ensure all mandatory orders are entered correctly. For your own learning, conduct a quick debriefing after each procedure to assess what you did well and what you can improve. There's always room for growth, and every case offers a learning opportunity. This reflection is a key to your procedural skill development.

Types of Procedures

Procedures occur in various settings, including in-office, outpatient procedural suites (like for LPs), the ED, inpatient bedsides, and emergency scenarios. These can be further categorized by the following:

- Type of anesthesia (none, topical, local, moderate sedation, deep sedation, general)
- Purpose (screening, palliation, diagnosis, treatment, research)
- Need for implant placement
- Involvement of industry
- Degree of invasiveness
- Technical difficulty
- Risk level
- Urgency
- Frequency (routine versus rare or experimental)

While we can't cover every variation, understanding the main principles is key. Each setting presents unique considerations for trainees before, during, and after the procedure, which aren't always obvious. These include differences in patient counseling, instruments, team composition, hands-on opportunities, and post-procedure management.

Many skilled attendings take as much pride in the seemingly simple, routine procedures as they do in complex ones. Paying attention to detail is crucial, even in common procedures like paracentesis or central line insertion. Attendings want you to strive for the same level of precision, understanding that it takes practice. Therefore, never dismiss an attending's suggestion, even if you feel confident in your skills.

It's also important to distinguish between procedures performed on aware versus unaware patients (due to sedation or anesthesia). When patients are aware, specific professionalism and calming techniques are essential, as discussed in the next section.

Patient Interactions

Adapt to the Patient

In procedures like outpatient pain management injections, patient interactions are crucial from the start. Each patient is unique—some relaxed, others anxious; some talkative, others quiet; and some confident, others deferential. While remaining authentic, adapt your tone and message to each individual. This *gut-check and gear shift*, learned through experience, is invaluable.

Instill Confidence

Build confidence and address concerns by demonstrating knowledge of the patient's case through chart review and fluent discussion of the procedure. If they've had negative experiences, understand what happened and offer reassurance. Emphasize the competence of the entire care team.

It's harder for trainees to instill confidence due to their higher rate of uncertainty. Preparation is key. Balance confidence with honesty, avoiding overconfidence or timidity. If a patient requests an attending, respect their wishes and learn from observing.

Promote Relaxation

In procedures like pain management injections, where patients are awake and receive local anesthetic, ensure they are relaxed. Even slight movements can complicate the procedure. Tailor your communication—some want play-by-play updates during the procedures, others distraction. With proper technique and reassurance, patients often barely notice the procedure. Nervous patients require extra reassurance and calm confidence.

Remember that the approach differs from procedures under general anesthesia. While professionalism is always essential, awake patients require specific attention to reassurance and communication.

Procedural Skill Development

Procedural Memory

When learning a new procedure, your working memory is heavily taxed.[673] You're constantly thinking, doing, questioning, and second-guessing. This process is naturally awkward, especially with beginner anxiety. It's normal to feel overwhelmed at first—no one expects you to be an instant expert. That's why it's crucial to be receptive to feedback.

As you improve, brain activation shifts from the prefrontal cortex (working memory) to the basal ganglia and cerebellum. Your skills become more automatic, smoother, faster, and less reliant on working memory.[673] Experienced proceduralists may even enter a state of "flow," making difficult tasks seem effortless, like a concert pianist performing flawlessly.[47]

Active physical and mental involvement is essential; observation is a good starting point but insufficient for independent practice. Think of it like being a passenger in a car your whole life—you'd still struggle to drive. The only way to learn a procedure is to *do* it. Remember, supervising a new resident is like teaching a teenager to drive—some anxiety and intervention are natural. Learning procedures takes time, so don't be discouraged if a senior physician takes over to keep things moving.

Kinesthetic, visual, and declarative memory all contribute to procedure execution. For example, in interventional radiology, navigating a needle by feel teaches you intimate knowledge of anatomy—what it looks and feels like. Experts can even detect subtle anatomical features by feel alone.

Caveats

The adage *see one, do one, teach one* is better phrased as *see several, do many, then teach many*. Trainees, especially those lacking confidence, often underestimate their procedural potential with time, experience, and the right guidance.

Here's a critical caveat, though: both correct and incorrect techniques become ingrained through practice. Practicing the wrong approach is counterproductive and hard to unlearn. While clumsiness is expected, ensure your technique is fundamentally sound. Also, remember that not all cases are suitable for new trainees due to complexity, patient acuity, or other factors.

Learning About Procedures Versus Learning How to Do Procedures

Sometimes, the goal is to learn *about* a procedure, not *how* to perform it. Ideally, trainees and staff should have a shared understanding of this objective. However, the more involved you are in the entire process, the more you'll learn. Prepare as if you were going to perform the procedure, and clearly communicate your learning goals to both yourself and the attendings.

Note

1   "Minor details have been altered for anonymity, but the general message is not materially altered."

41

Pathology and Radiology

Vance T. Lehman, Julia S. Lehman

Most trainees will not become pathologists or radiologists. However, pathology, laboratory medicine, and radiology are pillars of the practice of medicine. To best serve your patients, you should learn the basic principles as you progress through your clinical training. This chapter provides a high-level introduction to many concepts you should focus on.

Pathology

Some authors have expressed concern that foundational knowledge of pathology has suffered with the introduction of integrated medical school curricula, putting more onus on trainees to learn proactively.[140] Later during clinical rotations, however, it is best to think about pathology in an integrated fashion rather than to relegate it to a free-standing pathology rotation. Even if you do not directly interpret pathology specimens in your ultimate career, you should understand the common terminology, basic processes involved with tissue preparation and interpretation, limitations, and role of clinical correlation.

Various Tissues and Specimens

There are various tissue and body fluid specimens that may be submitted for pathology interpretation: biopsy specimens (usually sent in formalin for permanent fixation and hematoxylin and eosin (H&E) staining, though depending on the clinical context, potentially submitted in saline for frozen section interpretation, etc.), excision specimens (typically after diagnosis has been confirmed histopathologically by biopsy or other diagnostic techniques), fine-needle aspirates, bone marrow biopsy specimens, and others.

H&E-Stained Slides Provide Considerable Information

Diagnosis often can be rendered from H&E-stained slides alone. While this may be the case for certain neoplasms, infections and inflammatory conditions, there are areas in which clinical or radiologic correlation is required for definitive diagnosis. It can be tremendously helpful when clinicians understand how the histopathologic changes in tissue reflect disease pathogenesis. In some cases, clinicians must integrate histopathologic findings with clinical, laboratory and radiographic information to make rational treatment decisions, even when insufficient data are available to make a diagnosis with certainty.

DOI: 10.1201/9781003633389-45

Ancillary Tests Are Needed in a Variety of Cases

In certain cases, various ancillary tests may be required for diagnostic confirmation. For example, the cellular origin of a poorly differentiated neoplasm can be determined via a panel of immunohistochemical stains, which may include melanocytic markers (e.g., MART-1, SOX10, S100), keratinocyte markers (e.g., AE1/AE3, OSCAR, p63), endothelial cell markers (e.g., CD31, ERG), lymphocyte markers (e.g., leukocyte common antigen, CD3 for T-cells, CD20 for B-cells), or muscle markers (e.g., desmin, smooth muscle actin). However, virtually no stain is entirely sensitive or specific, so caution should be taken before arriving at a diagnosis based on immunophenotype alone.

When various histopathologic features (such as the presence of abscesses or granulomas) suggest infection, special stains can be requested to evaluate for fungus (e.g., GMS, PAS stains), mycobacteria (e.g., Fite, AFB stains), bacteria (e.g., Gram stain), and others.

Ancillary studies may also be requested to assist with prognosis of certain conditions. For example, newly diagnosed breast cancer is often evaluated with ER, PR, Her2, and Ki67 for prognostication and therapeutic decision-making. Molecular studies are also becoming part of standard of care in various facets of pathology practice. For example, in severely atypical melanocytic neoplasms, molecular assays such as chromosomal microarray, fluorescence in situ hybridization (FISH), or next-generation sequencing studies, may be requested to help determine the potential biologic behavior of the neoplasm.

In increasingly frequent scenarios, special studies are ordered to triage treatment options. For example, demonstrating a BRAFV600E mutation by immunohistochemical staining in Langerhans cell histiocytosis may predict therapeutic response to a BRAF-inhibitor.

Key Takeaways

Some advanced tests may not be available at your institution and may need to be sent to a specialized reference laboratory. It is important to understand motivations for ordering specialized tests, as these tests may be ordered at academic centers for educational purposes but are not necessarily medically necessary or likely to eventuate in a change in patient management. Typically, these educational studies are billed to a departmental discretionary fund rather than to the patient's insurance. Resource utilization must be balanced against ensuring high-quality, safe patient care.

Pathology Reports Take Time

Preparing pathology reports can take time. This delay in the turnaround time can be due to the need for recuts, additional stains, and second opinions, for example. Depending on the nature of the biopsy and the clinician's question, the pathology report may take various forms. In general, there is a diagnostic line and a comments section. The *diagnostic line* generally includes the most precise diagnosis or diagnostic classification that can be rendered based on the findings. In some cases, the diagnostic line contains descriptive information only, in which case a differential diagnosis (often, with rationale) in the *comments section* is useful. Further studies (e.g., tissue cultures) or treatments (e.g., re-excision with appropriate surgical margins) can be recommended in the comments section. For certain malignancies, standardized synoptic reporting is often facilitated using templates.

Pathologic Diagnosis Is Not Aways Ground Truth

Pathologic diagnosis is not always ground truth. If the pathology report does not fit with the clinical presentation, it is not only acceptable but prudent to contact the signing pathologist to discuss the case. Usually, she will welcome the opportunity to review the situation in light of all available information, to ensure that no error was made.

Pathology is Going Digital

In recent years, the digital revolution has transformed the landscape of many areas of medicine, including pathology. For centuries, pathologists had to hunch over microscopes, with trainees crowding around accessory microscope heads in academic centers. Now, pathology slides can be scanned and converted into digital images, to be viewed on high-resolution monitors. For early adopters of the technology, digital pathology has enabled more comfortable ergonomics, simplified archiving, and facilitated remote work. Modern pathology holds promise to become a great flexibility career option.

Radiology

Like pathology, radiology is best learned in an integrated fashion in training. Doing so provides context and, unless you pursue a radiology residency, radiology rotations are too intermittent and short to provide full benefit. Also, like pathology, radiology is a broad topic, and there is too much to cover comprehensively here. Instead, we'll focus on a few basic principles that medical trainees can use.

Imaging Basics

Modern digital radiographic images are not photographs from exposed film but rather represent mathematically processed information derived from complex physical interactions of an imaging source with body tissue and exogenous contrast agents. Thus, the precise techniques used for source application, source detection, and processing impact image quality and also introduce approximations, limitations, and artifacts. Imaging examinations are thus an imperfect representation of reality. When there are questions about whether an imaging finding is real or what modality is best to answer a specific clinical question, it can be useful to consult a radiologist.

New Technology Hype (Appeal to Novelty)

There is a constant influx of new technology, often delivered in a package decorated with a ribbon of hype. Some clinicians might wonder why not every patient is scanned at 7 Tesla MRI or with photon-counting CT, for example. Being at the cutting edge of imaging technology, studies such as these are often presumed to be better than standard of care.

In truth, however, new technology may offer advantages for certain applications but may have a neutral or even disadvantageous impact in other applications. Access to new technology can be limited or expensive, and not all patients might be candidates. All old technology was once new. In general, it is best not to get distracted by the newest technology available but instead to focus on how best to answer the precise clinical questions being asked.

The Main Purposes of Medical Imaging

We'll now address two key questions that should be asked before ordering or interpreting medical imaging: (1) what information is needed, and (2) what type of examination is best? For the first question, consider that medical imaging can be used for many purposes, not all of which are routinely reflected in radiology reports.

Types of Information from Imaging Examinations

Beyond diagnostic confirmation, additional reasons for imaging include cancer screening, cancer staging, hybrid image fusion, procedure planning, intra-operative/intra-procedural guidance, research, and forensic purposes, for example. These can be further subcategorized. For instance, planning could be done on a routine exam, a stereotactic planning exam, a radiation planning exam, or with imaging processing such as creation of special reformats, 3D images, or 3D printed models.

In addition, the lines drawn between imaging and therapeutic interventions are becoming blurred with an evolving field known as *theranostics*, which employs nuclear medicine probes that can be used for both diagnosis and targeted rational treatment, depending on the precise radioisotope used.

Which Imaging Examination Is Best?

Addressing which imaging examination is ideal for a given clinical indication is a vast topic, with answers that are often non-determinant and situation specific. Key considerations include diagnostic accuracy needed, availability, local interpretation expertise, cost, radiation, safety, and urgency. The American College of Radiology publishes detailed evidence-based, up-to-date appropriateness criteria for many common imaging indications. For a given indication, the appropriateness of several imaging modalities are provided, demonstrating that there is often not a single acceptable answer.

For unusual indications, it is helpful to consult with local radiologists. They can provide information about the available examinations, local expertise, and diagnostic accuracy. Local capability depends on factors beyond modality availability. For example, certain types of MRIs can only be performed with certain software packages or other protocol programming, even if the hardware is present. In addition, some invasive tests (e.g., certain types of angiography or advanced myelography) are not available at all locations. Finally, referral to another institution is occasionally needed, and radiologists should be able to provide guidance.

When ordering imaging examinations, it is important to ensure that all critical clinical information and questions to answer are included on the examination indications.

Understanding Radiology Reports

Regardless of your ultimate career choices, you will likely need to read and understand radiology reports. There are two basic formats: templates or free form. Both have their place and their proponents. As medicine becomes ever more complex, there may be an uptick in templated reports. Templates serve as a checklist for the radiologist, can include built-in scoring systems, and make it easy to find specific information in the report for clinical or research purposes. Some radiologists include standardized scoring systems, such as Brain Tumor Reporting and Data System (BT-RADS).

Pitfalls of Templates

However, templated reports (in radiology and elsewhere) can be rigid and awkward to read. For basic cases, they can also just become lists of normal findings. Templates risk obscuring the key findings and/or diluting the clinical correlation and thinking if not used judiciously. They can auto-populate sections with misinformation or items that were not truly assessed (this is also a common problem with pre-populated physical examination templates).

Some radiologists view templates as a crutch for those who have not mastered the art of high-quality report generation. Finally, some trainees in radiology or elsewhere create poorly constructed templates that are hard to read or contain too much distracting or irrelevant information.

Radiology Language is Often Not Standardized

Though many have advocated adoption of standardized language in radiology reports, this practice has not caught on widely. Thus, the selection of words and reporting style vary among radiologists and institutions. Most reports include both *Findings* and *Impression* sections. Any critical information for diagnosis and follow-up should be included in the impression, though sometimes, you will find it buried in the findings instead. Further, depending on the clinical scenario, the *Findings* section may include relevant information too.

Some imaging findings require standardized follow-up based on vetted criteria. An example is an incidentally discovered pulmonary nodule. A report may include specific follow-up criteria in a dedicated section that incorporates nodule size, imaging features, and clinical information. Many findings that might need further evaluation, however, do not fit neatly into well-defined follow-up criteria.

While most reports will provide a differential diagnosis and clinical impression, some will remain descriptive. There are many potential reasons for this, most of which depend on the anticipated primary audience for the report and the specific findings. Sometimes, the significance of the findings is unclear, and the radiologist does not want to box a clinician in a corner. In this case, sometimes an off-line discussion with the radiologist is useful.

42

Social Determinants of Health

Vance T. Lehman, Mark L. Wieland

Introduction

Nineteenth-century physician Rudolf Virchow's observations on the dominant role of social factors in disease laid the foundation for integrating social determinants of health (SDOH) into medicine. In the United States, the 1910 *Flexner Report* solidified the biomedical model's dominance for decades. A key turning point came in 1977, when Dr. George Engel advocated for the biopsychosocial model.[674] Recently, medical education has increasingly emphasized SDOH, as evidenced by their inclusion in student evaluations and MCAT social science questions.

Decades after Engel's proposal, the biomedical model still dominates medical curricula. Consequently, trainees may undervalue SDOH in clinical care and deprioritize learning about them.[406,675] Unfortunately, this may be to the detriment of their future patients who would benefit from holistic care. In addition, medical students may learn to depersonalize patients with unmet social needs as a hidden curriculum effect.[407] Here, we'll briefly review the key concepts, challenges, and practical methods of addressing SDOH.

Defining and Understanding SDOH

The discussion of SDOH is complex due to varying definitions, models, and contributing factors. A 2008 WHO commission identified numerous daily living conditions and structural resource allocations impacting health outcomes. These factors can be classified as nonstructural (intermediate) or structural (systemic).[1] Nonstructural factors include education level, living conditions, occupation, and healthcare access, while structural factors encompass taxation, social policies, gender equity, and political empowerment.[676]

Unlike the biomedical model's focus on individual-level disease determinants, SDOHs emphasize *distal determinants*—both individual and structural. Socioeconomic status (SES), encompassing income/wealth, education, and occupation, is a key driver of SDOH.[678] There are other potential fundamental drivers upstream and/or distinct from SES. For example, structural racism independently impacts health.[679] Family dynamics, childhood experiences, social support, and self-determination also significantly contribute.[680]

How do social factors affect health? Thimm-Kaiser et al. describe eight mechanisms of SDOH, summarized in a comprehensive model.[681] For example, *biological embedding* occurs when SDOHs are associated with detectable changes in biologic states, such as the volume of

DOI: 10.1201/9781003633389-46

certain brain structures or levels of certain hormones. A key consideration here is *allostatic load*, the cumulative effects of chronic stress that result in numerous biological responses (e.g., elevated cortisol levels) and increase the risk of many clinical conditions (e.g., cardiovascular disease, pre-eclampsia, and depressive symptoms).[682]

Addressing SDOH Clinically

While addressing SDOH involves social, community, and organizational levels, this section focuses on the individual level. Several approaches can facilitate action on SDOH in clinical practice. Specifically, we'll briefly introduce a few ways to help do this using the general methods to assess, refer, advocate, and consult.

In clinic, the first step is to assess for SDOHs with a population- and patient-context approach[680,681] by asking relevant questions in an empathetic and culturally acceptable manner.[680] While it takes extra time, incorporating these questions improves diagnosis, avoids unnecessary (and time-consuming) investigations, and builds patient trust.[680] For example, understanding a patient's domestic situation is crucial in addressing chronic pain aggravated by abuse.

It is also important to know local resources for optimal patient referral,[680,681] such as shelters, support groups, housing support organizations, nutritional assistance programs, and more. It is helpful to establish a clinical support team (or, as a trainee, become familiarized with any preexisting teams) that is well-connected to these resources.[683] Physicians should also advocate for patient access to these resources.[680]

To facilitate this approach, there are established questionnaires with questions such as "Do you ever have difficulty making ends meet at the end of the month?" to screen for poverty.[680,684,685] There is also a variety of online point of care *clinical decision aides* available for reference in clinic.[680] One early example is the CLEAR toolkit (https://www.mcgill.ca/clear/download#English), which provides example questions relevant for community health along the major domains of SDOH and methods of implementation in over a dozen languages. Numerous additional clinical decision aids to facilitate interventions for specific situations including by population and specific SDOHs have also been developed.[680]

The Centers for Medicare and Medicaid Services (CMS) recommends implementing the Accountable Health Communities Health Related Social Needs Screening Tool. The tool screens for five core domains, which became mandatory for inpatients in 2024: housing, food, transportation, utilities, and safety. Eight supplemental domains include financial strain, employment, social support, education, physical activity, substance use, mental health, and disability.

Additional strategies include grouping appointments (clinical, radiological, laboratory) for patients with limited transportation.[677] For patients with lower literacy or communication skills, ensure clear written and oral communication.[677] This includes educational and health promotional pamphlets and patient-directed reports and electronic correspondence.

It is also essential to consider medical costs to patients, especially for patients from a lower SES. Refer patients with unmet needs to evidence-based interventions, such as community health workers for diabetes management.[686] These core tenets of medical practice do not only apply in primary care; all medical providers should be mindful of social context when caring for patients.

Key Takeaways

SDOHs are dynamic, complex, and context-dependent. The mechanisms of SDOH's impact on health, including the interplay of proximal and structural causes, are sometimes unclear. In other words, patient management is complex. While an in-depth analysis is outside the scope of this book, the basic concepts of such complexity are explored further in Chapter 48.

Note

1 Some resources define social determinants of health as those acting on individuals at a community level and structural determinants of health as those that act at a societal level (e.g., racism, class).[677]

43

Evaluations and Feedback

Vance T. Lehman

Why Third-Year Clinical Evaluations Matter Most in Medical School

Third-year clinical evaluations (or pre-match evaluations in highly integrated programs) are largely subjective and poorly standardized, as discussed below. Attendings sometimes seem to assign grades (usually a B or Pass) based on subjective observations, with little objective data or clearly stated expectations. Attendings may fail to clearly communicate expectations, understand your learning style, assess your knowledge base, provide timely feedback, or define *honors* criteria. Unfortunately, attendings often receive insufficient training on how to teach and assess trainees. However, remember that a slow start or one poor evaluation does not determine your long-term trajectory.

Third-year evaluations encompass multiple assessments. Beyond the formal grade, evaluation comments hold weight and are reviewed during residency or even future fellowship applications. With purely P/F pre-clinical grades, your clinical performance becomes paramount. Further, P/F scoring of USMLE Step 1 has increased the importance of Step 2 scores of clinical knowledge. Clinical rotations are typically the final step of your residency application, so they are heavily weighted from the perspective of performance trends, too. This marks the beginning of a career increasingly reliant on subjective evaluations.

Evaluations

You Have Primary Responsibility

While attendings share responsibility for your training, most will place responsibility squarely on you. Unlike professional sports, where coaches face accountability for poor performance, attendings often lack similar accountability. Therefore, you must proactively identify learning objectives and manage your experience.

Identifying Your Evaluators

Understand who contributes to your evaluations. On a clinical service, the evaluation will be posted under the attending's name, and the attending might be the primary source of your evaluation. Residents, fellows, and sometimes other staff also significantly contribute. Remember that you should always be in interview mode. Selective performance based on perceived importance of others who are present is risky.

 DOI: 10.1201/9781003633389-47

You Can't Predict Easy Versus Tough Evaluators

You should be aware that the toughest, scariest attendings in person can be softies on formal evaluations and the *nicest* attendings in person are sometimes the most brutal. We just cannot predict how authority figures will act behind closed doors. Remember that many of history's most ruthless figures were described as shy, unimpressive, or ordinary in their personal encounters. People can be unpredictable.

Several factors can compromise the validity of evaluations. Evaluator burnout can lead to superficial or homogenous evaluations.[687] Many evaluators fail to systematically assess learners' knowledge and skills.

Understanding Evaluation Components

Understand the grading breakdown, often 50% clinical evaluation and 50% examination, with adjustments for observed structured clinical examinations (OSCE). Study for examinations; the material benefits both clinical service and USMLE Step 2 preparation, but tailor your study plan to rotation-specific expectations and workload. Determine if the examination is standardized or institution-specific; if the latter, identify specific learning objectives.

Both grades and narrative comments appear on the MSPE and influence residency and fellowship applications. Given institutional grade variations, comments are crucial for admissions committees. Even limited negative comments can be detrimental to an application. Therefore, strong clinical performance is essential, even in shelf-exam-heavy rotations with limited narrative comments.

The Impossibility of a Perfect Evaluation

There's a good reason you cannot have the perfect evaluation. Here's the little secret—attendings all have different ideas on practice and wouldn't even give their own colleagues a perfect evaluation. They can't always live up to their own standards either, so some wouldn't even give themselves a perfect evaluation. Even if it were possible to agree on a definition of perfect, there would still be countless ways to be imperfect. Therefore, a flawless evaluation is impossible.

Responding to Feedback

Receptiveness to constructive feedback is imperative. Unreceptiveness has several negative consequences. That is, trainees miss out on the primary message; instead of moving on, the attendings now remember the episode and label the trainee as stubborn, arrogant, or plainly unreceptive. Future feedback may be anonymous, relayed through the PD, or absent altogether.

Ineffective Responses to Feedback

Several common responses undermine feedback effectiveness. The first is a defensive tone, body language, or verbalized language. Responses like "of course" or "I knew that" should be avoided; focus on learning from the feedback instead. Even mild defensiveness can lead to indirect future feedback.

Ego threat often hinders learning from failures (as discussed in Chapter 24). That said, certain actions can improve the reception of constructive feedback. Demonstrating effort, commitment, and respect increases the likelihood of receiving positive feedback. It is also useful to view your feedback as a normal distribution. Most feedback will reflect reality, with some positive and negative outliers. This perspective helps us avoid dwelling on the negative.

Take seriously any constructive feedback from the PD or other staff, even if it seems like only a gentle reminder. The first time the topic is broached might be gentle, kind, and might even be (mis)interpreted as a suggestion. An understated approach may reflect various factors, including leniency, maintaining positive relationships, and individual personality. Don't assume low-key feedback is merely a suggestion. If you fail to respond, the next discussion could be more serious.

Express appreciation to your attending and other teachers at the end of each day. Clearly express your commitment to success and request feedback. If you are struggling to manage constructive feedback, consider talking to your PD or a mentor to help put it in perspective.

Absent Feedback

Many staff avoid providing constructive feedback. Reasons for this range from apathy, gamesmanship, lack of skill, cowardice, lack of anonymized process, to reaction to previous retaliation from trainees (recall Maitland Jones). Today, providing genuine feedback requires vulnerability from the attending. It is a true act of kindness. While this is largely out of our control, actively seeking feedback and responding favorably can help offset staff reluctance to provide it.

Mixed Feedback

Mixed feedback from different staff on the same rotation is common. In such cases, careful navigation is essential. When this simply reflects variable staff preferences, it is usually best to try to accommodate those of your current attending. Ignoring more substantial feedback, however, can be perceived as defiance. Instead, accept responsibility and express your commitment to improvement.

Some staff give uniformly positive feedback while others routinely error on the negative side. Positive or negative evaluations of the same performance can be justified based on subjective weighting of factors. Furthermore, a small subset of attendings error on the side of positive feedback to curry favor.

Once Bitten, Twice Shy Syndrome

A natural response to negative feedback is to avoid similar situations in the future. Perhaps it is a type of patient admission, procedure, giving a presentation, reading a type of radiology examination, and so forth. Avoiding future challenges, however, is counterproductive and reflects poorly on your receptiveness to feedback.

Providing Constructive Feedback

Though you will receive more feedback than you deliver during training, you should also develop effective feedback delivery skills. You will eventually provide feedback to medical students and team members—positive, neutral, or negative. Effective feedback is intentional, timely, consistent, high-quality, and focused on improvement, not judgment. Focus on objective observations without assuming intentions. In addition, there are some specific steps and strategies you can consider.

High-quality feedback begins with establishing trust and systematically assessing performance. That aside, once you think that you need to provide feedback, it helps to start with a few essential questions:

- Is feedback necessary? Do you have credible, objective evidence of a pattern or a serious single incident? Consider potential misunderstandings or missing information.
- If feedback remains warranted, are you the appropriate person to deliver it?
- Is the recipient appropriate? Direct feedback is usually best, but exceptions exist.

If feedback is needed, set the stage for feedback delivery.

- Substantive feedback should ideally be delivered privately, in person (consider involving another authority for serious matters). Giving serious constructive feedback in front of others is problematic. Defensiveness and blame can replace productive conversation, leaving the recipient feeling undermined. While spontaneous feedback is sometimes necessary, avoid *gotcha* moments.
- Constructive feedback for the little things is usually best done with a light-hearted approach. For example, "Can I offer a tip based on my experience?" A friendly tone minimizes defensiveness.
- Table 43.1 lists situations requiring caution or avoidance of negative feedback.

Ensuring follow-through on improvement efforts is challenging. Your feedback for others may be unrecognized as feedback, but following the previous steps minimizes this risk. Requesting self-appraisals and action plans ensures feedback is received and followed up on.

What's more, feedback is often ignored, even by those who desire it.[688] A major reason is that the recipients often do not know how to apply the feedback.[688] Therefore, it helps to discuss implementation methods in addition to relationship building and goal setting. These goals can often be framed as aiming for the next level. Encourage self-reliance through bidirectional conversations emphasizing growth, motivation, and initiative.

Additionally, low-quality, perception-based feedback diminishes its impact. Specific feedback is more impactful than vague comments like *good job* or *try harder*. Clearly state whether feedback is objective or subjective, specifying objective metrics.

Ideally, feedback is based off explicitly stated expectations that can either be reinforced or, less preferably, introduced while giving feedback. Base your subjective appraisals on ample examples and facts, not just perceptions. This approach is more convincing, acceptable, and less likely to provoke negative responses.

Table 43.1 Times to Be Careful Giving Negative Feedback

You do not know the recipient very well
Your information is incomplete, indirect, retrospective, and/or based on a small, selected input sample
You would not be receptive to a similar category of feedback directed to you (if needed)
You do not model (i.e., are being hypocritical) or have experience doing a similar topic that you are commenting on ·
You are not ready to help the recipient grow and improve in response

In addition, convey unconditional positive regard, especially when performance expectations are unmet. Judgmental feedback is less effective, and you cannot know the recipient's mindset. Wherever this mindset is, you might knock them down a notch; the effect is relative. People often mask emotional struggles well; negative feedback can be unexpectedly detrimental to their self-image. Therefore, be direct but sensitive.

While strategies like the *6:1 positive-to-negative ratio* and the *feedback sandwich* exist, they aren't always practical. A 6:1 ratio is excessive and provides insufficient useful information. The feedback sandwich feels unnatural if genuine positive comments are lacking. A *Harvard Business Review* article even dismisses the feedback sandwich, advocating for a tactful, transparent approach.[689] That said, coupling positive and negative feedback can be effective for minor issues. For this, ensure all feedback is genuine, appropriate, and tactfully delivered.

Finally, the *One Minute Manager* offers practical feedback strategies and is a fast read. It provides methods for delivering quick, effective feedback. Its methods include normalization, positive regard, expectation setting, and belief in the recipient's ability.

Rotation Feedback

Rotation or classroom feedback differs from personal performance feedback. Trainees sometimes base rotation evaluations on anticipated evaluations rather than providing honest feedback. Trainees too often hesitate to offer constructive suggestions. The most common problem may be failing to provide feedback at all.

Problematic Feedback

Feedback can be ineffective, counterproductive, or weaponized. Feedback is also a difficult topic to study broadly and objectively. These problems stem partly from medicine's subjective, narrative feedback structure. Following the earlier feedback guidelines can mitigate these problems.

Characteristics of Ineffective Feedback

Ineffective feedback includes giving it to the wrong person, lacking positive regard, omitting action plans, or being too subtle. Subjective feedback is also inherently problematic. It often relies on *social comparisons* rather than objective standards. It's susceptible to labeling and biases (halo effect, recency bias, demographic biases, personality biases).[690]

Evaluator mood and fatigue can affect evaluations. Grade distributions vary among evaluators, reflecting differing metrics and low inter-rater reliability. Evaluators may extend negative feedback for a given trainee from one area to others. Subjective evaluations can also create a perception of injustice for the recipient.[691]

Nevertheless, this competitive environment relies on relative social comparisons. Evaluators inevitably compare your performance to your peers; many of your peers strive for excellence, so you must too to achieve top marks. As attendings may lack time for systematic assessment, you may need to proactively demonstrate your competencies.

While you can't control your attending's mood, poor performance can negatively impact it. Preparation, helpfulness, and a positive attitude are beneficial. Expect occasional unjust evaluations; for minor issues, it is usually best to consider it to be just one perspective and move on. Only egregiously unjust evaluations warrant review by the Dean or PD.

Counterproductive Aspects of Feedback

Counterproductive feedback also manifests in various ways. Harsh feedback can trigger negative self-perception and self-doubt. Remember the normal curve range of feedback; disproportionately focusing on negative feedback, especially with a fixed mindset, is counterproductive.

Staff and activity evaluations filled out by trainees are important but can also be counterproductive. Excessive evaluation requests (e.g., for every lecture) reflect commoditization. This creates a conflict of interest, discouraging staff from pushing you beyond your comfort zone.

Remember too that you may not be qualified to judge staff competence or teaching relevance. I've seen trainees give mediocre evaluations to excellent lectures by world experts. This likely reflects trainees' inability to appreciate the lecture's relevance and value. Provide honest evaluations but stay humble and avoid overly negative feedback.

Weaponization of Feedback

While less common, weaponized feedback—an abuse of office politics—deserves mention. The feedback system can be manipulated to unfairly hinder internal promotions, particularly for perceived competitors. Alternatively, negative feedback may reflect passive aggression. Distinguish between harsh but genuine feedback and weaponized feedback; if unfairly targeted, consider escalating the issue.

44

Conferences, Medical Societies, and Industry

Vance T. Lehman

Multidisciplinary Conferences

Internal multidisciplinary conferences are at the heart of complex medical decision-making, bringing together physicians from various specialties to discuss challenging patient care decisions. Initially, the content may seem unfamiliar. Often held early or late in the day, trainee participation is typically passive and ungraded (beyond attendance). As a result, it can be easy to tune out. However, tuning out represents a significant missed opportunity.

Initially, don't aim to grasp every detail or follow every line of reasoning. That would be impossible given the fast pace and highly technical commentary. Instead, focus on understanding the process and key takeaways. This is also a golden opportunity to learn about the different roles of various specialists and team members and how they all fit together. Observe *how* complex decisions are made and the factors influencing treatment plans.

For example, while pathology often provides the gold standard diagnosis, nuances exist. The final diagnosis may rely on an integration of clinical, pathologic, and radiologic factors. Even straightforward decisions can be complicated by unrealistic patient goals, difficult home situations, substance abuse, or psychiatric issues. Many decisions are personalized, reflecting judgment and ethical considerations.

Observe the decision-making processes of attending physicians. This may reveal gaps in the literature discussed and the limitations of current treatment options. Note the role of common considerations like smoking and anticoagulation in surgical decisions. Integrate key concepts into your studies but avoid getting bogged down in details.

During residency or fellowship, trainees may begin participating in multidisciplinary conferences. For this, thorough preparation is essential. While some attendants may comment on the fly, presenters should prepare. This involves understanding the clinical features, reviewing relevant literature, and preparing a concise yet comprehensive presentation. Even with thorough preparation, unexpected questions may arise. Don't worry about occasional unprepared answers (unless it becomes a recurring issue). It will be quickly forgotten.

DOI: 10.1201/9781003633389-48

National Conferences and Medical Societies

Conference Purpose and Planning

While internal conferences provide valuable experience, national meetings offer broader opportunities for professional development. Many programs support trainee attendance, especially for presentations, with some offering limited time. While enjoyable, remember these are professional development opportunities, not vacations. Trainees who misuse institutional resources for meetings risk being blacklisted.

This also forfeits the key benefits of attendance. Poor attendance or excessive time spent with vendors distributing free samples will be noticed. Also, avoid posting leisure activities on social media during conference attendance (remember someone is covering your clinical responsibilities).

Plan and budget your time. Attend a significant portion of the meeting, considering how your attendance reflects on your professionalism. Check the dress code beforehand. If it is business casual, do not show up in shorts and a Hawaiian T-shirt. If you are giving a presentation, attend your entire session; walking out the door immediately after the talk is inappropriate. Book your hotel room early to secure a reservation. While conference hotels may offer discounts, explore nearby, more affordable options.

Maximizing Your Research Output

Maximize the dissemination of your research findings and unique case studies at national meetings. Research projects can lead to enduring educational presentations and meeting attendance. However, avoid presenting the same work at multiple national conferences (unless it's a truly groundbreaking discovery). This could negatively impact your relationships with attendings (future letter writers, sponsors, and references).

Oral Presentations Have Greater Impact

When submitting abstracts to national meetings, remember that oral presentations generally have greater impact than posters. National meeting presentations offer low-stakes practice and learning opportunities for oral presentation skills. Observe experienced presenters. Notice how they speak, their body language, tone, and slide formats. Take note of professional etiquette like expressing gratitude and providing contact information for questions.

Types of Conferences

When selecting national meetings to attend, distinguish between large, general conferences and smaller, specialized ones. Once you've chosen a specialty, attending both types of conferences is beneficial. Larger conferences offer prestige and broader expertise, but networking may be more challenging. In comparison, smaller conferences offer greater early involvement and networking with local leaders. Smaller conferences offer excellent learning and networking opportunities, often connecting you with individuals involved in larger conferences. Conferences offer networking opportunities with other training programs, providing valuable information and potential allies.

Understand the conference's purpose beforehand. Conferences may focus on education, research, or advocacy, for example. Some may be a mix of all three. Many conferences are sponsored by medical societies. After choosing a specialty, consider joining a medical society and getting involved. This is a great way to network and stay current. While some societies may have industry ties, they remain valuable resources.

Industry Relationships

Both at national meetings and during clinical rotations, you'll encounter industry representatives. While their information is inherently biased toward their company, they provide essential details on medical devices, software, and medications. Collaboration with industry is essential for maintaining current skills and technology. Industry representatives can also offer insights into practice trends. Industry collaboration is crucial for translating research into practice. Therefore, positive industry relationships are essential.

Physicians may receive industry compensation for consultation or research. This raises ethical concerns, but proper management and disclosure support compensation. Trainee reporting of industry support on conflict-of-interest statements is questionable, however. Why would industry support non-board-certified trainees if not for undue influence? Financial relationships are publicly accessible via the Sunshine Act (https://openpaymentsdata.cms.gov/. Nonetheless, many research articles fail to disclose COIs for various reasons.[692] Authors attribute this to vague interpretations of "relevant" information and systemic issues.[693]

45

Applying to Residency or Other Positions

Vance T. Lehman

Selections, Subjectivity, and Fairness in Medical Training

Medical school and residency selection, like college admissions, involve various factors with both positive and negative consequences. In *The Chosen*, Jerome Karabel provides compelling evidence that incorporating subjective measures like extracurricular activities or interview performance into the admissions process for Ivy League universities in the early 20th century was a clear mechanism to enable discrimination.[694] Therefore, while not intentionally discriminatory today, the inclusion of intangible qualities introduces the possibility of bias and chance for applicants to medical school and other post-secondary programs.

Regardless of fairness, application trends are notable. The increasing prevalence of P/F grades and USMLE Step 1 scores elevates the importance of other factors: extracurricular activities, school reputation, and other CV details. One study showed that the social or ideological nature of extracurricular activities influences applicant rankings.[695] Mentioning avid golfing and extensive travel, for instance, are perfectly fine but might signal a social affiliation to the interviewers that "I'm one of you." Eliminating such influences is difficult.

Moreover, the average number of abstracts, publications, and presentations for medical students matching into dermatology increased from 14.7 in 2018 to 20.9 in 2022.[696] As traditional metrics (grades, standardized test scores) decline, these other metrics will gain importance. Notice that these factors reflect a hidden curriculum related to the conflict theory of education (Chapter 18).

Choosing a Specialty

Objective and Subjective Factors

Specialty choice is highly personal. Objective considerations include competitiveness, training length, lifestyle, procedural availability, clinic volume, telemedicine opportunities, fellowship options, and job prospects. Niche specialties generally have greater geographic limitations. Family medicine offers broad practice settings, unlike transplant surgery, which requires specialized equipment and centers, for example.

DOI: 10.1201/9781003633389-49

Intangible factors include intuition and external influences. While intuition is important, consider the daily realities of the job, not just the theory. For example, if you dislike deep listening and conversation, clinical psychiatry may not be your best choice, even if you have a theoretical interest. Also, avoid making gut decisions when you are in an unusually good or bad mood. For example, while a 12-hour transplant might be exhilarating, revisit your feelings after prolonged exposure to the specialty.

Several other factors influence specialty selection. Specialty subcultures and personality fit can influence specialty choice.[697] Orthopedics, pathology, and dermatology conferences each reveal highly distinct cultures, for instance. As we learned, many specialties also remain segregated by gender. However, don't exclude specialties simply because you don't fit a stereotype.

Furthermore, attending messaging may subtly signal prestige for certain procedures (e.g., neurosurgery).[698] You should resist prestige-driven choices; prioritize your own goals. In addition, lack of exposure to specialties like pathology or radiology is a cited drawback to trainee recruitment.[140] Think outside the box and proactively seek out information about all the potential specialties, exposure, and mentorship to make your best-informed decision.

Specialty Forecasts and Anxieties

Specialty practice environments will evolve. Younger physicians demand for improved work-life integration such as part-time employment, shorter work weeks, job sharing, and telemedicine will likely continue to mold the landscape of medical practice in many specialties.[699] However, predicting specialty trajectories requires caution (discussed further in Chapter 48). While much will change like use of AI and other technology, the core aspects of medicine will likely remain consistent. *Lindy's Law* suggests that established practices tend to endure. Therefore, radical systemic change is unlikely.

Professional anxieties over possible disruptors will also persist, even though these do not always materialize. Interestingly, many current concerns in medicine (corporatization, technological disruption, declining public perception, erosion of the physician-patient relationship, over-specialization) mirror those of half a century ago.[136] Technological advancements (written records, printing press, telephones, television) have historically sparked concerns about cultural and intellectual erosion, despite often bringing positive change.[700] Thus, while some disruptions will come, wise physicians avoid letting anxieties have undue influence over career decisions.

Grades and the MSPE

While a variety of considerations matter, grades remain important. Many PDs cite third-year grades as most important, despite limited evidence of predictive validity.[701] In fact, these grading schemes are so variable among different sites that meaningful comparison of applicants is nearly impossible.[702]

The MSPE compiles student grades, test scores, and comments. Despite standardization efforts (e.g., outstanding, excellent, good), the format remains inconsistent. One study identified over 32 adjectives for overall performance, highlighting inconsistencies across evaluations.[701] The meaning of these descriptors also varies, and sometimes, even when coded, the real meaning is not revealed in the letter.[703] Numerical scores may also be unreliable and likely promote quantitative bias. What's more, schools have a conflict of interest, incentivized to minimize negative descriptions to showcase successful placements.[703]

Therefore, expect inherent biases and inconsistencies in the process. Your third-year grades, while imperfect, significantly impact competitiveness and program selection. Don't take rejections personally since this inherent randomness exists. Finally, PDs may rely on factors beyond objective performance (school reputation, stated interest, connections).

Letters of Recommendation

Limitations of the Process

Residency and fellowship applications require letters of recommendation, intended to add a human element beyond numerical scores. While you likely waive your right to review them, understanding the process is helpful.[704]

Letters of recommendation may not accurately reflect your ability for several reasons. The format and content vary considerably, despite standardization efforts. Some letters merely reiterate CV information, lacking insightful analysis. Furthermore, letter writers have an inherent conflict of interest, as applicant success reflects on their program.

What's even more important is that letter writers may be concerned about legal ramifications of providing a lackluster evaluation. In fact, it has been said that litigation concerns in the United States have ensured that the "predictive validity of personal references in the U.S. has fallen to almost zero."[705] This hesitancy to offer negative feedback results in incomplete, exaggerated, or vague letters. Therefore, true feedback often occurs informally (e.g., a phone call), through letter writers or other known contacts.

Letters often employ coded language that requires interpretation. This inconsistent code is difficult to decipher, however. This code generally interprets 'good' as lower third, 'very good' as middle third, "excellent" as top third, and "outstanding" as top 10%. Claims that an applicant is "in the top 10% of students I have ever worked with," are ambiguous, however; the applicant could be a true stand-out, or possibly just well-liked.

Requesting Letters of Recommendation

Resources exist to guide you in requesting letters of recommendation (including AMA website posts).[706] Remember that every interaction with your mentor is essentially an informal interview; so always present your best self. Consistent professionalism simplifies the letter-request process. Choose letter writers who know you well, are enthusiastic, and can provide specific, positive feedback on your abilities and qualities.

Missing any of these elements risks an unfavorable letter. Evaluators interpret omissions as lack of endorsement. Omitting comments on ability or personal strengths weakens an application. Weak letters can harm your matching chances. In fact, lukewarm ambivalent statements in an application are generally considered a red flag. Therefore, when requesting a letter, confirm the writer can provide a strong recommendation.

Avoiding Application Exaggeration

Aim for a strong application but avoid embellishment. Personal statements should accurately reflect the number of peer-reviewed publications listed on the CV. Listing non-peer-reviewed or informally published works as scientific publications can come across as deceptive. Also, be thoroughly familiar with your research experience and publications. As first author, you must know the paper thoroughly and have general topic knowledge. As a middle author, you must be able to clearly articulate your contributions.

While less critical, any listed hobbies are open to discussion. Common hobbies include fitness, cooking, reading, family time, music, gaming, travel, and pet care. These are more compelling if linked to humanitarian or insightful experiences. In addition, passion-driven volunteering is more impactful than merely checking a box. Be sure to highlight any leadership roles.

Do not exaggerate your hobbies since this can diminish your credibility. Also, you should generally avoid highly unusual hobbies (e.g., hula-hooping, eraser collecting).

The Importance of Interview Performance

General Principles

Your interview performance is crucial, especially given the current emphasis on P/F grading and testing. Interviews offer a chance to showcase your strengths and compensate for any perceived disadvantages. Thorough preparation is essential for successful interviews. Despite its basic importance, many medical interviewees are unprepared. Numerous preparation resources are readily available.

Every interaction, from initial contact to final thank-you, is part of the interview process. In-person interviews typically include meals with residents, department tours, and campus visits. Interactions with program coordinators and administrative staff are also part of the interview. Maintain professional, respectful email communication, using appropriate pleasantries and minimizing informal language. Maintain professional conduct throughout.

In addition, prioritize adequate sleep in the days leading up to the interview, especially if sleep will be short the night before. Arrive well-informed about the program and interviewers. Research the program website and interviewer backgrounds. Maintain a respectful and engaged demeanor with all staff. Present your best professional self. Review basic etiquette (including table manners) and arrive punctually. Wear professional attire. Address attendings formally (Dr. X) during residency and fellowship interviews.

Preinterview Dinners

Remember that informal settings remain part of the interview process; maintain professional conduct. Programs consider your behavior at informal events. Put your phone away. Avoid alcohol. Avoid ordering red sauce or messy plates.

The Formal Interview

The literature strongly supports structured over unstructured interviews. However, many physicians conduct unstructured interviews and lack formal interview training. Therefore, prepare for various interview formats.

Answer questions directly and completely, without dominating the conversation. Maintain a friendly yet professional tone. Avoid name-dropping. Make a good impression even for less-preferred programs; you might change your mind, they'll remember you for future applications, and you may interact with them later. Avoid criticizing other programs. Interviewers may have connections; criticizing programs, specialties, or individuals reflects poorly on you. Some interviewers may try to elicit negative comments.

Be open about yourself but maintain professionalism. Support all claims with evidence. For example, don't claim that you have high research aspirations without relevant experience. Demonstrate an understanding of basic ethical principles (some questions may center on these) and a commitment to beneficence and hard work. Focus on how you can benefit the program, not just how the program could benefit you.

Expect challenging questions and program-specific discussions. Prepare stories illustrating patient care, challenges overcome, and responses to failure. For example, some interviewers may use aggressive questioning techniques. If this occurs, maintain a calm, respectful composure. Expect unexpected questions (e.g., "Who would you have lunch with?") to assess your spontaneous thinking; your approach matters more than the specific answer. Ensure your answers align with the program's focus; specifically avoid expressing interest in areas where the program is weak.

Prepare thoughtful questions for the interviewers; you'll inevitably be asked, and lack of questions can be perceived negatively. Show curiosity to avoid prematurely ending the conversation. Avoid both curt and overly verbose responses. Frame questions to demonstrate your research in the program and interest, not to interrogate the interviewer.

Other Considerations

Take notes immediately after each interview. Ensure your social media presence is professional. Remember, perfection isn't expected. Thoughtful, prepared responses demonstrating interpersonal skills suffice. If you don't receive an interview invitation, a note of interest may help if you have a realistic target program. Initial rejection may reflect randomness; programs prefer enthusiastic candidates.

For virtual interviews, optimize your computer setup. Check lighting, camera angle, distance (avoid close-ups), background, and noise.

Post-Interview Communication

The NRMP code of conduct prohibits PDs from soliciting post-interview communication to influence applicant rankings.[707] However, information exchange remains permissible. Over 90% of applicants and programs engage in post-interview communication, often initiated by mentors, sponsors, or programs.[707] Communication ranges from thank-you notes to expressions of ranking intent.

Unfortunately, dishonest intentions, while anecdotal, do occur. Dishonesty damages future opportunities. Furthermore, program communication styles vary widely. Thus, you should avoid overinterpreting communication or lack thereof.

Ranking Residency Programs

Only Insiders Know for Sure

Ranking residency programs is a highly personal yet crucial career decision. This section explores less obvious considerations. First, insider knowledge is essential for understanding residency programs. Any program has areas for improvement, but critical issues can be closely guarded. Thus, online forums are generally unreliable sources of insider information. Casual acquaintances are also unlikely to be sources of reliable information. Lunch conversations with residents provide limited insight to major problems. Without close insider contacts, it is difficult to discern critical drawbacks to a program.

The Limitations of University Reputation and NIH Funding

Avoid conflating residency and university reputations. A University's reputation doesn't perfectly reflect medical school or individual residency program quality. Further, residency programs at a given hospital vary widely in quality. Many programs highlight NIH funding. Remember that NIH funding reflects research success, not necessarily educational quality. High funding may indicate resources, attract strong faculty, and offer exposure to complex cases. Program prestige, while useful for CVs, doesn't directly reflect educational quality. However, funded researchers may have limited clinical time. Be aware that renowned researchers may have limited trainee interaction. Conversely, educators may be more engaged with trainees. These educators may publish on clinical and educational topics.

Important Information to Ascertain

Tactfully seek informal information about potential program drawbacks. Consider the following:

1. **Assess the fellow-resident dynamic**. Do fellows limit resident opportunities? Observe informal interactions and casually inquire with residents.
2. **Assess scutwork**. Scutwork encompasses noneducational, time-consuming tasks. Patient care tasks (e.g., documentation) are not scutwork; teamwork is essential. Scutwork includes tasks for non-physician staff, attendings, and those inappropriate for trainees. Inquire about daily tasks and time spent on noneducational activities.
3. **Assess call frequency, intensity, and sleep patterns**. Estimate call volume (pages, admits, cases). Avoid implying a preference for minimal workload. Casually inquire about call schedules, experiences, and support systems.
4. **Inquire about significant changes during resident training**. Inquire about anticipated changes (workload, benefits, leadership), but negative changes may not be revealed. Use past experiences as a guide, recognizing that change is possible.
5. **Assess the program's connections to regional practices**. Review recent graduate career paths.
6. **Avoid extensive questioning about external moonlighting**, as opinions on the topic vary widely. Also, avoid such questions during formal interviews. Moonlighting opportunities vary and may be unstated. In some programs, these opportunities are managed by resident subgroups.

Additional considerations include the following:

- Salaries (though the cost of living varies more)
- Commute time
- Balance of oversight versus independence
- Hospital culture
- Residency climate (e.g., collegial or cutthroat)
- Ties to specific fellowships or private practices
- Region/weather
- Proximity to your support network
- Employment opportunities for a partner
- Family friendliness (especially if you anticipate having children during residency)

Trainees often prioritize independence, but a *balanced* level of responsibility is arguably more important. Finally, you might consider if a program offers certain fellowship programs you are likely to consider.

Doximity Rankings

Finally, Doximity rankings influence program fill rates.[708] Be aware that current and recent alumni residents with Doximity profiles can participate in the Doximity survey. Thus, self-ranking introduces inherent bias and conflict of interest. Furthermore, smaller or newer programs may be disadvantaged by this ranking system. While the Doximity site offers a treasure trove of valuable information, you must consider the methodology and source. Other hospital ranking systems, while helpful, are also imperfect.

Conclusion

Congratulations, with this information in hand, you have completed Part IV and should be well-equipped to apply the basic principles of understanding and managing the hidden curriculum in the clinical settings. As a final step, however, it is useful to briefly synthesize the highlights and examine how these apply in the quest to becoming an expert in the complex medical environment, the focus of Part V.

Part V

Mastery

46

Synthesizing the Hidden Curriculum

Vance T. Lehman

Why It Holds the Key to Success

A 2022 systematic review explored the traits that attending physicians believe make a resident excellent.[709] The top traits were communication, knowledge, professionalism, and leadership.[709] Additional traits included warm personality, empathy, motivation, and curiosity.[709]

Notice that these qualities are often deeply intertwined with a hidden curriculum—the unspoken expectations, invisible challenges, and stealth influences of training. This book has explored this critical, yet often overlooked, aspect of medical education in depth. Let's briefly synthesize our findings and understand why mastering the hidden curriculum is essential for success, why it exists, and how to manage it.

In sum, savvy navigation of the hidden curriculum is crucial for trainee success for several reasons:

- **Formal Curriculum Limitations**. The formal medical curriculum does not adequately teach you how to *learn* medicine. For example, trainees are often not taught effective learning strategies, the importance of collective knowledge, or how to prioritize learning material. While the formal curriculum is rigid and riddled with gaps, the hidden curriculum is organic, nimble, and more encompassing.
- **Uneven Playing Field**. Similar trainees giving commensurate effort can experience drastically different outcomes, even when following the same formal curriculum. This is because some trainees may use highly effective learning strategies, employ superior gamesmanship, or benefit from attendings' biases and attention.
- **Historical Context Matters**. The formal curriculum underemphasizes historical influences on controversies in medical education. For example, understanding the factors underlying the replication crisis and related debates is crucial.
- **Real Expectations Versus Formal Objectives**. The hidden curriculum reflects what people, including your attendings, *really* expect, which often differs from formal learning objectives. For example, research-heavy programs may formally require one research project, but attendings expect more.
- **Subjective Evaluations**. Professional evaluations, starting with clinical rotations, impact career trajectories but are largely subjective. Rotation evaluations are skewed by attendings' personal expectations.
- **Untaught Skills**. Many useful skills for success are not formally taught, such as basic logic or negotiation tactics.
- **Real-World Experience**. Most trainees lack real-world work experience. Acquiring professional skills early confers an advantage.

DOI: 10.1201/9781003633389-51

- **Stealth Influences**. The hidden curriculum imparts strong influences that can fundamentally change you in ways you might not recognize. For example, trainees conform to norms and are taught to don a "*cloak of competence*."[14]
- **Ripple Effects**. Since every topic of the hidden curriculum is connected, one small change can have widespread ripple effects. For example, improved EC can enhance learning, well-being, negotiation ability, leadership, and patient care.
- **Accountability and Incentive**. The single person with the most vested interest in your success is you. You cannot count on the system to bring you everything you need to succeed on a silver platter.

Where the Hidden Curriculum Comes from and How to Manage It

Creating this book was like piecing together a complex puzzle, requiring a broad view of the human condition, our societal and professional environment, and historical factors that shape the hidden curriculum. Historical factors include several key historical influencers such as William Halsted who have had outsized enduring impacts. There are others too worth recognizing even though we did not explore their impact in depth (Figures 46.1 and 46.2).[533,535,710]

The proximate sources of the hidden curriculum, such as interpersonal interactions, operate within this historical context. This exploration extended beyond traditional teachings, drawing on disciplines like organizational psychology, social psychology, communication, and philosophy. Every topic in this book is like a puzzle piece and interconnected when looking at the big picture.

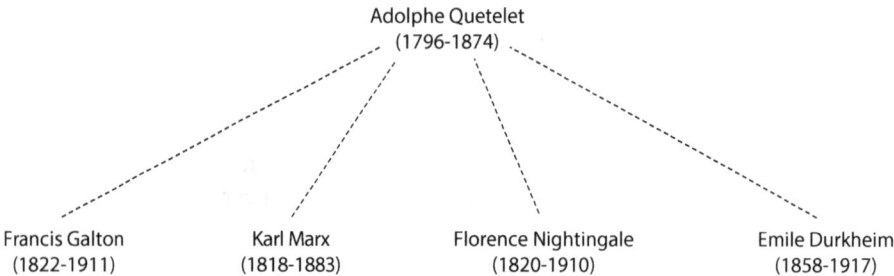

Adolphe Quetelet
(1796-1874)

| Francis Galton | Karl Marx | Florence Nightingale | Emile Durkheim |
| (1822-1911) | (1818-1883) | (1820-1910) | (1858-1917) |

Figure 46.1 The enduring outsized influence of small networks of people. Today, we remain under the heavy influence of disproportionately influential individuals who lived centuries ago, some of whom are not widely mentioned or recognized in medical education. The enduring influence often starts with a direct impact of one influential person on other key impactful individuals. Consider the Belgian astronomer and mathematician Adolphe Quetelet, who could be considered the forefather of modern social and behavioral sciences. He thought that the range of errors seen in astronomical measurements could apply to ranges of human traits, thus planting the seed of the concept of the normal curve (which was formalized later). He directly influenced Francis Galton (a pioneer of statistics who also coined the term eugenics), Karl Marx (a promulgator of conflict theory), Florence Nightingale (a nurse known for sanitation reforms and applied statistics), and Emile Durkheim (a pioneer of sociology who defined the basic tacit expectations, described the functional definition of religion, and explored societal influences on suicide among other things). Through multiple channels, Adolphe Quetelet had a profound, enduring effect on science and medicine.[533,710]

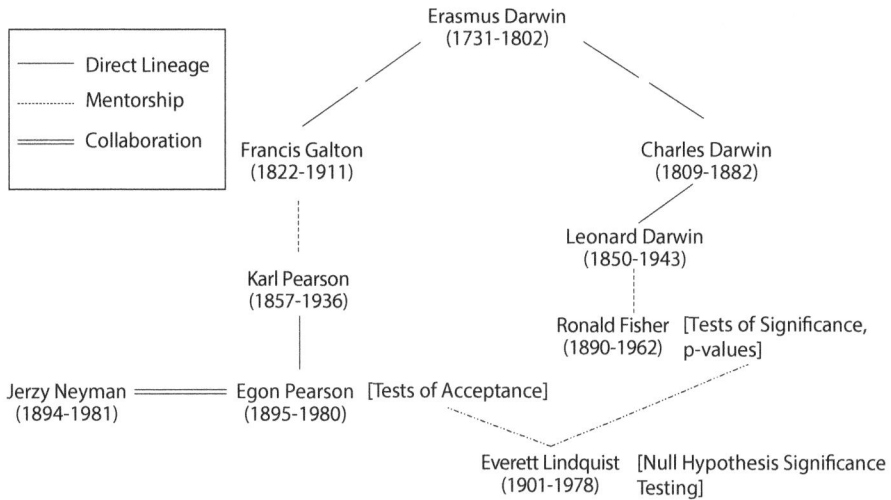

Figure 46.2 Another example of the enduring impact of key influential individuals, tracing a lineage (genetic, mentor-based, and collaboration-based) that shows the origins of modern statistical tests.[535] Many of the individuals in this chain were prominent proponents of highly problematic eugenic viewpoints. Erasmus Darwin was a prominent physician and intellectual of his day. He was grandfather to both Charles Darwin and Francis Galton. Galton has been called the "grandfather" of statistics, as he used new statistical methods to study heredity and coined the term "eugenics," with the aim of improving humanity with selective breeding. His protégé Karl Pearson invented many new statistical techniques still in use today, while the younger Ronald Fisher formally described p-values and statistical testing. Karl Pearson's son, Egon Pearson, and his collaborator Jerzy Neyman introduced statistical acceptance. The concepts of Fisher and Neyman-Pearson were reconciled and adapted to NHST, first by Lindquist. Additional methods to overcome the limitations of this approach have continued to be described.

One challenge for us was the inconsistent definition of the hidden curriculum, which has been viewed from many angles. This likely stems from the many forces influencing our professional experiences, often operating beneath the surface. While this book focused mostly on external forces, we also considered internal forces like self-expectations and defense mechanisms to cope with uncomfortable experiences (e.g., dark humor) and ego defense (e.g., denial). All these facets have the potential to significantly impact your professional trajectory.

The good news is that you can increase your control by understanding these hidden forces and implementing tactics centered around the six central strategies. While each strategy has specific applications in medicine, they also draw on insights from diverse fields. Similar advice has been offered in other arenas. For example, Dale Carnegie, citing Henry Ford, stated, "If there is any one secret of success, it lies in the ability to get the other person's point of view."[176]

But you can achieve even more. Gaining that incremental edge requires work, effort, and planning. However, hard work and effort are not synonymous with misery; in fact, they are often the opposite. The more invested you are (while maintaining balance), the more enjoyable and rewarding training becomes. This also requires humility: acknowledging your biases and areas for improvement and recognizing that your ego can be your greatest obstacle. While some trainees may have natural talents in certain areas, no one can reach their full potential in medicine without effort and planning.

This brings us to the final message: reading this book and understanding the information is necessary, but not sufficient. The six core strategies require deliberate practice in the real world to be effective—that is, to be translated into expertise. It's possible to know what to do but fail to act. So, what can you do?

Everyone is unique, and there's no single road map. Start by tackling the basic, easy things first. Then, focus on one or two areas at a time, making a deliberate daily effort. Everything you see, say, write, and do is an opportunity to master these strategies.

47

Becoming an Expert

Vance T. Lehman

Mastering the hidden curriculum can help you gain the wisdom and skills needed to become an expert. This chapter will explore key concepts to help you achieve this goal. To do this, we'll connect many key topics, focusing on the value of multidisciplinary knowledge, the nature of wisdom, continued professional growth, and the importance of environment and mindset.

The Value of Multidisciplinary Knowledge

While the formal curriculum equips trainees with direct professional skills, it focuses less on building a foundation for wisdom. Consider how Kuhn reimagined the nature of science and scientific revolutions. Stepping outside of a one-dimensional scientific analysis, he integrated concepts from sociology, history, philosophy, and science to provide a more complete and insightful viewpoint.[527]

Kuhn believed that the narrow pedagogy of formal textbook teachings indoctrinates and misleads science students, leaving them stuck in the dominant paradigm.[527] Textbooks (or modern equivalents), he said, shortchange historical nuances, downplaying past and present uncertainty. They also attempt to prop up a few heroes we can aspire to be like, but this is misleading since discoveries are rarely made in isolation or at a single time point.

There are parallels in medicine, as the formal curriculum and medical textbooks can understate historical influences and oversimplify many things. While comprehensive textbooks (or their equivalents) are preferable to shortcut learning methods, it is useful to view their contents through a multidisciplinary lens and in historical context.

I have attempted to lay such groundwork in this book, with often-untaught information from many disciplines like organization psychology, history, communication studies, complexity science (next chapter), and much more. This approach provides a richer background that is enormously helpful for understanding how medicine evolves and how it fits into the big picture of society and our patients' lives. This perspective is at the heart of general medical wisdom.

Wisdom

Applying Multidisciplinary Knowledge

Building upon this concept of integrating diverse perspectives, we now turn to a deeper exploration of wisdom in medical practice. Specifically, wisdom implies that physicians are familiar with the relevant social, psychological, philosophical, and ethical contexts of medicine. Medicine is not pure science but a more complex discipline created to serve societal needs and,

DOI: 10.1201/9781003633389-52

more directly, the needs of the patient before you. A rich background helps physicians manage uncertainty and nuance, think logically, see through hype and premature predictions, and interpret literature deeper than the headline message. This wisdom is one element that helps separate a physician from a technical professional.

Beyond the general considerations of humanity topics, your individual history matters too. As you approach problems, whether in research or clinical settings, recall that our observations and viewpoints are *theory-laden* in that we view them through the lens of past experiences and education (Chapter 26). Thus, we should remain aware of our individual environment, viewpoints, and biases that could affect our approach to patient care.

Meditation and Mindfulness

Another important avenue to wisdom and compassion is meditation and mindfulness. One of the goals of these practices is achieving higher levels of wisdom, including of the hidden forces that societal complexity, coincidence, and evolutionary biology exert on those around us.[122] Through this wisdom, we can understand life stressors; relinquish unrealistic illusions of control; clarify our priorities and values; and improve our compassion. In other words, one thing we can do through mindful reflection is set a framework to contextualize information.

Wisdom Is Different than Information

Wisdom, however, is different than information. Having information or knowledge does not ensure that you have the judgment to assess its validity and to know if or how to apply it. Recall that experience is the catalyst that converts information to knowledge and knowledge to wisdom.

In addition, it takes wisdom to know how to manage information overload, one of the major challenges facing us today.[711] We must manage an information deluge of learning resources, websites, meetings, emails, in-box messages, and more.[712-714] Information overload has been associated with stress, burnout, difficulty finding important information, and impaired decision-making.[712-714] A wise approach manages knowledge using hierarchy of learning material, optimized literature search strategies, EBM, problem-solving strategies, and productivity measures.

In sum, your patients and society will expect that you are wise. When you appraise a situation and offer a recommendation, they rightfully assume a lot of background knowledge and experience underlies the decision. With the rise of disinformation and distrust in higher institutions, physician credibility and wisdom are as important as ever.

Some Professionals Plateau, and Others Become Experts

We already highlighted the importance of active learning and deliberate practice, but let's now consider how easy it is for deliberate practice to wane over time with a brief analogy. Let's say at the beginning of a training program your goal is to arm curl 25 pounds with perfect form for 2 sets of 10 repetitions. You start at 12 pounds, move up to 15, then 20, and by the end of training you are doing 25 pounds just as you had hoped. Then, when you leave training, you are less accountable to coaches, and you can get by doing just 20 pounds for the repetitions, so that is what you do. Then, no matter how many years you spend doing it, you will likely lose ground over time.

The same concept is true in medicine. Some of us will plateau or even experience a decline in ability at some point in our careers, while others will defy the notion of a professional ceiling effect and continue to improve.[716] It turns out that this difference is not accounted for by pure innate talent or the number of hours of practice. The reasons are similar to the arm curl analogy.

If you stop pushing yourself, you will plateau. Our natural tendency is to take this path of least resistance, and this temptation is heightened by the temptation of delayed gratification after years of sacrifice. Remember, achieving expertise takes many years of continued effort, even after formal training is complete.

These experts generally practice and excel at two categories of cognitive processes.[716] The first category is pattern recognition for commonly encountered scenarios. In clinical medicine, these patterns are part of *clinical schemas* that develop with experience and are aligned with System 1 thinking. The second category is refined problem-solving skills for novel scenarios and are aligned with System 2 thinking.

The Importance of Environment and Mindset

Practice Environment

In addition, it helps to practice in an environment that fosters System 2 thinking through clinical challenges, but even then, there is not enough feedback from clinical encounters alone.[716] Thus, you need supplemental challenges that push you beyond prior boundaries. It is also important to be available as a consultant to colleagues when they encounter challenging patient care dilemmas in your area of expertise. Further, just as chess masters study the moves of other chess masters, master clinicians study the practices of other master clinicians.[716]

Fortunately, you can gain expertise through different paths in a variety of environments. For example, physicians who serve rural areas might not see as many rare conditions but may develop expertise in serving the broad needs of their local population and their individual patients. The common thread in all instances though, from rural primary care to subspecialized metropolitan medicine, is complexity.

Mindset

Beyond your environment, simply identifying as someone who pursues expertise in a field is a key step. Cutting-edge performance also incorporates many other concepts we have discussed. These include active participation in multidisciplinary conferences, national or international meetings, critical appraisal of the literature, and teaching. Your aptitude for decision-making strategies like using System 2 thinking for difficult cases or self-audits of biases risk becoming stale without deliberate measures.

Conclusion

Overall, becoming an expert in medicine requires years of deliberate practice in part because it is a highly complex discipline. We introduced the idea of deliberate practice in Chapter 3 on learning and that of complexity in medical decision-making in Chapter 5. Next, in our last chapter, we'll look deeper into the often-neglected topic of complexity and why it matters in medical practice.

48

Complexity, Connections, and Chaos

Vance T. Lehman

Now that we have explored the topics of the hidden curriculum, imagine yourself in a few common scenarios:

- During the first year of medical school, you memorize the microscopic chemical composition of amino acids in proteins and the microanatomical structure of sarcomeres in muscle (along with many other basic science concepts) but are unsure how these explain the clinically applicable properties of proteins or muscles. Beyond short-term memorization for the test, you never quite sort it out and so forget a lot of the details along the way.
- During the first year of medical school, you memorize a vast number of anatomic structures one by one—for example, blood vessels and major airway channels—but are not taught the big picture patterns about why the larger systems work so efficiently. You briefly notice there are similarities to other things in nature like tree branches but cannot determine why this might be.
- During your early clinical rotations, you are considering a career in radiology, but you overhear an attending predict that the specialty will be extinct within a decade because of AI, so you start considering other options. A few years later, radiology is flourishing, and you, having gone another route, wonder if you have chosen the best-fit field for your career.
- During your early clinical rotations, you do one thing well at the beginning of a rotation (arriving the first day prepared, with notes and enthusiasm), make a great first impression, and have a subsequent series of positive experiences, opening doors to additional opportunities. Among these is the opportunity to be mentored by an esteemed and well-connected attending in this area. The attending gladly uses these connections to set you up with important collaborative projects and influential people at various other institutions.
- During residency, you are evaluating a patient in clinic with several chronic conditions. These all seem important to treat, but you pick one you think is the best to prioritize with the most aggressive treatment. However, the patient has an allergy to the first-line treatment for this condition. The second-line treatment has potential to exacerbate his other chronic conditions. You look to the evidence, but all the RCTs have very strict inclusion criteria and cannot provide a clear answer to the best treatment approach in this unique situation.

What these (and most) scenarios and topics in this book have in common is *complexity*.

 DOI: 10.1201/9781003633389-53

Basic Complexity Concepts

Medical training is far more complex than what is formally taught, and this complexity permeates every aspect of the hidden curriculum. Understanding and managing this complexity is crucial for success in modern medicine. For decades, medical education has emphasized reductionist thinking, breaking down problems into their smallest components and assuming that understanding the parts will reveal the whole. Complexity science is a reaction to reductionism, focusing on the broader effects.

Challenges Arising from Reductionism

While reductionism has its place, over-reliance on this approach presents several challenges:

1) **Information Overload**. The sheer volume of detail to memorize becomes overwhelming.
2) **Lack of Clinical Relevance**. It's often unclear how specific details apply to daily clinical practice.
3) **Inability to Explain Macroscopic Properties**. Details often fail to explain properties of complex systems, such as self-organization and emergence (discussed in the following section).

In fact, reductionism sometimes leads us astray. For instance, antioxidants show promise for cancer prevention in the laboratory, but antioxidant supplementation has not borne out for this purpose in real-life studies.[717] Furthermore, traditional thinking often idealizes problems, portraying them as solvable with predictable outcomes and linear dose-response curves, for example. With complexity, problems do not always have a perfect solution; there is no predictable repetition of conditions, and there may be sudden changes in state or exponential effects.

Sources of Complexity

Complexity arises from a combination of three main factors: (1) nonlinearity, (2) uncertainty, and (3) interdependence. Physicians often think linearly, but few things in medicine are truly linear.[718,719] Linear systems are additive (the sum of the individual components equals the whole), proportional (double the dose, double the effect), and amenable to reductionist analysis. Complex, nonlinear systems, like those in biology exhibit none of these properties. Furthermore, complex systems have areas of uncertainty. However, with complexity, even small areas of uncertainty can amplify and have widespread effects due to non-linearity and interconnectedness with other areas, eroding determinism.

To understand these effects in more depth, consider that nonlinearity results from threshold effects, feedback mechanisms, complex interconnections, or situations where an output becomes an input (like pathogen replication, for example). Furthermore, feedback mechanisms can be inhibitory and stabilizing or excitatory and amplifying. For example, recall the inverted U-curve of learning versus arousal, the nonlinear returns on work done in so-called greedy jobs, or the natural limitations humans have in understanding the exponential spread of some infectious diseases like COVID-19.[718]

Many other examples in medicine range from a U-shaped association between BMI and all-cause mortality to complex exponential relationships between social media use and negative impact on well-being.[612,720] The butterfly effect reflects that nonlinear processes can amplify a minuscule uncertainty (or difference) to momentous changes in outcome.

Basic Features of Complex Systems

Complex systems are comprised of multiple interdependent parts functioning as networks *without central organization*. These networks tend toward certain states called *attractors*. Complex systems can *self-organize* and acquire *emergent properties* that are difficult to predict from the individual components. Examples of self-organization include bacterial colony formation, protein folding, and the organization of cellular contents. Examples of emergent properties include consciousness (which cannot be fully explained by studying individual neurons) and the phenotypes of *multimorbidity* (which cannot be fully characterized as the sum of individual diseases).[683]

Networks

Complex systems often function as networks, with nodes connected by lines (called edges). One example is the *small world network*, where connections are neither completely regular nor completely random. Components have relatively low degrees of separation but few direct contacts (Figure 48.1).[721,722] Think of it this way: though you likely don't know your country's leader directly, you're probably only a few degrees of separation away from each other.

The small world network model also acknowledges that some individuals, like influencers or established professionals, have more connections than others. This explains the power of well-connected mentors and social media. To collaborate with someone, you don't need a direct connection; a mutual contact will suffice. This model also helps explain other important

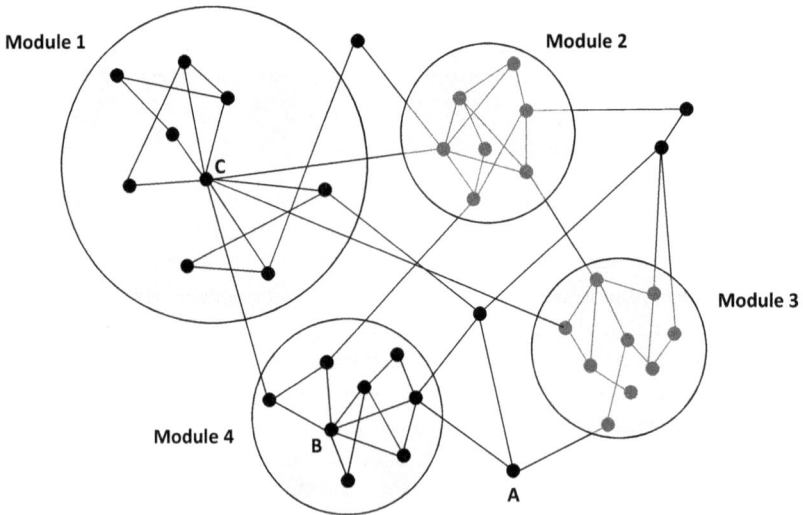

Figure 48.1 An example of a small world network. The black circles are nodes and lines are edges. The nodes could represent people, brain regions, etc. while the lines represent connections. The small world network is not entirely random but not entirely regular either. There is a short average path length from one node to another (degrees of separation) and areas of clustering (gray circles, also called modules). While most connections occur in clusters within a module (among neighbors), there are a few connections between modules too. Even a few long-distance connections from one module to another can help create a small world network. Node A, as an example, is six or fewer connections removed from any other node. Node B is a *provincial hub*, such as a local celebrity. Node C is a *connector hub* that links several modules.

topics you will encounter in your career, ranging from how rumors spread to how brain networks work.[723]

Fractals: Scale-Free Patterns in Space and Time

From a geometric perspective, complexity often generates, and reflects, fractals—self-similar patterns at different scales. Consider the branching airways: zoom in, and you'll see a similar, smaller branching pattern throughout the lung parenchyma. Zoom in again, and the pattern repeats. Fractals are abundant in anatomy and physiology, forming blood vessels, airways, urinary collecting systems, cardiac nerve pathways, heart rate variability patterns, and brain wave activity.[711,724,725] They're also found in epidemiological patterns of seasonal infectious diseases.[711]

Fractal organization is spatially efficient, allowing a large surface area to be compacted into a small space with effective distribution.[711] Fractal physiology reflects adaptability, such as a healthy heart's ability to handle different stress levels. Fractal patterns are also information-efficient, allowing DNA sequences to prescribe general self-similar patterns instead of every detail. This concept helps us understand biology on multiple levels.

The Unpredictability of Open Systems

Complexity analysis recognizes the impact of operating within *open systems*. *Closed systems* are isolated from outside influence, while open systems are subject to external factors. In medicine, we almost always deal with open systems. This means we can't know or control all the influences for a given situation, leading to unexpected and variable effects.

Unintended Consequences and Forecasts

A key outcome of complexity is unintended consequences. Just as weather, economic, or political forecasts have limitations, complexity leads to unpredictable results in medicine. While foresight can prevent some unintended consequences, those arising from complexity are inherently unpredictable.[726] Medical training is rife with examples of such unintended consequences, from the *Flexner Report* to P/F grading schemes and well-being initiatives. While we can't always manage these consequences, awareness is key.

Experts have also made inaccurate predictions, such as the claim that radiologists' jobs would disappear due to AI.[727] Even medical insiders, top scientists, and other leaders in the field struggle to predict the future. Implementation of gene therapies was slower than expected due to unforeseen complexities.[728]

As another example, while we can guess at trends like increased technology, transitions to minimally invasive or noninvasive interventions, and molecular diagnostics, the future of any specialty is uncertain. Consider vascular interventional radiology: once a field threatened by vascular surgeons, it has flourished due to innovations like targeted chemotherapy. Vascular surgeons, disrupted by interventional radiology, adapted and thrived. Molecular imaging, once seemingly stagnant, is now transforming medicine through theranostics.

Subspecialization Is a Double-Edged Sword

Medicine has responded to increasing complexity with increasing subspecialization.[519] While offering benefits, such as expertise in specific conditions and improved outcomes, subspecialization also has drawbacks. Benefits include in-depth knowledge, access to experts, and potentially better outcomes. Subspecialization also provides clarity on the limits of medical knowledge.

A major drawback is that subspecialization creates trade-offs between general and narrow knowledge. Specialists may overlook diagnoses outside their expertise, and care gaps can arise when patients are treated by multiple specialists. Subspecialization can also hinder innovation by limiting cross-fertilization of ideas. A historical example of cross-fertilization of ideas was when Dr. Walter Dandy pioneered pneumoencephalography, a revolutionary method to assess intracranial mass effect with introduction of air into the ventricles, during a less-specialized era, after observing free air on an abdominal radiograph.[131]

Navigating Subspecialization and Information Overload

Increasing subspecialization presents several challenges for trainees, including the following:

- **Choosing a Specialty**. Carefully consider your desired degree of specialization, as this decision will significantly impact your career. There are now more choices than ever and it is difficult to know about all of the possibilities when you select a residency. The need to determine your desired degree of specialization is also greater than ever.
- **Balancing Knowledge**. There are no definitive guides to help us maintain a balance between general and specialized knowledge.
- **Practicing Teamwork**. The need for effective teamwork skills for patient care and research is greater than ever, as multiple specialists must work together, including the need to share perspectives to promote cross-fertilization of ideas and to take measures to manage knowledge gaps.

The ever-increasing volume of medical information is impossible to master. To manage this challenge:

- **Manage Your Hierarchy of Knowledge**. Prioritize information based on its relevance to your practice.
- **Stay Current**. Read the latest issues of flagship journals and attend major conferences.
- **Utilize Synthesis Resources**. Identify reliable sources for meta-analyses, expert opinions, and review articles.
- **Review General Medical Journals**. Read journals like *NEJM* and *Mayo Clinic Proceedings* for high-quality educational content.

Complex Diagnoses

Medical analyses are now *informed by* guidelines, clinical decision support, and AI, but the final determinations are still very human. However, even when there is high-quality evidence such as RCTs to guide clinical decision making, it can still be challenging to weigh the pros and cons of different interventions for a given clinical situation. Specifically, the inclusion/exclusion criteria of RCTs are often so stringent that the results have limited applicability to patients with multimorbidity.

To address such situations, clinicians can rely on the heuristics of System 1 thinking to make their best experience-based recommendation based on the constellation of clinical considerations. However, this approach has potential to lead clinicians astray. Alternative approaches include using complexity principles or other advanced analyses like medical decision analysis.[729]

A special case of complexity in medicine though is managing situations that are not found in any textbook or literature search, because the presentation is atypical. This is where we need to check that we are using System 2 problem-solving mode. These situations arise because of innumerable possible afflictions, pathologic variants, comorbidities, and points of inter-individual variability. There are many rare conditions (aka *zebras*) that while individually are unlikely to occur, still crop up commonly, because there are many zebra possibilities, diagnostic methods are constantly improving, and available literature is never entirely up to date.

Occasionally, a zebra should be the favored diagnosis. In radiology, when we see something that is completely pathognomonic, albeit rare, there is no real differential diagnosis. For example, on imaging, I've seen a teratoma (a benign tumor containing heterotopic tissues) in a highly unusual anatomic location. While I second-guessed the diagnosis initially due to the atypical anatomic site, I realized that the only entity with those particular radiographic features is teratoma. So that's what I called it. And pathology evaluation after removal confirmed that's what it was.

In general though, for classic or atypical presentations alike, it is useful to consider the approach of proof by reasonable elimination of alternative possibilities. Medical education tends to overemphasize classic presentations, and we can overfit a clinical scenario into our clinical schemas if we do not consider other diagnoses. This means we should consider uncommon possibilities but maintain a high threshold to favor them over common ones.

In real life, patients often have multiple conditions, or *multimorbidity*, and as mentioned, the patterns of disease findings or types of treatments may not be a simple sum of the individual diagnoses.[683,730–732] These patients often have (or develop) mental health considerations as well.[733] Medical guidelines tend to focus on single, rather than multimorbid, states, but the sum of all guideline recommendations for a patient with multiple comorbidities is often suboptimal, resulting in polypharmacy, fragmented delivery of care, and overly burdensome follow-up schedules.[733] As we mentioned in Part I, with the current system care of such complex patients relies on street smarts in addition to book smarts.

Complexity and Evidence

Complexity in medicine and related sciences has important implications for statistical analysis, research methodology, and EBM. As mentioned, there are debates over modern applications of NHST and falsification in complex situations. Additionally, the usefulness of pure academic principles in real life has been questioned in many areas, including negotiation, engineering, economics, investing, and medicine.[111,500,734] From this viewpoint, the value of academic theory over real-life experience is often overblown.

Regardless, it turns out that the analytic techniques used in EBM were originally designed to be relatively simple and thus accessible to the typical clinician. In fact, the first guidelines published in 1993 included only two measures to assess study strength of evidence and two to assess risk of bias.[735] However, many new measures have since been introduced as an attempt to refine these assessments. A potential problem is that these new tools are complex, risking lower author compliance.[734] Thus, some authors have called for a return to a simpler EBM approach.[733] For now, it may be best to understand the overarching concepts but leave the details to scientific methods experts.

The Widespread Impact of Complexity in Medicine

In medicine, we face a host of complex challenges. When I first wrote this chapter, I attempted to construct a table of all the areas we can understand better through the lens of complexity that I uncovered while researching this book. This list included topics in education, organizational/business studies, medical practice, and more. I had to stop when the list hit several dozen. In the end, I realized that it is difficult to find a topic in this book that is not complex.

I did not begin writing this book with complexity in mind; it bubbled to the surface organically. So, my message to you is this: the sooner you understand the basic principles of complexity, the sooner you will see how it impacts your experience in medicine on many fronts. Interestingly, the study of complexity science *simplifies* a great many things. That is, nature and life have a way of producing the same patterns—like emergence or fractals described earlier—in many different settings.

In fact, this is the structure of life and human interactions. By excluding these concepts, the medical curriculum can lead us astray, down the erroneous path of never-ending reductionism and forgetting. This is not to say that details do not matter, because they can be critical. It is just that the big picture, organization, and final effects often matter more. To further make the point, here is just one additional common pattern in complexity that needs mention—a *hierarchical nested organization*.

Nested Hierarchies

Once you recognize that hierarchy is found in biological materials like DNA and bone, for example, it becomes much easier to remember both the fine details and the final function. On the molecular scale, one pattern found is twists and turns, such as the double helix of DNA or the triple helix of collagen in bone. On larger scales, there is another layer of folding and organization such as the packing of DNA around histones and organization of collagen fibers within osseous lamellae. At larger scales, there are chromosomes and osteons, respectively.

Nested hierarchy allows for incredibly efficient packing, interweaving of composites, and exquisite structural properties that engineers could only dream of. The resultant mineral-protein composite structure of bone has both strength to resist deformation under stress and toughness to resist fracture, features that are typically trade-offs in man-made products.[734] Glass, for example, is strong but brittle, while a rubber band is weak but fracture resistant.[734] DNA, on the other hand, has far more information-carrying capacity than any state-of-the-art computer chip.[736] While the molecular bonds matter, the final effects of structural stability and information are most important.

Additionally, notice that nested hierarchies are found in other social structures and broader concepts discussed in this book, like culture and change.

Chaos and The Butterfly Effect

The concept of chaos and complexity are related, but chaos describes something specific.[737] In brief, chaos finds that even a few deterministic rules can collectively create a system that superficially looks entirely random and *chaotic* but truly has an underlying order.[711]

This order may be a strange attractor governed by fractal geometry in which two very similar starting conditions that differ by no more than a rounding error can diverge drastically through nonlinear effects and interdependence. The technical term for this is *sensitive dependence on initial conditions*, but colloquially, this has become known as the butterfly effect.

Recall our opening scenario of you and Claire dashing for the airport amid a traffic jam. Claire, who made it to her medical school interview thanks to just one piece of insider knowledge, could experience further career-altering or life-altering downstream effects as a result. Perhaps she is connected to a mentor who sparks an interest in a field she had not previously considered but turns out to be a perfect fit. She goes on to publish extensively in this field, is frequently invited to deliver international talks, and makes a landmark discovery. No one can ever access every perfect opportunity at every fork in the road, but certainly, daily parallels arise when trainees do just one small thing right that finds that first domino and leads to large rewards later.

Our scenario is not an extreme reflection of the sensitive dependence on initial conditions. Missing a flight is a bit more than a small rounding error. Still, the important message is that relatively minor situations can amplify over time. The more steps you can take, large or small, to stack the deck in your favor, the better your odds are of a final favorable outcome.

We discussed some other possible butterfly effects too. The initial conditions of our modern training paradigm set up by the *Big Four* (introduced in Chapter 6) still have a resounding influence today, for example. If they had taken a different philosophy, the *Flexner Report* and other downstream effects might have been entirely different. More immediately, we have many opportunities to recalibrate our *initial conditions* during training, as it is a time of many life changes. And finally, the impact of first impressions, labels, and rumors, certainly seems like a setup for butterfly effects.

Perhaps how chaos relates to career expectations though is the most fitting final message about complexity.[738] We live and work in an open system and cannot possibly know, much less control, all the factors that affect our personal and professional success. Thus, a pragmatic approach is to brace for unforeseen effects.

Some setbacks will inevitably occur and, when they do, we cannot let the unforeseeable aspects control us and allow our self-confidence and self-image to deteriorate.[736] Conversely, while we deserve to celebrate our successes, we should be careful not to become complacent by overattributing all to pure talent.[738] Chaos tells us that, after we have done everything possible to turn things in our favor, we should accept that some things are ultimately out of our control and learn to take them in stride.

Key Takeaways

So, here are four things to keep in your back pocket:

- Complexity does not mean randomness but instead points to patterns. These are seen as fractals or as emergent, self-organizing, and network properties, for example. These same patterns are found across disciplines from medicine to meteorology and beyond. Once you recognize these patterns, you will start to find them all around.
- A complex situation—whether it is multimorbidity, a team dynamic, or anything else—is not the sum of its parts, but instead something new.
- When we need to solve problems because our simplified models are insufficient, we may need to consider complexity to find solutions.
- Approximations and small variances do not always cancel during a process but instead can amplify, leading to widely divergent outcomes via the butterfly effect.

Conclusion

Your Hero Journey

In his book on storytelling *The Writer's Journey*, Christopher Vogler describes the steps the define hero stories that transcend time and cultures.[739] In brief, the main character has a calling to leave her normal, comfortable life for an adventure. Reluctant to accept the calling, she is convinced only with the encouragement and guidance of a mentor. She faces mountainous challenges, often culminating in the discovery and defeat of a hidden foe. After overcoming the challenges, she achieves elevated status as a member of an exclusive group. In the end, she returns home enlightened and transformed and can use her newfound abilities for the benefit of her people.

This archetypal journey, while seemingly fantastical, resonates broadly with the experiences of medical trainees and parallels several key concepts in this book. Having a calling (yes, despite the controversy mentioned earlier, I still believe that medicine is a calling), encountering overt and hidden challenges, realizing the need to seek guidance from experienced mentors, and, finally, making a transformation. I hope this book has helped clear away the brush—the hidden curriculum—from the often overgrown, windy, and unmarked pathway of your journey and has revealed ways to unlock personal and professional success.

References

1. Bruni R. The most important thing I teach my student isn't on the syllabus. *The New York Times*. 2024. https://www.nytimes.com/2024/04/20/opinion/students-humility-american-politics.html

2. Lawrence C, et al. The hidden curricula of medical education: A scoping review. *Acad Med* 2018. doi: 10.1097/acm.0000000000002004

3. Pourbairamian G, et al. Hidden curriculum in medical residency programs: A scoping review. *J Adv Med Educ Prof* 2022. doi: 10.30476/jamp.2021.92478.1486

4. Brosnan SF, et al. Mechanisms underlying responses to inequitable outcomes in chimpanzees, Pan troglodytes. *Anim Behav* 2010. doi: 10.1016/j.anbehav.2010.02.019

5. Lehmann LS, et al. Hidden curricula, ethics, and professionalism: Optimizing clinical learning environments in becoming and being a physician: A position paper of the American College of Physicians. *Ann Intern Med* 2018. doi: 10.7326/m17-2058

6. Braschi E, et al. Evidence-based medicine, shared decision making and the hidden curriculum: A qualitative content analysis. *Perspect Med Educ* 2020. doi: 10.1007/S40037-020-00578-0

7. Kentli FD. Comparison of hidden curriculum theories. European Journal of Educational Studies. *Eur J Edu Stud* 2009. https://www.researchgate.net/publication/265989584_Comparison_of_hidden_curriculum_theories

8. Gable R. *The Hidden Curriculum: First Generation Students at Legacy Universities*. Princeton: Princeton University Press; 2021. ISBN: 9780691216614

9. Moss DM. The hidden curriculum of legal education: Toward a holistic model for reform journal of dispute resolution. *Journal of Dispute Resolution*. 2013. https://scholarship.law.missouri.edu/jdr/vol2013/iss1/3/

10. Hafferty FW. Beyond curriculum reform: Confronting medicine's hidden curriculum. Academic Medicine. *Academic Medicine*; 1998. doi: 10.1097/00001888-199804000-00013

11. Becker HS, et al. *Boys in White: Student Culture in Medical School*. Chicago: University of Chicago Press; 1961. ISBN: 9781412818865

12. Merton RK. *The Student-Physician: Introductory Studies in the Sociology of Medical Education*. Oxford: Oxford University Press; 1957. ISBN: 9780674366824

13. Shem S. *House of God*. New York City: Delta Trade Paperbacks; 2003. ISBN: 9780385337380

14. Haas J, et al. Cl the professionalization of medical students: Developing competence and a cloak of competence. *Symbol Int* 1977. doi: 10.1525/si.1977.1.1.71

15. Haas J, et al. Ritual evaluation of competence: The hidden curriculum of professionalization in an innovative medical school program. *Work Occup* 1982. doi: 10.1177/0730888482009002001

16. Hafferty FW, et al. The Hidden Curriculum and Anatomy Education. In: Chan LK, et al., editors. *Teaching Anatomy: A Practical Guide*. Cham: Springer International Publishing; 2015. p. 339–349. 978-3-319-08930-0

17. Hafferty FW, et al. The hidden curriculum, ethics teaching, and the structure of medical education. *Acad Med* 1994. doi: 10.1097/00001888-199411000-00001

18. Rauf A, et al. Development and validation of a questionnaire about hidden curriculum in medical institutes: A pilot study. *Front Med (Lausanne)* 2023. doi: 10.3389/fmed.2023.996759

19. Papadakis MA, et al. Unprofessional behavior in medical school is associated with subsequent disciplinary action by a state medical board. *Acad Med* 2004. doi: 10.1097/00001888-200403000-00011

20. Rist RC. Student social class and teacher expecatations: The self-fulfilling prophecy in ghetto education. *Harvard Educational Review*. Fall 2000. https://faculty.washington.edu/rsoder/EDUC305/310RistHarvardEdReview.pdf

21. Zazulia AR, et al. *Teach Learn Med* 2014. doi: 10.1080/10401334.2014.945028

22. MacLeod A. *Med Teach* 2014. doi: 10.3109/0142159X.2014.907876

23. Chen PW. *The New York Times*. 2009. https://www.nytimes.com/2009/01/30/health/29chen.html

24. Stanek A, et al. Depictions of the hidden curriculum in medical television programs. *BMC Med Educ* 2015. doi: 10.1186/s12909-015-0437-8

25. Ewen S, et al. Exposing the hidden curriculum influencing medical education on the health of Indigenous people in Australia and New Zealand: The role of the Critical Reflection Tool. *Acad Med* 2012. doi: 10.1097/ACM.0b013e31823fd777

26. Galam E. Becoming doctor: Highlight the hidden curriculum. Medical error as an example. *Presse Med* 2014. doi: 10.1016/j.lpm.2013.06.031

27. Hao F, et al. Construction of hidden curriculum in the academic experience inheritance of distinguished TCM veteran doctors. *Zhongguo Zhen Jiu* 2019. doi: 10.13703/j.0255-2930.2019.11.024

28. Howick J, et al. Towards an empathic hidden curriculum in medical school: A roadmap. *J Eval Clin Pract* 2024. doi: 10.1111/jep.13966

29. Kang YJ, et al. The hidden hurdles of clinical clerkship: Unraveling the types and distribution of professionalism dilemmas among South Korean medical students. *BMC Med Educ* 2024. doi: 10.1186/s12909-024-05115-9

30. Karnieli-Miller O. Caring for the health and well-being of our learners in medicine as critical actions toward high-quality care. *Isr J Health Policy Res* 2022. doi: 10.1186/s13584-022-00517-w

31. Keis O, et al. How do German medical students perceive role models during clinical placements ("Famulatur")? An empirical study. *BMC Med Educ* 2019. doi: 10.1186/s12909-019-1624-9

32. Kulkarni P, et al. Medical education in India: Past, present, and future. *APIK J Int Med* 2019. doi: 10.4103/AJIM.AJIM_13_19

33. Ludwig B, et al. The search for attitude-a hidden curriculum assessment from a central European perspective. *Wien Klin Wochenschr* 2018. doi: 10.1007/s00508-018-1312-5

34. Mahood SC. Medical education: Beware the hidden curriculum. *Journal* 2011. PMID: 21918135.

35. Mulder H, et al. Addressing the hidden curriculum in the clinical workplace: A practical tool for trainees and faculty. *Med Teach* 2019. doi: 10.1080/0142159x.2018.1436760

36. Murakami M, et al. The perception of the hidden curriculum on medical education: An exploratory study. *Asia Pac Fam Med* 2009. doi: 10.1186/1447-056x-8-9

37. Nakamura A, et al. Impact of group work on the hidden curriculum that induces students' unprofessional behavior toward faculty. *BMC Med Educ* 2024. doi: 10.1186/s12909-024-05713-7

38. Safari Y, et al. The role of hidden curriculum in the formation of professional ethics in Iranian medical students: A qualitative study. *J Educ Health Promot* 2020. doi: 10.4103/jehp.jehp_172_20

39. Silveira GL, et al. The influences of the hidden curriculum on the professional identity development of medical students. *Health Prof Educ* 2019. doi: 10.1016/j.hpe.2018.07.003

40. Swanzen R, et al. Navigating the hidden curriculum: Reflections from graduates of a multidisciplinary postgraduate diploma in pediatric palliative care. *J Palliat Med* 2024. doi: 10.1089/jpm.2023.0470

41. Villanueva M. *Medical Training as a Transformative Experience: An Analysis of Doctorhood to Question the Professional Identity Formation Paradigm. Tapuya: Latin American Science, Technology and Society.* Tapuya: Latin American Science, *Technology and Society.* 2020. doi: 10.1080/25729861.2020.1754043

42. Atherley A, et al. Medical students' socialization tactics when entering a new clinical clerkship: A mixed methods study of proactivity. *Acad Med* 2022. doi: 10.1097/acm.0000000000004627

43. Young DG. *Wrong: How Media, Politics, and Identity Drive Our Appetite for Misinformation.* Baltimore: Johns Hopkins University Press; 2023. ISBN: 9781421447759

44. Brown PC, et al. *Make It Stick: The Science of Successful Learning.* Cambridge: The Belknap Press of Harvard University Press; 2014. ISBN: 9780674729018

45. Just M, et al. Watching the human brain process information. *Nieman Reports.* 2010. https://niemanreports.org/watching-the-human-brain-process-information/

46. Gardner H. *Frames of Mind: The Theory of Multiple Intelligences.* New York City: Basic Books Inc.; 1983. ISBN: 9780133306149

47. Goleman D. *Emotional Intelligence: The 25th Anniversary Edition.* New York City: Bantam Books; 2020. ISBN: 9780553383713

48. Visser BA, et al. Putting multiple intelligences theory to the test. *Intelligence* 2006. doi: 10.1016/j.intell.2006.02.004

49. White ND, et al. Goals in lifestyle medicine prescription. *Am J Lifestyle Med* 2020. doi: 10.1177/1559827620905775

50. Bjork RA, et al. Self-regulated learning: Beliefs, techniques, and illusions. *Annu Rev Psychol* 2013. doi: 10.1146/annurev-psych-113011-143823

51. Bickerdike A, et al. Learning strategies, study habits and social networking activity of undergraduate medical students. *Int J Med Educ* 2016. doi: 10.5116/ijme.576f.d074

52. Dandavino M, et al. Why medical students should learn how to teach. *Med Teach* 2007. doi: 10.1080/01421590701477449

53. Khalil MK, et al. Learning and study strategies correlate with medical students' performance in anatomical sciences. *Anat Sci Educ* 2018. doi: 10.1002/ase.1742

54. Martin IG, et al. Benefiting from clinical experience: The influence of learning style and clinical experience on performance in an undergraduate objective structured clinical examination. *Med Educ* 2000. doi: 10.1046/j.1365-2923.2000.00489.x

55. Mattick K, et al. Approaches to learning and studying in medical students: Validation of a revised inventory and its relation to student characteristics and performance. *Med Educ* 2004. doi: 10.1111/j.1365-2929.2004.01836.x

56. McManus IC, et al. Clinical experience, performance in final examinations, and learning style in medical students: Prospective study. *BMJ* 1998. doi: 10.1136/bmj.316.7128.345

57. Reid WA, et al. Relationship between assessment results and approaches to learning and studying in Year Two medical students. *Med Educ* 2007. doi: 10.1111/j.1365-2923.2007.02801.x

58. Dunlosky J, et al. Improving students' learning with effective learning techniques: Promising directions from cognitive and educational psychology. *Psychol Sci Public Interest* 2013. doi: 10.1177/1529100612453266

59. Immordino-Yang MH. Implications of affective and social neuroscience for educational theory. *Educ Philos Theory* 2011. doi: 10.1111/j.1469-5812.2010.00713.x

60. Mason HRC, et al. First-generation and continuing-generation college graduates' application, acceptance, and matriculation to U.S. medical schools: A national cohort study. *Med Educ Online* 2022. doi: 10.1080/10872981.2021.2010291

61. Thomas MH, et al. Learning by the keyword mnemonic: Looking for long-term benefits. *J Exp Psychol Appl* 1996. doi: 10.1037/1076-898X.2.4.330

62. Wang V. Killer loans—college debt triggers depression and suicide. *Salon.* 2019. https://www.salon.com/2019/06/01/killer-loans-college-debt-triggers-depression-and-suicide_partner/

63. Lakhlifi C, et al. Illusion of knowledge in statistics among clinicians: Evaluating the alignment between objective accuracy and subjective confidence, an online survey. *Cogn Res Princ Implic* 2023. doi: 10.1186/s41235-023-00474-1

64. Schwartzstein RM, et al. Saying goodbye to lectures in medical school — Paradigm shift or passing fad? *N Engl J Med* 2017. doi: 10.1056/NEJMp1706474

65. Eliseev ED, et al. Understanding why searching the internet inflates confidence in explanatory ability. *Appl Cogn Psychol* 2023. doi: 10.1002/acp.4058

66. Mills CM, et al. Knowing the limits of one's understanding: The development of an awareness of an illusion of explanatory depth. *J Exp Child Psychol* 2004. doi: 10.1016/j.jecp.2003.09.003

67. Baldi E, et al. The inverted "u-shaped" dose-effect relationships in learning and memory: Modulation of arousal and consolidation. *Nonlinearity Biol Toxicol Med* 2005. doi: 10.2201/nonlin.003.01.002

68. Ericsson KA, et al. The role of deliberate practice in the acquisition of expert performance. *APA PsycNet* 1993. doi: 10.1037/0033-295X.100.3.363

69. Smolen P, et al. The right time to learn: Mechanisms and optimization of spaced learning. *Nat Rev Neurosci* 2016. doi: 10.1038/nrn.2015.18

70. Sundem G. Everything you thought you knew about learning is wrong. How, and how not, to learn anything. *Psychology Today.* 2012. https://www.psychologytoday.com/us/blog/brain-candy/201201/everything-you-thought-you-knew-about-learning-is-wrong

71. Graves MF, et al. Effects of previewing difficult short stories on low ability junior high school students' comprehension, recall, and attitudes. *Read Res Q* 1983. doi: 10.2307/747388

72. Brame CJ. Effective educational videos: Principles and guidelines for maximizing student learning from video content. *CBE Life Sci Educ* 2016. doi: 10.1187/cbe.16-03-0125

73. Ploetzner R, et al. When learning from animations is more successful than learning from static pictures: Learning the specifics of change. Instructional Science. *Instr Sci* 2021. doi: 10.1007/s11251-021-09541-w

74. Amadieu F, et al. The attention-guiding effect and cognitive load in the comprehension of animations. *Comput Hum Behav* 2011. doi: 10.1016/j.chb.2010.05.009

75. Clemmons KR, et al. Educational videos versus question banks: Maximizing medical student performance on the united states medical licensing examination step 1 exam. *Cureus* 2023. doi: 10.7759/cureus.38110

76. Luo C, et al. Cl does youtube provide qualified patient education videos about atrial fibrillation? *Front Public Health* 2022. doi: 10.3389/fpubh.2022.925691

77. Senzaki S, et al. Reinventing flashcards to increase student learning. *Psychol Learn Teach* 2017. doi: 10.1177/1475725717719771

78. Kirschner PA, et al. An analysis of the failure of constructivist, discovery, problem-based, experiential, and inquiry-based teaching. *Educ Psychol* 2006. doi: 10.1207/s15326985ep4102_1

79. Szymczak JE, et al. Training for efficiency: Work, time, and systems-based practice in medical residency. *J Health Soc Behav* 2012. doi: 10.1177/0022146512451130

80. Rankin CH, et al. Habituation revisited: An updated and revised description of the behavioral characteristics of habituation. *Neurobiol Learn Mem* 2009. doi: 10.1016/j.nlm.2008.09.012

81. Sharot T, et al. Why people fail to notice the horrors around them. *The New York Times*. 2024. https://www.nytimes.com/2024/02/25/opinion/brain-habituation-horrors.html

82. Garrett N, et al. The brain adapts to dishonesty. *Nat Neurosci* 2016. doi: 10.1038/nn.4426

83. Professional Identity Formation. 2025. https://www.aacp.org/article/professional-identity-formation

84. Vaidyanathan B. Professional socialization in medicine. *AMA J Ethics* 2015. doi: 10.1001/virtualmentor.2015.17.02.msoc1-1502

85. Fiske ST, et al. What does the schema concept buy us? *Personal Soc Psychol Bull*. 1980. doi: 10.1177/014616728064006

86. Piaget J, et al. The Psychology of the Child. *The Psychology of the Child*. New York City: Basic Books; 1969. ISBN: 9780465095001

87. Taylor SE, et al. Schematic Bases of Social Information Processing. *Schematic Bases of Social Information Processing*. Social Cognition. London: Routledge; 2022. pp. 89–134. ISBN: 9781003311386

88. Underman K, et al. Emotional socialization in twenty-first century medical education. *Soc Sci Med* 2016. doi: 10.1016/j.socscimed.2016.05.027

89. Chakravorty T. Fat shaming is stopping doctors from helping overweight patients—here's what medical students can do about it. *BMJ* 2021. doi: 10.1136/bmj.n2830

90. Walker M. *Why We Sleep*. New York City: Penguin Books; 2017. ISBN: 9780141983769

91. de Sousa D, et al. Munchausen syndrome and Munchausen syndrome by proxy: A narrative review. *Einstein (Sao Paulo)* 2017. doi: 10.1590/s1679-45082017md3746

92. Banay GL. An introduction to medical terminology I. Greek and latin derivations. *Bull Med Libr Assoc* 1948. PMID: 16016791.

93. Wulff HR. The language of medicine. *J R Soc Med* 2004. doi: 10.1177/014107680409700412

94. Brüssow H. What is health? *Microb Biotechnol* 2013. doi: 10.1111/1751-7915.12063

95. Sartorius N. The meanings of health and its promotion. *Journal* 2006. PMID: 16909464.

96. Scully JL. What is a disease? *EMBO Rep*. 2004. doi: 10.1038/sj.embor.7400195

97. Ayers DM, et al. *English Words: From Latin and Greek Elements*, Second Edition. Second Edition Revised and Explanded ed. Tucson: The University of Arizona Press; 1986. ISBN: 9780816508990

98. Kottow MH. A medical definition of disease. *Med Hypotheses* 1980. doi: 10.1016/0306-9877(80)90085-7

99. Stanbrook MB. Addiction is a disease: We must change our attitudes toward addicts. *Can Med Assoc J* 2012. doi: 10.1503/cmaj.111957

100. Tikkinen KAO, et al. What is a disease? Perspectives of the public, health professionals and legislators. *BMJ Open* 2012. doi: 10.1136/bmjopen-2012-001632

101. Disease. 2024. https://www.cancer.gov/publications/dictionaries/cancer-terms/def/disease

102. Rosen H. Is obesity a disease or a behavior abnormality? Did the AMA get it right? *Mo Med* 2014. PMID: 30323513.

103. Luli M, et al. The implications of defining obesity as a disease: A report from the Association for the Study of Obesity 2021 annual conference. *EClinicalMedicine* 2023. doi: 10.1016/j.eclinm.2023.101962

104. Cosgrove L, et al. Financial ties between DSM-IV panel members and the pharmaceutical industry. *Psychother Psychosom* 2006. doi: 10.1159/000091772

105. Cosgrove L, et al. Mental health as a basic human right and the interference of commercialized science. *Journal* 2020. PMID: 32669789.

106. Kitsis EA. The pharmaceutical industry's role in defining illness. *Virtual Mentor* 2011. doi: 10.1001/virtualmentor.2011.13.12.oped1-1112

107. Quinlan MM, et al. Wehy one mom battles to change the term "incompetent cervix." Shifting medical language from shame to accuracy. *Psychology Today*. 2021. https://www.psychologytoday.com/us/blog/medical-humanities-mamas/202105/why-one-mom-battles-to-change-the-term-incompetent-cervix

108. Nickel B, et al. Words do matter: A systematic review on how different terminology for the same condition influences management preferences. *BMJ Open* 2017. doi: 10.1136/bmjopen-2016-014129

109. Goldman B. Derogatory slang in the hospital setting. *AMA J Ethics* 2015. doi: 10.1001/virtualmentor.2015.17.2.msoc2-1502

110. Kahneman D. *Thinking, Fast and Slow*. New York City: Farrar, Straus and Giroux; 2011. ISBN: 978037427563

111. Groopman J. *How Doctors Think*. Boston: Houghton Mifflin Company; 2007. ISBN: 9780618610037

112. Krawczyk D. *Reasoning: The Neuroscience of How We Think*. San Diego: Academic Press; 2018. ISBN: 9780128092859

113. Nesse RM, et al. Making evolutionary biology a basic science for medicine. *Proc Natl Acad Sci* 2010. doi: 10.1073/pnas.0906224106

114. Hidaka BH, et al. The status of evolutionary medicine education in North American medical schools. *BMC Med Educ* 2015. doi: 10.1186/s12909-015-0322-5

115. Power ML, et al. Integrating evolution into medical education for women's health care practitioners. *Evol Med Public Health* 2020. doi: 10.1093/emph/eoaa009

116. Harris EE, et al. Evolutionary explanations in medical and health profession courses: Are you answering your students' "why" questions? *BMC Med Educ* 2005. doi: 10.1186/1472-6920-5-16

117. Dunsworth HM. Origin of the genus homo. *Evol: Educ Outreach* 2010. doi: 10.1007/s12052-010-0247-8

118. Smith D, et al. Cooperation and the evolution of hunter-gatherer storytelling. *Nat Commun* 2017. doi: 10.1038/s41467-017-02036-8

119. Harari YN. *Sapiens: A Brief History of Humankind*. New York City: Harper; 2025. ISBN: 9780063422018

120. Harari YN. *Homo Deus: A Brief History of Tomorrow*. New York City: Harper; 2017. ISBN: 9780062464316

121. Wrangham R. *The Goodness Paradox: The Strange Relationship Between Virtue and Violence in Human Evolution*. New York City: Vintage Books; 2019. ISBN: 9781101970195

122. Sood A. Mindfulness Redesigned for the Twenty-First Century: Let's Not Cage the Hummingbird. *A Mindful Path to Resilience*. Rochester: Global Center for Resiliency and Wellbeing; 2018. ISBN: 9780999552506

123. Konrath SH, et al. Changes in dispositional empathy in American college students over time: A meta-analysis. *Personal Soc Psychol Rev* 2011. doi: 10.1177/1088868310377395

124. Murphy JM. Psychiatric labeling in cross-cultural perspective. *Science* 1976. doi: 10.1126/science.1251213

125. Barrett D. *Supernormal Stimuli: How Primal Urges Overran Their Evolutionary Purpose*. New York City: W. W. Norton & Company; 2010. ISBN: 9780393068481

126. Peoples HC, et al. Cl hunter-gatherers and the origins of religion. *Hum Nat* 2016. doi: 10.1007/s12110-016-9260-0

127. Lerner G. *The Creation of Patriarchy*. New York City: Oxford University Press; 1986. ISBN: 9780195051858

128. Amanpour C. Top relationship expert: 'Are we becoming a different species?'. 2023. https://www.cnn.com/videos/tv/2023/11/11/esther-perel-amanpour.cnn

129. Cochran G, et al. *The 10,000 Year Explosion: How Civilization Accelerated Human Evolution*. New York City: Basic Books; 2009. ISBN: 9780465020423

130. Hawking S. *Brief Answers to the Big Questions*. London: John Murray Press; 2018. ISBN: 9781473695986

131. Imber G. *Genius on the Edge: The Bizarre Double Life of Dr.* William Stewart Halsted. Fort Lauderdale: Kaplan Publishing; 2010. ISBN: 9781607146278

132. Rae A. Osler vindicated: The ghost of Flexner laid to rest. *Journal* 2001. PMID: 11450285.

133. Duffy TP. The flexner report—100 years later. *Journal* 2011. PMID: 21966046.

134. Barkin SL, et al. Unintended consequences of the flexner report: Women in pediatrics. *Pediatrics* 2010. doi: 10.1542/peds.2010-2050

135. Laws T. How should we respond to racist legacies in health professions education originating in the flexner report? *AMA Journal of Ethics*. 2021. https://journalofethics.ama-assn.org/article/how-should-we-respond-racist-legacies-health-professions-education-originating-flexner-report/2021-03

136. Mizrahi T. *Getting Rid of Patients: Contradictions in the Socialization of Physicians*. New Brunswick: Rutgers University Press; 1986. ISBN: 9780813511283

137. *Institute of Medicine Committee on Optimizing Graduate Medical Trainee Hours and Work Schedule to Improve Patient Safety. Resident Duty Hours: Enhancing Sleep, Supervision, and Safety*. In: Ulmer C, et al., editors. Washington (DC): National Academies Press (US); 2009. ISBN: 9780309127769

138. ACGME Task Force on Quality Care and Professionalism. *The ACGME 2011 Duty Hour Standards: Enhancing Quality of Care, Supervision, and Resident Professional Development* https://www.acgme.org: Accreditation Council for Graduate Medical Education; 2011. Available from: https://www.acgme.org/globalassets/pdfs/jgme-monograph1.pdf

139. Quintero GA, et al. Integrated medical curriculum: Advantages and disadvantages. *J Med Educat Curri Develop* 2016. doi: 10.4137/jmecd.S18920

140. Buja LM. Medical education today: All that glitters is not gold. *BMC Med Educ* 2019. doi: 10.1186/s12909-019-1535-9

141. Olsen LD. *Curricular Injustice: How U.S. Medical Schools Reproduce Inequalities*. New York City: Columbia University Press; 2024. ISBN 9780231207874

142. Spiess JP, et al. Survey of pass/fail grading systems in US doctor of pharmacy degree programs. *Am J Pharm Educ* 2022. doi: 10.5688/ajpe8520

143. Hill E, et al. You've got to know the rules to play the game: How medical students negotiate the hidden curriculum of surgical careers. *Med Educ* 2014. doi: 10.1111/medu.12488

144. Habiger Institute for Catholic Leadership. *The Heart of Culture: A Brief History of Western Education*. St. Paul: Cluny Media LLC; 2020. ISBN: 9781950970599

145. Puchner M. *Culture: The Story of Us, from Cave Art to K-Pop*. New York City: W. W. Norton & Company; 2023. ISBN: 9781324074502

146. Engel JM. Why Does Culture 'Eat Strategy For Breakfast'? *Forbes Leadership* 2018. https://www.forbes.com/sites/forbescoachescouncil/2018/11/20/why-does-culture-eat-strategy-for-breakfast/?sh=2836da471e09

147. Schein EH. *The Corporate Culture Survival Guide, New and Revised Edition*. San Francisco: Jossey-Bass; 2009. ISBN: 9780470293713

148. Brodell R. 2025. *Personal Communication*.

149. Meeks LM, et al. Wellness and work: Mixed messages in residency training. *J Gen Intern Med* 2019. doi: 10.1007/s11606-019-04952-5

150. Garfield ZH, et al. Investigating evolutionary models of leadership among recently settled Ethiopian hunter-gatherers. *Leadersh Q* 2020. doi: 10.1016/j.leaqua.2019.03.005

151. From Foraging to Farming: The 10,000-year Revolution. 2012. https://www.cam.ac.uk/research/news/from-foraging-to-farming-the-10000-year-revolution

152. Leavitt HJ. *Top Down: Why Hierarchies are Here to Stay and How to Manage Them More Effectively*. Boston: Harvard Business School Press; 2005. ISBN: 9781591394983

153. Koski JE, et al. Understanding social hierarchies: The neural and psychological foundations of status perception. *Soc Neurosci* 2015. doi: 10.1080/17470919.2015.1013223

154. Meisner OC, et al. Amygdala connectivity and implications for social cognition and disorders. *Handb Clin Neurol* 2022. doi: 10.1016/b978-0-12-823493-8.00017-1

155. Vanstone M, et al. Medical student strategies for actively negotiating hierarchy in the clinical environment. *Med Educ* 2019. doi: 10.1111/medu.13945

156. Vanstone M, et al. Thinking about social power and hierarchy in medical education. *Med Educ* 2022. doi: 10.1111/medu.14659

157. Catmull E, et al. *Creativity, Inc.: Overcoming the Unseen Forces That Stand in the Way of True Inspiration*. New York City: Random House; 2014. ISBN: 9780812993011.

158. Zimbardo P. *The Lucifer Effect: Understanding How Good People Turn Evil*. New York City: Random House Trade Paperbacks; 2008. ISBN: 9780812974447

159. Scott-Bottoms S. The dirty work of the Stanford Prison Experiment: Re-reading the dramaturgy of coercion. *Incarceration* 2020. doi: 10.1177/2632666320944316

160. Cialdini RB. *Influence, New and Expanded: The Psychology of Persuasion*. New York City: Harper Business; 2021. ISBN: 9780062937650

161. Frankl VE. *Man's Search For Meaning*. Boston: Beacon Press; 2006. ISBN: 9780807014271

162. The BBC *Prison Study*. 2008. http://www.bbcprisonstudy.org/index.php

163. Franzen A, et al. The power of social influence: A replication and extension of the Asch experiment. *PLoS1* 2023. doi: 10.1371/journal.pone.0294325. PMID 38019779.

164. Beran TN, et al. Observational study of conformity in yet another medical learning environment: Conformity to preceptors during high-fidelity simulation. *Adv Med Educ Pract* 2023. doi: 10.2147/amep.S427996

165. Grendar J, et al. Experiences of pressure to conform in postgraduate medical education. *BMC Med Educ* 2018. doi: 10.1186/s12909-017-1108-8

166. Burnum JF. The physician as a double agent. *N Engl J Med* 1977. doi: 10.1056/NEJM197708042970513

167. Levine RJ. Clinical trials and physicians as double agents. *Yale J Biol Med* 65, 65–74. 1992. PMID: 1519378.

168. Shortell SM, et al. Physicians as double agents: Maintaining trust in an era of multiple accountabilities. *JAMA* 1998. doi: 10.1001/jama.280.12.1102

169. Thomas LR, et al. Charter on physician well-being. *JAMA* 2018. doi: 10.1001/jama.2018.1331

170. Porter J, et al. Revisiting the time needed to provide adult primary care. *J Gen Intern Med* 2023. doi: 10.1007/s11606-022-07707-x

171. US DoHaHS. *Physical Activity Guidelines for Americans*, 2nd Edition. https://odphp.health.gov/: U.S. Department of Health and Human Services, 2018.

172. Dillon K. *HBR Guide to Office Politics: Rise Above Rivalry, Avoid Power Games, Build Better Relationships*. Boston: Harvard Business Review Press; 2015. ISBN: 9781625275325

173. Voss C, et al. *Never Split the Difference: Negotiating as if Your Life Depended on It*. New York City: Penguin Books; 2016. ISBN: 9781847941497

174. Cote C. 2023. https://online.hbs.edu/blog/post/strategies-for-conflict-resolution-in-the-workplace

175. Patterson K, et al. *Crucial Conversations: Tools for Talking When the Stakes are High*. New York City: McGraw-Hill; 2012. ISBN: 9780071771320

176. Carnegie D. *How to Win Friends & Influence People*. Uttar Pradesh: Manjul Publishing House; 2017. ISBN: 9788183227896

177. Grant A. *Think Again: The Power of Knowing What You Don't Know*. New York City: Viking; 2021. ISBN: 9781984878106

178. Coleman PT. *The Five Percent: Finding solutions to seemingly impossible conflicts*. New York City: Public Affairs; 2011. ISBN: 9781586489212

179. Vedantam S. Learning from your mistakes. 2023. https://hiddenbrain.org/podcast/learning-from-your-mistakes/

180. Pickren W. Indian J *Psychiatry* 2007. doi: 10.4103/0019-5545.37318

181. Ayers S, et al. *Psychology for Medicine & Healthcare*, Third Edition. London: SAGE Publications Ltd.; 2021. ISBN: 9781526496829

182. Weseley AJ, et al. *AP Psychology Premium, 2022-2023: Comprehensive Review with 6 Practice Tests + an Online Timed Test Option*. New York City: Simon and Schuster; 2022. ISBN: 9781506278513

183. Coppini S, et al. Experiments on real-life emotions challenge Ekman's model. *Sci Rep* 2023. doi: 10.1038/s41598-023-36201-5

184. Ekman P. Are there basic emotions? *Psychol Rev* 1992. doi: 10.1037/0033-295X.99.3.550

185. Ekman P, et al. What is meant by calling emotions basic. *Emot Rev* 2011. doi: 10.1177/1754073911410740

186. Gu S, et al. A model for basic emotions using observations of behavior in drosophila. *Front Psychol* 2019. doi: 10.3389/fpsyg.2019.00781

187. Tracy JL, et al. Four models of basic emotions: A review of ekman and cordaro, izard, levenson, and panksepp and watt. *Emot Rev* 2011. doi: 10.1177/1754073911410747

188. Ekman P. 2024. https://www.paulekman.com/blog/cultural-differences-in-emotional-expressions/

189. Barrett LF, et al. Emotional expressions reconsidered: Challenges to inferring emotion from human facial movements. *Psychol Sci Public Interest* 2019. doi: 10.1177/1529100619832930

190. Hogeveen J, et al. Alexithymia. *Handb Clin Neurol* 2021. doi: 10.1016/b978-0-12-822290-4.00004-9

191. Damour L. *Untangled: Guiding Teenage Girls Through the Seven Transitions into Adulthood*. New York City: Ballantine Books; 2016. ISBN: 9780553393057

192. Personality. 2018. https://dictionary.apa.org/personality

193. Van Edwards V. *Captivate: The Science of Succeeding with People*. New York City: Penguin Publishing Group; 2017. ISBN: 9780399564499

194. Grant A. 2015. https://medium.com/@AdamMGrant/mbti-if-you-want-me-back-you-need-to-change-too-c7f1a7b6970

195. Big 5 Personality Traits. 2025. https://www.psychologytoday.com/us/basics/big-5-personality-traits

196. Brooks D. *How to Know A Person: The Art of Seeing Others Deeply and Being Deeply Seen*. New York City: Random House; 2023. ISBN: 9780593230060

197. Confessore N. Cambridge analytica and facebook: The scandal and the fallout so far. *The New York Times*. 2018. https://www.nytimes.com/2018/04/04/us/politics/cambridge-analytica-scandal-fallout.html

198. Cain S. *Quiet: The Power of Introverts in a World That Can't Stop Talking*. New York City: Crown; 2013. ISBN: 9780307352156

199. Laney MO. *The Introvert Advantage: How Quiet People Can Thrive in an Extrovert World*. New York City: Workman Publishing Company; 2002. ISBN: 9780761123699

200. Pasca R. Person-Environment Fit Theory. In: Michalos AC, editor. *Encyclopedia of Quality of Life and Well-Being Research*. Dordrecht: Springer Netherlands; 2014. p. 4776–4778. ISBN: 978-94-007-0753-5

201. The Founding Physicians. 2024. https://www.hopkinsmedicine.org/about/history/history-of-jhh/founding-physicians

202. Cameron JL, et al. William stewart halsted: Letters to a young female admirer. *Ann Surg* 2001. doi: 10.1097/00000658-200111000-00018

203. Harvard Business Review. *HBR's 10 Must Reads on Managing People*. Boston: Harvard Business Review Press; 2011. ISBN: 9781422158012

204. Bloom P. *Against Empathy: The Case for Relational Compassion*. New York City: Ecco Books; 2016. ISBN: 9780062339348

205. Greene R. *The 48 Laws of Power*. London: Penguin Books; 2000. ISBN: 9780140280197

206. Muthuri RNDK, et al. Determinants of happiness among healthcare professionals between 2009 and 2019: A systematic review. *Humanit Soc Sci Commun* 2020. doi: 10.1057/s41599-020-00592-x

207. Anderman EM, et al. Motivation, Learning, and Instruction. In: Wright JD, Ed-in-Chief, editor. *International Encyclopedia of the Social & Behavioral Sciences*. Second Edition. Amsterdam: Elsevier Ltd.; 2015. p. 928-35. ISBN: 9780080970875

208. Fogg BJ. *Tiny Habits: The Small Chages That Change Everything*. Eugene: Harvest House Publishers; 2021. ISBN: 9780358362777

279

209. Faries MD. Why we don't "just do it": Understanding the intention-behavior gap in lifestyle medicine. *Am J Lifestyle Med*. 2016. doi: 10.1177/1559827616638017

210. Bischof G, et al. Motivational interviewing: An evidence-based approach for use in medical practice. *Dtsch Arztebl Int* 2021. doi: 10.3238/arztebl.m2021.0014

211. Clear J. *Atomic Habits: An Easy & Proven Way to Build Good Habits & Break Bad Ones*. 1st Edition. Garden City Park: Avery; 2018. ISBN: 9780735211292

212. Khoddam R. 2017. https://www.psychologytoday.com/us/blog/the-addiction-connection/201708/the-myth-of-motivation

213. Goldin C. *Career & Family: Women's Century-Long Journey Toward Equity*. Princeton: Princeton University Press; 2021. ISBN: 9780691201788

214. Boyle P. *AAMCNews*. 2022. https://www.aamc.org/news/nation-s-medical-schools-grow-more-diverse

215. Adler PA, et al. Socialization to gender roles: Popularity among elementary school boys and girls. *Sociol Educ* 1992. doi: 10.2307/2112807

216. Bejerano AR, et al. Learning masculinity: Unmasking the hidden curriculum in science, technology, *Eng Math Courses* 2015. doi: 10.1615/JWomenMinorScienEng.2015011359

217. Booher-Jennings J. Learning to label: Socialisation, gender, and the hidden curriculum of high-stakes testing. *Br J Sociol Educ* 2008. doi: 10.1080/01425690701837513

218. Cassese EC, et al. A hidden curriculum? Examining the gender content in introductory-level political science textbooks. *Polit Gend* 2013. doi: 10.1017/S1743923X13000068

219. Chen ESL, et al. Gender socialization in Chinese Kindergartens: Teachers' contributions. *Sex Roles* 2011. doi: 10.1007/s11199-010-9873-4

220. Cvencek D, et al. Math-gender stereotypes in elementary school children. *Child Dev* 2011. doi: 10.1111/j.1467-8624.2010.01529.x

221. Denny KE. Gender in context, content, and approach: Comparing gender messages in girl scout and boy scout handbooks. *Gend Soc* 2011. doi: 10.1177/0891243210390517

222. Dersch A-S, et al. Exploring the nature of teachers' math-gender stereotypes: The math-gender misconception questionnaire. *Front Psychol* 2022. doi: 10.3389/fpsyg.2022.820254

223. Gansen HM. Push-ups versus clean-up: Preschool teachers' gendered beliefs, expectations for behavior, and disciplinary practices. *Sex Roles*. 2019. doi: 10.1007/s11199-018-0944-2

224. Grace K, et al. The socialization of gender-based aggression: A case study in cambodian primary schools. *Sex Roles* 2020. doi: 10.1007/s11199-019-01091-3

225. Hilliard LJ, et al. Differing levels of gender salience in preschool classrooms: Effects on children's gender attitudes and intergroup bias. *Child Dev* 2010. doi: 10.1111/j.1467-8624.2010.01510.x

226. Lee JFK. A hidden curriculum in Japanese EFL textbooks: Gender representation. Linguistics and Education. *Linguist Educ* 2014. doi: 10.1016/j.linged.2014.07.002

227. Mkuchu SGV. *Gender Roles in Textbooks as a Function of Hidden Curriculum in Tanzania Primary Schools [Dissertation]*. University of South Africa, Pretoria, South Africa 2004.

228. Nasri B, et al. The gendered socialization of girls and boys in tunisian schools. *Sci Res* 2023. doi: 10.4236/oalib.1110027

229. Osieja H. Year. https://library.iated.org/view/OSIEJA2018EDU

230. Petruchenia HH, et al. 2014. https://www.researchgate.net/publication/339236720_Gender_issues_of_Ukrainian_higher_education

231. Phan A, et al. Gender stereotypes as hidden curriculum: A case of Vietnamese English textbooks. *Int J Educ* 2021. doi: 10.17509/ije.v14i1.30553

232. Smith DS, et al. Gender Norm Salience Across Middle Schools: Contextual Variations in associations between gender typicality and socioemotional distress. *J Youth Adolesc* 2018. doi: 10.1007/s10964-017-0732-2

233. van de Rozenberg TM, et al. Hidden in plain sight: Gender bias and heteronormativity in dutch textbooks. *Educ Stud* 2023. doi: 10.1080/00131946.2023.2194536

234. Vu MT, et al. Gender, critical pedagogy, and textbooks: Understanding teachers' (lack of) mediation of the hidden curriculum in the EFL classroom. *Lang Teach Res* doi: 10.1177/13621688221136937

235. Wafa D. Reinforced stereotypes: A case study on school textbooks in Egypt. *J Int Women's Stud* 2021. https://vc.bridgew.edu/jiws/vol22/iss1/22/

236. Grace MK. Parting ways: Sex-based differences in premedical attrition. *Soc Sci Med* 2019. doi: 10.1016/j.socscimed.2019.04.030

237. Witherspoon EB, et al. When making the grade isn't enough: The gendered nature of premed science course attrition. *Educ Res* 2019. doi: 10.3102/0013189x19840331

238. Arsever S, et al. A gender biased hidden curriculum of clinical vignettes in undergraduate medical training. *Patient Educ Couns* 2023. doi: 10.1016/j.pec.2023.107934

239. Cheng LF, et al. Learning about gender on campus: An analysis of the hidden curriculum for medical students. *Med Educ* 2015. doi: 10.1111/medu.12628

240. Phillips CB.Student portfolios and the hidden curriculum on gender: Mapping exclusion. *Med Edu* 2009. doi: 10.1111/j.1365-2923.2009.03403.x

241. Turbes S, et al. The hidden curriculum in multicultural medical education: The role of case examples. *Acad Med* 2002. doi: 10.1097/00001888-200203000-00007

242. Lempp H, et al. The hidden curriculum in undergraduate medical education: Qualitative study of medical students' perceptions of teaching. *BMJ* 2004. doi: 10.1136/bmj.329.7469.770

243. Brown MEL, et al. Exploring the perceptions of senior medical students on gender and pain: A qualitative study of the interplay between formal and hidden curricula. *BMJ Open*. 2024. doi: 10.1136/bmjopen-2023-080420

244. Patrick-Smith M, et al. Medical student perceptions of gender and pain: A systematic review of the literature. *BMC Med* 2024. doi: 10.1186/s12916-024-03660-0

245. Anderson KJ. Women Are Wonderful, but Most Are Disliked. *Modern Misogyny: Anti-Feminism in a Post-Feminist Era*. Oxford: Oxford University Press; 2014. p. 106–137. ISBN: 9780199328178

246. Horowitz A. Sons and daughters as caregivers to older parents: Differences in role performance and consequences. *The Gerontologist* 1985. doi: 10.1093/geront/25.6.612

247. Parker K, et al. On gender differences, no consensus on nature vs. nurture. *Pew Research Center*. 2017. https://www.pewresearch.org/social-trends/2017/12/05/on-gender-differences-no-consensus-on-nature-vs-nurture/

248. Parker K, et al. Americans see men as the financial providers, even as women's contributions grow. *Pew Research Center*. 2017. https://www.pewresearch.org/short-reads/2017/09/20/americans-see-men-as-the-financial-providers-even-as-womens-contributions-grow/

249. Simmons R. *Odd Girl Out: The Hidden Culture of Aggression in Girls*, Revised Edition. Boston: Mariner Books Houghton Mifflin Harcourt; 2011. ISBN: 9780547520193

250. Eagly AH, et al. Gender stereotypes stem from the distribution of women and men into social roles. *J Pers Soc Psychol,*. 1984. doi: 10.1037/0022-3514.46.4.735

251. Ly DP, et al. Sex differences in time spent on household activities and care of children among US physicians, 2003-2016. *Mayo Clin Proc* 2018. doi: 10.1016/j.mayocp.2018.02.018

252. Schaeffer K. Among U.S. couples, women do more cooking and grocery shopping than men. *Pew Research Center* 2019. https://www.pewresearch.org/short-reads/2019/09/24/among-u-s-couples-women-do-more-cooking-and-grocery-shopping-than-men/

253. Jolly S, et al. Gender differences in time spent on parenting and domestic responsibilities by high-achieving young physician-researchers. *Ann Intern Med* 2014. doi: 10.7326/m13-0974

254. Isaac C, et al. Male spouses of women physicians: Communication, compromise, and carving out time. *Journal* 2013. PMID: 25419544.

255. Heilman ME. Gender stereotypes and workplace bias. *Res Organ Behav* 2012. doi: 10.1016/j.riob.2012.11.003

256. Axelson RD, et al. Assessing implicit gender bias in Medical Student Performance Evaluations. *Eval Health Prof* 2010. doi: 10.1177/0163278710375097

257. Filippou P, et al. The presence of gender bias in letters of recommendations written for urology residency applicants. *Urology* 2019. doi: 10.1016/j.urology.2019.05.065

258. Khan S, et al. Gender bias in reference letters for residency and academic medicine: A systematic review. *Postgrad Med J* 2021. doi: 10.1136/postgradmedj-2021-140045

259. Madera JM, et al. Gender and letters of recommendation for academia: Agentic and communal differences. *J Appl Psychol* 2009. doi: 10.1037/a0016539

260. Rojek AE, et al. Differences in narrative language in evaluations of medical students by gender and under-represented minority status. *J Gen Intern Med* 2019. doi: 10.1007/s11606-019-04889-9

261. Ross DA, et al. Differences in words used to describe racial and gender groups in Medical Student Performance Evaluations. *PLoS One* 2017. doi: 10.1371/journal.pone.0181659

262. Turrentine FE, et al. Influence of gender on surgical residency applicants' recommendation letters. *J Am Coll Surg* 2019. doi: 10.1016/j.jamcollsurg.2018.12.020

263. Yang SE, et al. Functional connectivity signatures of political ideology. *PNAS Nexus* 2022. doi: 10.1093/pnasnexus/pgac066

264. Hansen M, et al. Implicit gender bias among US resident physicians. *BMC Med Educ* 2019. doi: 10.1186/s12909-019-1818-1

265. Yan VX, et al. I forgot that you existed: Role of memory accessibility in the gender citation gap. *Am Psychol* 2025. doi: 10.1037/amp0001299

266. Salles A, et al. Estimating implicit and explicit gender bias among health care professionals and surgeons. *JAMA Netw Open* 2019. doi: 10.1001/jamanetworkopen.2019.6545

267. Maitra A, et al. Assessment of interruptive behavior at residency teaching conferences by gender. *JAMA Netw Open* 2021. doi: 10.1001/jamanetworkopen.2020.33469

268. Snyder K. How to get ahead as a woman in tech: Interrupt men. *Slate*. 2014. https://slate.com/human-interest/2014/07/study-men-interrupt-women-more-in-tech-workplaces-but-high-ranking-women-learn-to-interrupt.html

269. Boston SE, et al. Influence of speaker's gender on speaker introductions at the 2018 ACVS Surgical Summit. *Vet Surg* 2020. doi: 10.1111/vsu.13437

270. Davids JS, et al. Female representation and implicit gender bias at the 2017 American Society of Colon and Rectal Surgeons' Annual Scientific and Tripartite Meeting. *Dis Colon Rectum* 2019. doi: 10.1097/dcr.0000000000001274

271. Duma N, et al. Evaluating unconscious bias: Speaker introductions at an international oncology conference. *J Clin Oncol* 2019. doi: 10.1200/jco.19.01608

272. Files JA, et al. Speaker Introductions at Internal Medicine Grand Rounds: Forms of Address Reveal Gender Bias. *J Womens Health (Larchmt)* 2017. doi: 10.1089/jwh.2016.6044

273. Davuluri M, et al. Gender bias in medicine: Does it exist at AUA plenary sessions? *Urology* 2021. doi: 10.1016/j.urology.2020.05.012

274. Gharzai LA, et al. Speaker introductions at grand rounds: Differences in formality of address by gender and specialty. *J Womens Health (Larchmt)* 2022. doi: 10.1089/jwh.2021.0031

275. Huang CC, et al. Evaluating bias in speaker introductions at the American Society for Radiation Oncology Annual Meeting. *Int J Radiat Oncol Biol Phys* 2021. doi: 10.1016/j.ijrobp.2020.12.027

276. Van Osch K, et al. Evaluating implicit gender bias at Canadian otolaryngology meetings through use of professional title. *World J Otorhinol Head Neck Surg* 2024. doi: 10.1002/wjo2.96

277. Harvey JA, et al. Patient Use of Physicians' First (Given) name in direct patient electronic messaging. *JAMA Netw Open* 2022. doi: 10.1001/jamanetworkopen.2022.34880

278. Liddell SS, et al. Gender disparities in electronic health record usage and inbasket burden for internal medicine residents. *J Gen Intern Med* 2024. doi: 10.1007/s11606-024-08861-0

279. Rittenberg E, et al. Primary care physician gender and electronic health record workload. *J Gen Intern Med* 2022. doi: 10.1007/s11606-021-07298-z

280. Stroud L. Reflections on sexism in medicine. *Can Med Assoc J* 2020. doi: 10.1503/cmaj.74909

281. Yeung EYH. Sexism and racism in medical care: It depends on the context. *Can Med Assoc J* 2020. doi: 10.1503/cmaj.74905

282. Carnevale M, et al. Gender disparities in academic vascular surgeons. *J Vasc Surg* 2020. doi: 10.1016/j.jvs.2019.12.042

283. Cho E, et al. Gender disparity in authorship among orthopaedic surgery residents. *JB JS Open Access* 2024. doi: 10.2106/jbjs.Oa.24.00061

284. Eloy JA, et al. Gender disparities in research productivity among 9952 academic physicians. *Laryngoscope* 2013. doi: 10.1002/lary.24039

285. McDermott M, et al. Sex differences in academic rank and publication rate at top-ranked US neurology programs. *JAMA Neurol* 2018. doi: 10.1001/jamaneurol.2018.0275

286. McDonald JS, et al. Gender and radiology publication productivity: An examination of academic faculty from four health systems in the United States. *J Am Coll Radiol* 2017. doi: 10.1016/j.jacr.2017.04.017

287. Nguyen AX, et al. Gender gap in neurology research authorship (1946-2020). *Front Neurol* 2021. doi: 10.3389/fneur.2021.715428

288. Diamond SJ, et al. Gender Differences in Publication Productivity, Academic Rank, and Career Duration Among U.S. Academic Gastroenterology Faculty. *Acad Med* 2016. doi: 10.1097/acm.0000000000001219

289. Ence AK, et al. Publication productivity and experience: Factors associated with academic rank among orthopaedic surgery faculty in the United States. *J Bone Joint Surg Am* 2016. doi: 10.2106/jbjs.15.00757

290. Mutsaers A, et al. Research Productivity of Canadian Radiation Oncology Residents: A Time-Trend Analysis. *Curr Oncol* 2020. doi: 10.3390/curroncol28010003

291. Sebo P, et al. Gender gap in research: A bibliometric study of published articles in primary health care and general internal medicine. *Fam Pract* 2020. doi: 10.1093/fampra/cmz091

292. Reed DA, et al. Gender differences in academic productivity and leadership appointments of physicians throughout academic careers. *Acad Med* 2011. doi: 10.1097/ACM.0b013e3181ff9ff2

293. Campbell JC, et al. Collaboration metrics among female and male researchers: A 5-year review of publications in major radiology journals. *Acad Radiol* 2018. doi: 10.1016/j.acra.2017.12.034

294. Ellsworth BK, et al. Is there gender disparity in orthopedic surgery resident research productivity. *HSS J* 2024. doi: 10.1177/15563316221150934

295. Fang AC, et al. National awards and female emergency physicians in the United States: Is the "recognition gap" closing?. *J Emerg Med* 2021. doi: 10.1016/j.jemermed.2021.07.009

296. King JT, Jr., et al. Gender disparities in medical student research awards: A 13-year study from the yale school of medicine. *Acad Med* 2018. doi: 10.1097/acm.0000000000002052

297. Kuo LE, et al. Gender disparity in awards in general surgery residency programs. *JAMA Surg* 2020. doi: 10.1001/jamasurg.2020.3518

298. Lambert CM, et al. Addressing the gender gap in residency awards using a blinded selection process. *Neurol Educ* 2024. doi: 10.1212/NE9.0000000000200136

299. Silver JK, et al. Women physicians underrepresented in American Academy of Neurology recognition awards. *Neurology* 2018. doi: 10.1212/WNL.0000000000006004

300. Woldegerima N, et al. Gender differences in urology society award recipients. *Am J Surg* 2020. doi: 10.1016/j.amjsurg.2020.06.062

301. Pelley E, et al. When a specialty becomes "women's work": Trends in and implications of specialty gender segregation in medicine. *Acad Med* 2020. doi: 10.1097/acm.0000000000003555

302. Bakkensen JB, et al. Childbearing, infertility, and career trajectories among women in medicine. *JAMA Netw Open* 2023. doi: 10.1001/jamanetworkopen.2023.26192

303. Parekh R, et al. Medical students' experience of the hidden curriculum around primary care careers: A qualitative exploration of reflective diaries. *BMJ Open* 2021. doi: 10.1136/bmjopen-2021-049825

304. Nading MB. 'Beautiful' medicine: Gender segregation by medical specialty in Ukraine. *Med Anthropol Theory* 2022. doi: 10.17157/mat.9.1.5429

305. Hill E, et al. 'You become a man in a man's world': Is there discursive space for women in surgery? *Med Educ* 2015. doi: 10.1111/medu.12818

306. Liang R, et al. Why do women leave surgical training? A qualitative and feminist study. *Lancet* 2019. doi: 10.1016/S0140-6736(18)32612-6

307. Cater SW, et al. Bridging the gap: Identifying global trends in gender disparity among the radiology physician workforce. *Acad Radiol* 2018. doi: 10.1016/j.acra.2017.12.021

308. Kaye EC. One in four — The importance of comprehensive fertility benefits for the medical workforce. *N Engl J Med* 2020. doi: 10.1056/NEJMp1915331

309. Stentz NC, et al. Fertility and childbearing among american female physicians. *J Women's Health* 2016. doi: 10.1089/jwh.2015.5638

310. World Health Organization. *Infertility Prevalence Estimates, 1990-2021.* https://www.who.int/: World Health Organization, 2023. Contract No.: ISBN 978 92 4 006831 5.

311. Levy MS, et al. Psychosocial burdens associated with family building among physicians and medical students. *JAMA Intern Med* 2023. doi: 10.1001/jamainternmed.2023.2570

312. Veade A, et al. Investing in female physician fertility benefits to improve long-term physician retention. *Am J Obstet Gynecol* 2023. doi: 10.1016/j.ajog.2023.05.009

313. Marshall AL, et al. Physician fertility: A call to action. *Acad Med Acad Med* 2020. doi: 10.1097/acm.0000000000003079

314. Menon NK, et al. Association of physician burnout with suicidal ideation and medical errors. *JAMA Netw Open* 2020. doi: 10.1001/jamanetworkopen.2020.28780

315. Suicide Data and Statistics. 2024. https://www.cdc.gov/suicide/suicide-data-statistics.html

316. Dyrbye LN, et al. Burnout and suicidal ideation among U.S. medical students. *Ann Intern Med* 2008. doi: 10.7326/0003-4819-149-5-200809020-00008

317. Shanafelt TD, et al. Special report: Suicidal ideation among American surgeons. *Arch Surg* 2011. doi: 10.1001/archsurg.2010.292

318. Luse B, et al. The men's loneliness epidemic might not exist. *MPRnews* 2025. https://www.npr.org/2025/02/17/1263527043/its-been-a-minute-male-loneliness-epidemic-real

319. Carr PL, et al. Faculty perceptions of gender discrimination and sexual harassment in academic medicine. *Ann Intern Med* 2000. doi: 10.7326/0003-4819-132-11-200006060-00007

320. Caruso R, et al. Violence against physicians in the workplace: Trends, causes, consequences, and strategies for intervention. *Curr Psychiatry Rep* 2022. doi: 10.1007/s11920-022-01398-1

321. The Lancet. The structural roots of violence against female health workers. *Lancet* 2024. doi: 10.1016/S0140-6736(24)01864-6

322. Ayala-Burboa MO, et al. Workplace violence as a predictor of suicidal ideation in undergraduate internal physicians. *Rev Med Inst Mex Seguro Soc* 2024. doi: 10.5281/zenodo.13306721

323. Yun JY, et al. Associations among the workplace violence, burnout, depressive symptoms, suicidality, and turnover intention in training physicians: A network analysis of nationwide survey. *Sci Rep* 2023. doi: 10.1038/s41598-023-44119-1

324. Berg S. Medical boards probe mental health; doctors pause in getting help. *AMA Pract Manag Phys Health*. 2017. https://www.ama-assn.org/practice-management/physician-health/medical-boards-probe-mental-health-doctors-pause-getting-help

325. Leonhardt M. Researchers mostly have no idea what's contributing to the gender wage gap. *Fortune*. 2023. https://fortune.com/2023/03/14/gender-wage-gap-contributing-factors-discrimination/

326. Goldman AL, et al. Changes in physician work hours and implications for workforce capacity and work-life balance, 2001-2021. *JAMA Intern Med* 2023. doi: 10.1001/jamainternmed.2022.5792

327. Frank E, et al. Gender disparities in work and parental status among early career physicians. *JAMA Netw Open* 2019. doi: 10.1001/jamanetworkopen.2019.8340

328. Adesoye T, et al. Perceived discrimination experienced by physician mothers and desired workplace changes: A cross-sectional survey. *JAMA Intern Med* 2017. doi: 10.1001/jamainternmed.2017.1394

329. Halley MC, et al. Physician mothers' experience of workplace discrimination: A qualitative analysis. *BMJ* 2018. doi: 10.1136/bmj.k4926

330. Frank E, et al. Experiences of work-family conflict and mental health symptoms by gender among physician parents during the COVID-19 pandemic. *JAMA Netw Open* 2021. doi: 10.1001/jamanetworkopen.2021.34315

331. Moors AC, et al. Gendered impact of caregiving responsibilities on tenure track faculty parents' professional lives. *Sex Roles* 2022. doi: 10.1007/s11199-022-01324-y

332. Nishida S, et al. Dilemma of physician-mothers faced with an increased home burden and clinical duties in the hospital during the COVID-19 pandemic. *PLoS One* 2021. doi: 10.1371/journal.pone.0253646

333. Grant A. Work life with adam grant. 2024. https://podcasts.apple.com/au/podcast/beyond-breaking-the-glass-ceiling-with-julia/id1346314086?i=1000661579473

334. King's Global Institute for Women's Leadership. *Emerging Tensions? How Younger Generations Are Dividing On Masculinity and Gender Equality*. https://www.kcl.ac.uk/: King's College London, The Policy Institute, 2024.

335. Qiu L, et al. Fact-checking a Mogul's claims about avocado toast, millennials and home buying. *The New York Times*. 2017. https://www.nytimes.com/2017/05/15/business/avocado-toast-millennials.html

336. Mogg K. The 'lazy-girl job' is in right now. Here's why. *The Wall Street Journal*. 2023. https://www.wsj.com/articles/the-career-goal-of-the-moment-is-a-lazy-girl-job-f5075c4e?msockid=19b40ed4898960600ada1f4588fd617a

337. Lythcott-Haims J. *How to Raise an Adult: Break Free of the Overparenting Trap and Prepare Your Kid for Success*. New York City: Henry Holt and Company; 2016. ISBN: 9781250093639

338. Nierenberg AN. Nearly everyone gets as at Yale. Does that cheapen the grade? *New York Times*. 2023. https://www.nytimes.com/2023/12/05/nyregion/yale-grade-inflation.html

339. Rosenbaum L. Being well while doing well – distinguishing necessary from unnecessary discomfort in training. *N Engl J Med* 2024. doi: 10.1056/NEJMms2308228

340. Rosenbaum L. What do trainees want? The rise of house staff unions. *N Engl J Med* 2024. doi: 10.1056/NEJMms2308224

341. Rosenbaum L. Tough love – NOS episode 2.3. *N Engl J Med* 2024. doi: 10.1056/NEJMp2400690

342. Rosenbaum L. Revolutionary rumblings – NOS episode 2.1 *New England Journal of Medicine*. 2024. doi: 10.1056/NEJMp2303616, https://podcasts.apple.com/us/podcast/not-otherwise-specified/id1672610072

343. Philips AP, et al. Medical students aren't showing up to class. What does that mean for future docs? *MPRnews*. 2023. https://www.npr.org/sections/health-shots/2023/06/01/1179125090/medical-students-arent-showing-up-to-class-what-does-that-mean-for-future-docs

344. Francis A. Gen Z: The workers who want it all. 2022. https://www.bbc.com/worklife/article/20220613-gen-z-the-workers-who-want-it-all

345. PricewaterhouseCoopers. Millennials at work. *Reshaping the workplace*. https://www.pwc.com/: PricewaterhouseCoopers International Limited (PwC), 2011.

346. Welch S. For Gen Z, unemployment can be a blast. *WSJ*. 2023. https://www.wsj.com/lifestyle/careers/for-gen-z-unemployment-can-be-a-blast-employment-career-labor-generation-corporate-college-university-e24810ce

347. Gendron T, et al. Generational bias: Another form of ageism. *Int J Aging Hum Dev* 2024. doi: 10.1177/00914150231194244

348. Levy BR, et al. Age stereotypes held earlier in life predict cardiovascular events in later life. *Psychol Sci* 2009. doi: 10.1111/j.1467-9280.2009.02298.x

349. Zakaria F. *In Defense of a Liberal Education.* New York City: W. W. Norton & Company; 2015. ISBN: 9780393247688

350. Buklijas T. Surgery and national identity in late nineteenth-century Vienna. *Stud Hist Phil Biol Biomed Sci* 2007. doi: 10.1016/j.shpsc.2007.09.003

351. Robbins LL. The future of radiology. *Radiology* 1960. doi: 10.1148/74.3.485

352. Haidt J. *The Anxious Generation: How the Great Rewiring of Childhood Is Causing an Epidemic of Mental Illness.* New York City: Penguin Press; 2024. ISBN: 9780593655030

353. Twenge JM. *Generation Me - Revised and Updated: Why Today's Young Americans Are More Confident, Assertive, Entitled--and More Miserable Than Ever.* New York City: Atria Books; 2014. ISBN: 9781476755564.

354. Arnett JJ, et al. The dangers of generational myth-making: Rejoinder to twenge. *Emerg Adulthood* 2013. doi: 10.1177/2167696812466848

355. Rudolph CW, et al. Generations and generational differences: Debunking myths in organizational science and practice and paving new paths forward. *J Bus Psychol* 2021. doi: 10.1007/s10869-020-09715-2

356. Parker K. How pew research center will report on generations moving forward. 2023. https://www.pewresearch.org/short-reads/2023/05/22/how-pew-research-center-will-report-on-generations-moving-forward/

357. Carmody JB, et al. On step 1 Mania, USMLE Score reporting, and financial conflict of interest at the national board of medical examiners. *Acad Med* 2020. doi: 10.1097/acm.0000000000003126. PMID 31850948

358. US NCoEiE. *A Nation At Risk: The Imperative for Educational Reform : A Report to the Nation and the Secretary of Education, United States Department of Education.* Ann Arbor: University of Michigan Library; 1983. ISBN: 9781304100511

359. Smith R. Self esteem: The kindly apocylypse. *J Philos Educ* 2002. https://doi.org/10.1111/1467-9752.00261

360. Magness S. *Do Hard Things: Why We Get Resilience Wrong and the Surprising Science of Real Toughness.* New York City: HarperOne; 2022. ISBN: 9780063098619

361. Thaddeus M.College rankings whistleblower: Exposing inaccurate data was unpleasant but necessary. *CNN.* 2022. https://www.cnn.com/2022/09/22/opinions/columbia-ranking-inaccurate-data-thaddeus/index.html

362. Mamykina L, et al. How do residents spend their shift time? A time and motion study with a particular focus on the use of computers. *Acad Med* 2016. doi: 10.1097/acm.0000000000001148

363. Lee E, et al. Being well while doing well (comment). *N Engl J Med* 2024. doi: 10.1056/NEJMc2403542

364. Shurin SB. Being well while doing well (comment) *N Engl J Med* 2024. doi: 10.1056/NEJMc2403542

365. Keen WW. The ideal physician. *JAMA J Am Med Assoc* 1900. doi: 10.1001/jama.1900.24610250004002

366. Murthy DV. Surgeon General addresses growing stress and mental health struggles facing parents. *Journal.* 2024.

367. The Premed Competencies for Entering Medical Students. 2025. https://students-residents.aamc.org/real-stories-demonstrating-premed-competencies/premed-competencies-entering-medical-students

368. Donnelly LF, et al. The joint commission's ongoing professional practice evaluation process: Costly, ineffective, and potentially harmful to safety culture. *J Am Coll Radiol* 2024. doi: 10.1016/j.jacr.2023.08.031

369. Murphy B. Find better ways to do medical student clerkship grading. *AMA Medical Students Clinical Rotations.* 2023. https://www.ama-assn.org/education/medical-school-diversity/find-better-ways-do-medical-student-clerkship-grading

370. Bensing J, et al. What patients want. Patient Education and Counseling. *Patient Educ Couns* 2013. doi: 10.1016/j.pec.2013.01.005

371. Petrilli CM, et al. Understanding patient preference for physician attire: A cross-sectional observational study of 10 academic medical centres in the USA. *BMJ Open* 2018. doi: 10.1136/bmjopen-2017-021239

372. Lopez SJ. Why your physician should get serious about your happiness. 2013. https://www.huffpost.com/entry/why-your-physician-should_b_2900522

373. Griffin B et al. Parental career expectations: Effect on medical students' career attitudes over time. *Med Educ* 2019. PMID 30734329.

374. Liu S, et al. The effect of students' effort–reward imbalance on learning engagement: The mediating role of learned helplessness and the moderating-role of social support. *Front Psychol* 2024. doi: 10.3389/fpsyg.2024.1329664

375. Hall ET. *The Hidden Dimension.* Garden City: Anchor Books; 1969. ISBN: 9780385084765

376. Patterson ML, et al. Four misconceptions about nonverbal communication. *Perspect Psychol Sci* 2023. doi: 10.1177/17456916221148142

377. Mehrabian A, et al. Inference of attitudes from nonverbal communication in two channels. *J Consult Psychol* 1967. doi: 10.1037/h0024648

378. Mehrabian A, et al. Decoding of inconsistent communications. *J Pers Soc Psychol* 1967. doi: 10.1037/h0024532

379. Lapakko D. Communication is 93% nonverbal: An urban legend proliferates. *Commun Theater Assoc Minnesota J* 2015. doi: 10.56816/2471-0032.1000

380. Lowndes L. *How To Talk To Anyone: 92 Little Tricks for Big Success in Relationships*. New York City: McGraw-Hill; 2003. ISBN: 9780071418584

381. Kobayashi H, et al. Unique morphology of the human eye. *Nature* 1997. doi: 10.1038/42842

382. Shellenbarger S. WSJ: Just look me in the eye already. *Quantified*. 2013. https://quantified.ai/blog/wsj-just-look-me-in-the-eye-already/

383. Dal Monte O, et al. Widespread implementations of interactive social gaze neurons in the primate prefrontal-amygdala networks. *Neuron* 2022. doi: 10.1016/j.neuron.2022.04.013

384. Noah JA, et al. Real-time eye-to-eye contact is associated with cross-brain neural coupling in angular gyrus. *Front Hum Neurosci* 2020. doi: 10.3389/fnhum.2020.00019

385. Mayrand F, et al. A dual mobile eye tracking study on natural eye contact during live interactions. *Sci Rep* 2023. doi: 10.1038/s41598-023-38346-9

386. Kajimura S, et al. When we cannot speak: Eye contact disrupts resources available to cognitive control processes during verb generation. *Cognition* 2016. doi: 10.1016/j.cognition.2016.10.002

387. Ko CJ. *How to Improve Doctor-Patient Connection: Using Psychology to Optimize Healthcare Interactions*. New York City: Routledge; 2022. ISBN: 9780367769451

388. Ekman P. Fake smile or genuine smile? The importance of the Duchenne smile. 2024. https://www.paulekman.com/blog/fake-smile-or-genuine-smile/

389. Girard JM, et al. Reconsidering the duchenne smile: Indicator of positive emotion or artifact of smile intensity? *Int Conf Affect Comput Intell Interact Workshops* 2019. doi: 10.1109/acii.2019.8925535

390. Chartrand TL, et al. The chameleon effect: The perception-behavior link and social interaction. *J Pers Soc Psychol* 1999. doi: 10.1037//0022-3514.76.6.893

391. Wild B, et al. Why are smiles contagious? An fMRI study of the interaction between perception of facial affect and facial movements. *Psychiatry Res* 2003. doi: 10.1016/s0925-4927(03)00006-4

392. Schroeder J, et al. Handshaking Promotes Cooperative Dealmaking. Harvard Business School NOM Unit Working Paper No 14-117. 2014. https://papers.ssrn.com/sol3/papers.cfm?abstract_id=2443674

393. Stewart GL, et al. Exploring the handshake in employment interviews. *J Appl Psychol* 2008. doi: 10.1037/0021-9010.93.5.1139

394. Fred HL. Banning the handshake from healthcare settings is not the solution to poor hand hygiene. *Tex Heart Inst J* 2015. doi: 10.14503/thij-15-5254

395. Fisher R, et al. *Getting to Yes: Negotiating Agreement Without Giving In*, Third Edition. New York City: Penguin Books; 2011. ISBN: 9780143118756

396. Sullivan E, et al. Raising professionalism concerns as a medical student: Damned if they do, damned if they don't? *BMC Med Educ* 2024. doi: 10.1186/s12909-024-05144-4

397. Kelly J. Attractive people have a big advantage in the job interview. *Forbes*. 2021. https://www.forbes.com/sites/jackkelly/2021/11/04/attractive-people-have-a-big-advantage-in-the-job-interview/

398. Monrouxe LV, et al. Differences in medical students' explicit discourses of professionalism: Acting, representing, becoming. *Med Educ* 2011. doi: 10.1111/j.1365-2923.2010.03878.x

399. Krupat E, et al. Do professionalism lapses in medical school predict problems in residency and clinical practice? *Acad Med* 2020. doi: 10.1097/acm.0000000000003145

400. Olive KE, et al. Developing a physician's professional identity through medical education. *Am J Med Sci* 2017. doi: 10.1016/j.amjms.2016.10.012

401. Covey SR. *The 7 Habits of Highly Effective People: Powerful Lessons in Personal Change*. New York City: Free Press; 1990. ISBN: 9780671708634

402. Benbassat J. Role modeling in medical education: The importance of a reflective imitation. *Acad Med* 2014. doi: 10.1097/acm.0000000000000189

403. Glicken AD, et al. Addressing the hidden curriculum: Understanding educator professionalism. *Med Teach* 2007. doi: 10.1080/01421590601182602

404. Bandura A. Influence of model's reinforcement contingencies on the acquisition of imitative responses. *J Pers Soc Psychol* 1965. doi: 10.1037/h0022070

405. Billings ME, et al. The effect of the hidden curriculum on resident burnout and cynicism. *J Grad Med Educ* 2011. doi: 10.4300/jgme-d-11-00044.1

406. Connolly H. "They're training us to be helpless:" Medical student socialization around social determinants of health. *SSM -Qual Res Health* 2023. doi: 10.1016/j.ssmqr.2023.100327

407. Neumann M, et al. Empathy decline and its reasons: A systematic review of studies with medical students and residents. *Acad Med* 2011. doi: 10.1097/ACM.0b013e318221e615

408. Shaw MK, et al. Professionalism lapses and hierarchies: A qualitative analysis of medical students' narrated acts of resistance. *Soc Sci Med* 2018. doi: 10.1016/j.socscimed.2018.10.009

409. Arnold L. Responding to the professionalism of learners and faculty in orthopaedic surgery. *Clin Orthop Relat Res* 2006. doi: 10.1097/01.blo.0000224034.00980.9e

410. Brown MEL, et al. Exploring the hidden curriculum's impact on medical students: Professionalism, identity formation and the need for transparency. *Med Sci Educ* 2020. doi: 10.1007/s40670-020-01021-z

411. Torres Acosta MA, et al. The impact of underrepresented minority or marginalized identity status on training outcomes of MD-PhD students. *BMC Med Educ* 2023. doi: 10.1186/s12909-023-04399-7

412. Danckers M, et al. The sexual and gender minority (LGBTQ+) medical trainee: The journey through medical education. *BMC Med Educ* 2024. doi: 10.1186/s12909-024-05047-4

413. CBS/AP. CBS NEWS. Ohio hospital drops dress code requiring women to wear pantyhose. 2017. https://www.cbsnews.com/news/ohio-summa-health-drops-controversial-dress-code-requiring-women-wear-pantyhose/

414. American Medical Association. AMA Code of Medical Ethics: 9.3.1 Physician Health & Wellness. 2017. https://code-medical-ethics.ama-assn.org/sites/amacoedb/files/2022-08/9.3.1.pdf

415. Dyrbye LN, et al. Effect of a professional coaching intervention on the well-being and distress of physicians: A pilot randomized clinical trial. *JAMA Intern Med* 2019. doi: 10.1001/jamainternmed.2019.2425

416. Wilf-Miron R, et al. Health behaviors of medical students decline towards residency: How could we maintain and enhance these behaviors throughout their training. *Isr J Health Policy Res* 2021. doi: 10.1186/s13584-021-00447-z

417. Frank E, et al. Physician disclosure of healthy personal behaviors improves credibility and ability to motivate. *Arch Fam Med* 2000. doi: 10.1001/archfami.9.3.287

418. Howe M, et al. Patient-related diet and exercise counseling: Do providers' own lifestyle habits matter? *Prev Cardiol* 2010. doi: 10.1111/j.1751-7141.2010.00079.x

419. Hankir A, et al. Reducing mental health stigma in medical students and doctors towards their peers with mental health difficulties: A protocol. *Psychiatr Danub* 2020. PMID: 32890375.

420. Wilkinson E. Medical students face high levels of mental health problems but stigma stops them getting help. *BMJ* 2023. doi: 10.1136/bmj.p933

421. Dyrbye LN, et al. Medical licensure questions and physician reluctance to seek care for mental health conditions. *Mayo Clin Proc* 2017. doi: 10.1016/j.mayocp.2017.06.020

422. West CP, et al. Single item measures of emotional exhaustion and depersonalization are useful for assessing burnout in medical professionals. *J Gen Intern Med* 2009. doi: 10.1007/s11606-009-1129-z

423. Dyrbye LN, et al. Burnout among U.S. medical students, residents, and early career physicians relative to the general U.S. population. *Acad Med* 2014. doi: 10.1097/acm.0000000000000134

424. Dyrbye LN, et al. Residents' perceptions of faculty behaviors and resident burnout: A cross-sectional survey study across a large health care organization. *J Gen Intern Med* 2021. doi: 10.1007/s11606-020-06452-3

425. Trockel MT, et al. Assessment of physician sleep and wellness, burnout, and clinically significant medical errors. *JAMA Netw Open* 2020. doi: 10.1001/jamanetworkopen.2020.28111

426. Trockel MT, et al. Assessment of adverse childhood experiences, adverse professional experiences, depression, and burnout in US physicians. *Mayo Clin Proc* 2023. doi: 10.1016/j.mayocp.2023.03.021

427. Asken MJ. Physician burnout: Moral injury is a questionable term. *BMJ* 2019. doi: 10.1136/bmj.l2375

428. Dean W, et al. Reframing clinician distress: Moral injury not burnout. *Fed Pract* 2019. PMID: 31571807.

429. Kopacz MS, et al. It's time to talk about physician burnout and moral injury. *Lancet* 2019. doi: 10.1016/S2215-0366(19)30385-2

430. Shanafelt TD, et al. Executive leadership and physician well-being: Nine organizational strategies to promote engagement and reduce burnout. *Mayo Clin Proc* 2017. doi: 10.1016/j.mayocp.2016.10.004

431. Sood A. *That Makes Sense: Bite-sized resilience insights to lift your day.* Rochester: Global Center for Resiliency & Wellbeing; 2021. ISBN: 9781734737745

432. Werneburg BL, et al. Improving resiliency in healthcare employees. *Am J Health Behav* 2018. doi: 10.5993/ajhb.42.1.4

433. West CP, et al. Association of resident fatigue and distress with perceived medical errors. *JAMA* 2009. doi: 10.1001/jama.2009.1389

434. Kalm LM, et al. They starved so that others be better fed: Remembering Ancel Keys and the Minnesota experiment. *J Nutr* 2005. doi: 10.1093/jn/135.6.1347

435. Goebert D, et al. Depressive symptoms in medical students and residents: A multischool study. *Acad Med* 2009. doi: 10.1097/ACM.0b013e31819391bb

436. Seitz A. Loneliness poses health risks as deadly as smoking, U.S. surgeon general says. *PBS News Health*. 2023. https://www.pbs.org/newshour/health/loneliness-poses-health-risks-as-deadly-as-smoking-u-s-surgeon-general-says#:~:text=How%20do%20we%20design%20technology,15%20cigarettes%20daily%2C%20not%2012

437. Zakaria F. *Age of Revolutions*. New York City: W. W. Norton & Company; 2024. ISBN: 9780393239232

438. Kraemer KM et al. Mind-Body Skills Training to Improve Distress Tolerance in Medical Students: A pilot Study. Teaching and Learning in Medicine. 2016; 28(2) https://doi.org/10.1080/10401334.2016.1146605

439. About Jon Kabat-Zinn. 2025. https://jonkabat-zinn.com/about/

440. Van Dam NT, et al. Mind the hype: A critical evaluation and prescriptive agenda for research on mindfulness and meditation. *Perspect Psychol Sci* 2018. doi: 10.1177/1745691617709589

441. McDermott J, et al. Finding time and energy to exercise—5 tips for surgeons. *JAMA Surg* 2024. doi: 10.1001/jamasurg.2024.3400

442. Adams NE. Bloom's taxonomy of cognitive learning objectives. *J Med Libr Assoc* 2015. doi: 10.3163/1536-5050.103.3.010

443. Lee CD, et al. Nutrition in medicine – A new review article series. *N Engl J Med* 2024. doi: 10.1056/NEJMe2313282

444. Wong K. What did humans evolve to eat? *Sci Am Mag* 2024. doi: 10.1038/scientificamerican072024-6bq869CBW30IOM7mmJY81v

445. Sugimoto S, et al. Are future doctors prepared to address patients' nutritional needs? Cooking and nutritional knowledge and habits in medical students. *Am J Lifestyle Med* 2023. doi: 10.1177/15598276211018165

446. Pisaniello MS, et al. Effect of medical student debt on mental health, academic performance and specialty choice: A systematic review. *BMJ Open* 2019. doi: 10.1136/bmjopen-2019-029980

447. Walsemann KM, et al. Sick of our loans: Student borrowing and the mental health of young adults in the United States. *Soc Sci Med* 2015. doi: 10.1016/j.socscimed.2014.11.027

448. Jones JB, et al. *Portfolios Across the U.S. Wealth Distribution*. https://www.richmondfed.org/: Federal Reserve Bank of Richmond, 2023.

449. Dahle J. Why doctors get paid more in the US and why some people hate it. *The White Coat Investor*. 2023. https://www.whitecoatinvestor.com/why-us-doctors-get-paid-more/

450. Magnus SA, et al. Medical schools, affirmative action, and the neglected role of social class. *Am J Public Health* 2000. doi: 10.2105/ajph.90.8.1197

451. Lentz BF, et al. Why so many children of doctors become doctors: Nepotism vs. human capital transfers. *J Hum Resour* 1989. doi: 10.2307/145820

452. Following in Footsteps: Children of Physicians More Likely to Attend Medical School but No More Likely to Succeed. 2020. https://school.wakehealth.edu/-/media/wakeforest/school/files/about-the-school-of-medicine/wfjsm/journalsom_2020-physician-legacy---strowd.pdf?la=en

453. Zakaria F. Interview with Naftali Bennett; Interview with Finnish President Alexander Stubb. 2024. https://www.cnn.com/audio/podcasts/fareed-zakaria-gps/episodes/c961b2cc-9f75-11ee-a524-77412d04eb17

454. Nguyen M, et al. Temporal trends in childhood household income among applicants and matriculants to medical school and the likelihood of acceptance by income, 2014-2019. *JAMA* 2023. doi: 10.1001/jama.2023.5654

455. Talamantes E, et al. Closing the gap — Making medical school admissions more equitable. *N Engl J Med* 2019. doi: 10.1056/NEJMp1808582

456. Lepore G, et al. First-generation physicians: The pursuit of academic surgery. *Am J Surg* 2024. doi: 10.1016/j.amjsurg.2023.09.016

457. Robinson JA, et al. Increasing diversity in cardiothoracic surgery: First-generation medical students. *JTCVS Open* 2021. doi: 10.1016/j.xjon.2021.06.026

458. Romero R, et al. Understanding the experiences of first-generation medical students: Implications for a diverse physician workforce. *Acad Psychiatry* 2020. doi: 10.1007/s40596-020-01235-8

459. Havemann C, et al. Challenges facing first-generation college graduates in medical school: A qualitative analysis. *JAMA Netw Open* 2023. doi: 10.1001/jamanetworkopen.2023.47528

460. Chung H. Gender, flexibility stigma and the perceived negative consequences of flexible working in the UK. *Soc Indic Res* 2020. doi: 10.1007/s11205-018-2036-7

461. Christophers B, et al. First-generation physician-scientists are under-represented and need better support. *Nat Med* 2021. doi: 10.1038/s41591-021-01352-3

462. Southgate E, et al. Travels in extreme social mobility: How first-in-family students find their way into and through medical education. *Crit Stud Edu* 2017. doi: 10.1080/17508487.2016.1263223

463. Alves-Bradford J-M. Supporting first-generation medical students—Improving learning environments for all. *JAMA Netw Open* 2023. doi: 10.1001/jamanetworkopen.2023.47475

464. Fokas JA, et al. Opinion & special articles: Examining the hidden curriculum of medical school from a first-generation student perspective. *Neurology* 2023. doi: 10.1212/wnl.0000000000207174

465. Gallegos A, et al. Visibility & support for first generation college graduates in medicine. *Med Educ Online* 2022. doi: 10.1080/10872981.2021.2011605

466. Salinas KE, et al. The invisible minority: A call to address the persistent socioeconomic diversity gap in U.S. medical schools and the physician workforce. *Front Public Health* 2022. doi: 10.3389/fpubh.2022.924746

467. Conway-Hicks S, et al. Living in two worlds: Becoming and being a doctor among those who identify with "not from an advantaged background". *Curr Probl Pediatr Adolesc Health Care* 2019. doi: 10.1016/j.cppeds.2019.03.006

468. Garcia KA. An examination of the "giving back" asset of first-generation Latinx premedical students in an emerging Hispanic-serving institution. *J Divers High Educ* 2024. doi: 10.1037/dhe0000607

469. Garcia KA, et al. "Mamá en inglés se dice 'pre-med'": Bilingual Mexican-origin first-generation college undergraduates aspiring for medical careers. *Race Ethn Educ* 2024. doi: 10.1080/13613324.2024.2349879

470. Anyon J. Social class and the hidden curriculum of work. *J Educ* 1980. doi: 10.1177/002205748016200106

471. Balboni MJ, et al. Religion, spirituality, and the hidden curriculum: Medical student and faculty reflections. *J Pain Symptom Manag* 2015. doi: 10.1016/j.jpainsymman.2015.04.020

472. Rizzolo LJ. Human dissection: An approach to interweaving the traditional and humanistic goals of medical education. *Anat Rec* 2002. doi: 10.1002/ar.10188

473. Ferguson KJ, et al. Constructing stories of past lives: Cadaver as first patient: "Clinical summary of dissection" writing assignment for medical students. *Perm J* 2008. doi: 10.7812/tpp/07-145

474. Kumar Ghosh S, et al. Building professionalism in human dissection room as a component of hidden curriculum delivery: A systematic review of good practices. *Anat Sci Educ* 2019. doi: 10.1002/ase.1836

475. Bohl M, et al. Medical students' perceptions of the body donor as a "first patient" or "teacher": A pilot study. *Anat Sci Educ* 2011. doi: 10.1002/ase.231

476. Finkelstein P, et al. Post-traumatic stress among medical students in the anatomy dissection laboratory. Clinical Anatomy. *Clin Anat* 1990. doi: 10.1002/ca.980030308

477. Dueñas AN, et al. Uncovering hidden curricula: Use of dark humor in anatomy labs and its implications for basic sciences education. *Med Sci Educ* 2020. doi: 10.1007/s40670-019-00912-0

478. Escobar-Poni B, et al. The role of gross anatomy in promoting professionalism: A neglected opportunity! *Clin Anat* 2006. doi: 10.1002/ca.20353

479. Dehner LP. The medical autopsy: Past, present, and dubious future. *Mo Med* 2010. PMID: 20446515.

480. Hochberg MS. The doctor's white coat—An historical perspective. *Virtual Mentor* 2007. doi: 10.1001/virtualmentor.2007.9.4.mhst1-0704

481. Gillon R. White coat ceremonies for new medical students. *J Med Ethics* 2000. doi: 10.1136/jme.26.2.83

482. Wear D. On white coats and professional development: The formal and the hidden curricula. *Ann Intern Med* 1998. doi: 10.7326/0003-4819-129-9-199811010-00010

483. Russell PC. The white coat ceremony: Turning trust into entitlement. *Teach Learn Med* 2002. doi: 10.1207/s15328015tlm1401_13

484. Veatch RM. White coat ceremonies: A second opinion. *J Med Ethics* 2002. doi: 10.1136/jme.28.1.5

485. Karnieli-Miller O, et al. Cloak of compassion, or evidence of elitism? An empirical analysis of white coat ceremonies. *Med Educ* 2013. doi: 10.1111/j.1365-2923.2012.04324.x

486. Pronovost P. Why white coats should be optional. 2015. https://armstronginstitute.blogs.hopkinsmedicine.org/2015/12/18/why-white-coats-should-be-optional/

487. Askitopoulou H, et al. The relevance of the Hippocratic Oath to the ethical and moral values of contemporary medicine. Part I: The Hippocratic Oath from antiquity to modern times. *Eur Spine J* 2018. doi: 10.1007/s00586-017-5348-4

488. Riddick FA, Jr. The code of medical ethics of the American Medical Association. *Ochsner J* 2003. PMID: 22826677.

489. Strauss C, et al. What is compassion and how can we measure it? A review of definitions and measures. *Clin Psychol Rev* 2016. doi: 10.1016/j.cpr.2016.05.004

490. APA dictionary of psychology. *Empathy*. 2023. https://dictionary.apa.org/empathy

491. Cairns P, et al. The association between empathy and burnout in medical students: A systematic review and meta-analysis. *BMC Med Educ* 2024. doi: 10.1186/s12909-024-05625-6

492. Howick J, et al. Why might medical student empathy change throughout medical school? a systematic review and thematic synthesis of qualitative studies. *BMC Med Educ* 2023. doi: 10.1186/s12909-023-04165-9

493. Józsa L. [The establishment of the hospital-system in the Byzantine Empire]. *Orvostort Kozl* 2011. PMID: 22533247.

494. Yeo IS. The birth of hospital, asclepius cult and early christianity. *Uisahak* 2017. doi: 10.13081/kjmh.2017.26.3

495. Guiahi M, et al. Patient Views on Religious Institutional Health Care. *JAMA Netw Open* 2019. doi: 10.1001/jamanetworkopen.2019.17008

496. Durkheim E. *The Elementary Forms of Religious Life*. Oxford: Oxford University Press; Abridged edition; 2008. ISBN: 9780199540129

497. Koenig HG. Religion, spirituality, and medicine: How are they related and what does it mean? *Mayo Clin Proc* 2001. doi: 10.4065/76.12.1189

498. Bregman P. How (and Why) to Stop Multitasking. Harvard Business Review Time Management. *Harvard Business Review Time Management*. 2010. https://hbr.org/2010/05/how-and-why-to-stop-multitaski

499. Sydney Opera House Failed Project - What Can You Learn? 2017. https://blog.beyondsoftware.com/learning-from-failed-projects-sydney-opera-house

500. Taleb NN. *Antifragile: Things That Gain from Disorder (Incerto)*. New York City: Random House; 2012. ISBN: 9781400067824

501. Abobe Workfront. *The State of Work Report*, 2019 U.S. Edition. https://www.workfront.com/: 2019.

502. Allen D. *Getting Things Done: The Art of Stress-Free Productivity*. New York City: Penguin Books; 2015. ISBN: 9780143126560

503. Alpaio K. I tried 4 to-do list methods. Here's what worked. *Harvard Business Review*. 2021. https://hbr.org/2021/01/i-tried-4-to-do-list-methods-heres-what-worked

504. Loehr J, et al. *The Power of Full Engagement: Managing Energy, Not Time, Is the Key to High Performance and Personal Renewal*. New York City: Free Press; 2003. ISBN: 9780743226745

505. Schrager S, et al. Getting more done: Strategies to increase scholarly productivity. *J Grad Med Educ* 2016. doi: 10.4300/jgme-d-15-00165.1

506. Stulberg B, et al. *Peak Performance: Elevate Your Game, Avoid Burnout, and Thrive with the New Science of Success*. Emmaus: Rodale Books; 2017. ISBN: 9781623367930

507. Arleo EK. *First, Eat Your Frog: And Other Pearls for Professional Working Mothers*. Estes Park: Armin Lear Press Inc.; 2023. ISBN: 9781956450583

508. Schwartz AW, et al. Finding and doing what matters most: Five productivity strategies for physicians in academic medicine. *Med Teach* 2023. doi: 10.1080/0142159x.2022.2126762

509. Dux PE, et al. Isolation of a central bottleneck of information processing with time-resolved FMRI. *Neuron* 2006. doi: 10.1016/j.neuron.2006.11.009

510. Hirnstein M, et al. No sex difference in an everyday multitasking paradigm. *Psychol Res* 2019. doi: 10.1007/s00426-018-1045-0

511. Hirsch P, et al. Putting a stereotype to the test: The case of gender differences in multitasking costs in task-switching and dual-task situations. *PLoS One* 2019. doi: 10.1371/journal.pone.0220150

512. Paridon H, et al. Multitasking in work-related situations and its relevance for occupational health and safety: Effects on performance, subjective strain and physiological parameters. *Eur J Psychol* 2010. doi: 10.5964/ejop.v6i4.226

513. Szameitat AJ, et al. "Women are better than men"-public beliefs on gender differences and other aspects in multitasking. *PLoS One* 2015. doi: 10.1371/journal.pone.0140371

514. Linder JA, et al. Time of day and the decision to prescribe antibiotics. *JAMA Intern Med* 2014. doi: 10.1001/jamainternmed.2014.5225

515. Stec N, et al. A systematic review of fatigue in radiology: Is it a problem? *Am J Roentgenol* 2018. doi: 10.2214/ajr.17.18613

516. Gardner B, et al. Making health habitual: The psychology of 'habit-formation' and general practice. *Br J Gen Pract* 2012. doi: 10.3399/bjgp12X659466

517. Eskreis-Winkler L, et al. When Praise—Versus Criticism—Motivates Goal Pursuit. In: Brummelman EE, editor. *Psychological Perspectives on Praise*. London: Routledge; 2020. pp. 47–54. ISBN: 9780429327667

518. Karlsson N, et al. Ostrich effect: Selective attention to information. *J Risk Uncertain* 2009. doi: 10.1007/s11166-009-9060-6

519. Gawande A. *The Checklist Manifesto: How to Get Things Right*. New York City: Henry Holt and Company; 2010. ISBN: 9781429953382

520. Eskreis-Winkler L, et al. Not learning from failure-the greatest failure of all. *Psychol Sci* 2019. doi: 10.1177/0956797619881133

521. O'Keefe PA, et al. stop trying to 'find' your passion—There's a better way to love what you do. Recognizing that interests are malleable and can be developed can make us more resilient, open and creative. *Scientific American*

Magazine. 2023. https://www.scientificamerican.com/article/stop-trying-to-find-your-passion-theres-a-better-way-to-love-what-you-do/

522. King S. *On Writing: A Memoir of the Craft*. New York City: Scribner; 2000. ISBN: 9780684853529

523. Hye-Knudsen M, et al. How Stephen King writes and why: Language, immersion, emotion. *Orb Litt* 2023. doi: 10.1111/oli.12401

524. Hale C. *Sin and Syntax: How to Craft Wicked Good Prose*. New York City: Crown; 2013. ISBN: 9780385346894

525. Bossuyt PM, et al. Towards complete and accurate reporting of studies of diagnostic accuracy: The STARD initiative. *Clin Chem* 2003. doi: 10.1373/49.1.1

526. Bilgin C, et al. Journal selection primer for neuroradiology researchers. *Acad Radiol* 2023. doi: 10.1016/j.acra.2022.05.004

527. Kuhn TS. *The Structure of Scientific Revolutions*. 3rd Edition. Chicago: University of Chicago Press; 1996. ISBN: 9780226458083

528. Grant DC, et al. Psychoanalysis, science and the seductive theory of Karl Popper. *Aust N Zeal J Psychiatry* 2005. doi: 10.1080/j.1440-1614.2005.01602.x

529. Taran S, et al. Falsifiability in medicine: What clinicians can learn from Karl Popper. *Intensive Care Med* 2021. doi: 10.1007/s00134-021-06432-z

530. Pompeu FAMS. Why Pheidippides could not believe in the 'Central Governor Model': Popper's philosophy applied to choose between two exercise physiology theories. *Sports Med Health Sci* 2022. doi: 10.1016/j.smhs.2021.10.001

531. Robergs RA. Lessons from Popper for science, paradigm shifts, scientific revolutions and exercise physiology. *BMJ Open Sport Exerc Med* 2017. doi: 10.1136/bmjsem-2017-000226

532. Castillo M. The scientific method: A need for something better? *Am J Neuroradiol* 2013. PMID: 23370475

533. Clayton A. *Bernoulli's Fallacy: Statistical Illogic and the Crisis of Modern Science*. New York City: Columbia University Press; 2022. ISBN: 9780231199957

534. Bartos F, et al. Fair coins tend to land on the same side they started: Evidence from 350,757 flips. *Mathematics History and Overview*. 2023. https://arxiv.org/abs/2310.04153

535. Perezgonzalez JD.Fisher, neyman-pearson or NHST? A tutorial for teaching data testing. *Front Psychol* 2015. doi: 10.3389/fpsyg.2015.00223

536. Szucs D, et al. When null hypothesis significance testing is unsuitable for research: A reassessment. *Front Hum Neurosci* 2017. doi: 10.3389/fnhum.2017.00390

537. Wilcox RR. *Basic Statistics: Understanding Conventional Methods and Modern Insights*. Oxford: Oxford University Press; 2009. ISBN: 9780195315103

538. Conover WJ. *Practical Nonparametric Statistics*, Third Edition. Hoboken: John Wiley and Sons, Inc.; 1999. ISBN: 9780471160687

539. Wasserstein RL, et al. The ASA statement on p-values: Context, process, and purpose. *Am Stat* 2016. doi: 10.1080/00031305.2016.1154108

540. Austin PC, et al. Testing multiple statistical hypotheses resulted in spurious associations: A study of astrological signs and health. *J Clin Epidemiol* 2006. doi: 10.1016/j.jclinepi.2006.01.012

541. Scicurious. IgNobel Prize in Neuroscience: The dead salmon study. 2012. https://blogs.scientificamerican.com/scicurious-brain/ignobel-prize-in-neuroscience-the-dead-salmon-study/

542. Hardin CC, et al. Bayesian way. *NEJM Evid* 2023. doi: 10.1056/EVIDstat2300090

543. Brown PM. What is the logic in mixing data and beliefs? *Pharm Stat* 2007. doi: 10.1002/pst.256

544. Bernard C. Stop reproducing the reproducibility crisis. *eNeuro* 2023. doi: 10.1523/eneuro.0032-23.2023

545. Allen GE. Was Nazi eugenics created in the US? *EMBO Rep* 2004. doi: 10.1038/sj.embor.7400158

546. Da Silva SM, et al. Confronting the Legacy of Eugenics and Ableism: Towards anti-ableist bioscience education. *CBE Life Sci Educ* 2024. doi: 10.1187/cbe.23-10-0195

547. Sackett DL, et al. Evidence based medicine: What it is and what it isn't. *BMJ* 1996. doi: 10.1136/bmj.312.7023.71

548. Kyriacou DN. Evidence-based medical decision making: Deductive versus inductive logical thinking. *Journal* 2004. PMID: 15175207.

549. Guyatt G, et al. *Users' Guide to the Medical Literature*. 3rd Edition. New York City: McGraw-Hill Education; 2015. ISBN: 9780071790710

550. Ioannidis JPA. Why most published research findings are false. *PLoS Med* 2005. doi: 10.1371/journal.pmed.0020124

551. Carney DR, et al. Power posing: Brief nonverbal displays affect neuroendocrine levels and risk tolerance. *Psychol Sci* 2010. doi: 10.1177/0956797610383437

552. Carney DR. My position on "power poses". 2017. https://faculty.haas.berkeley.edu/dana_carney/pdf_my%20position%20on%20power%20poses.pdf

553. Ranehill E, et al. Assessing the robustness of power posing: No effect on hormones and risk tolerance in a large sample of men and women. *Psychol Sci* 2015. doi: 10.1177/0956797614553946

554. Al-Leimon O, et al. "Publish or Perish" paradigm and medical research: Replication crisis in the context of artificial intelligence trend. *Ann Biomed Eng* 2025. doi: 10.1007/s10439-024-03625-7

555. Kapoor S, et al. Leakage and the reproducibility crisis in machine-learning-based science. *Patterns* 2023. doi: 10.1016/j.patter.2023.100804

556. Sanbonmatsu DM, et al. The impact of complexity on methods and findings in psychological science. *Front Psychol* 2021. doi: 10.3389/fpsyg.2020.580111

557. Carlisle JB. False individual patient data and zombie randomised controlled trials submitted to Anaesthesia. *Anaesthesia* 2021. doi: 10.1111/anae.15263

558. Ioannidis JPA. Hundreds of thousands of zombie randomised trials circulate among us. *Anaesthesia* 2021. doi: 10.1111/anae.15297

559. O'Connell N, et al. Trials we cannot trust: Investigating their impact on systematic reviews and clinical guidelines in spinal pain. *J Pain* 2023. doi: 10.1016/j.jpain.2023.07.003

560. Hunter P. The reproducibility "crisis": Reaction to replication crisis should not stifle innovation. *EMBO Rep* 2017. doi: 10.15252/embr.201744876

561. Millar N, et al. Trends in the use of promotional language (Hype) in abstracts of successful national institutes of health grant applications, 1985-2020. *JAMA Netw Open* 2022. doi: 10.1001/jamanetworkopen.2022.28676

562. Pal L, et al. The women's health initiative: An unforgettable decade. *Menopause* 2012. doi: 10.1097/gme.0b013e31825397f0

563. Bloom JM. Vitamin D and incident fractures. *N Engl J Med* 2022. doi: 10.1056/NEJMc2211434

564. Cummings SR, et al. VITAL findings - a decisive verdict on vitamin D supplementation. *N Engl J Med* 2022. doi: 10.1056/NEJMe2205993

565. Fakheri RJ. Vitamin D Supplementation: To D or not to D? Mayo clinic proceedings. *Mayo Clin Proc* 2024. doi: 10.1016/j.mayocp.2024.01.003

566. Kallmes DF, et al. A randomized trial of vertebroplasty for osteoporotic spinal fractures. *N Engl J Med* 2009. doi: 10.1056/NEJMoa0900563

567. Rosen R. Vitamin D and incident fractures. *N Engl J Med* 2022. doi: 10.1056/NEJMc2211434

568. Klazen CA, et al. Vertebroplasty versus conservative treatment in acute osteoporotic vertebral compression fractures (Vertos II): An open-label randomised trial. *Lancet* 2010. doi: 10.1016/s0140-6736(10)60954-3

569. Manson JE, et al. Menopausal hormone therapy and health outcomes during the intervention and extended poststopping phases of the Women's Health Initiative randomized trials. *JAMA* 2013. doi: 10.1001/jama.2013.278040

570. Kamenova K, et al. Stem cell hype: Media portrayal of therapy translation. *Sci Transl Med* 2015. doi: 10.1126/scitranslmed.3010496

571. Maguire G. Therapeutics from adult stem cells and the hype curve. *ACS Med Chem Lett* 2016. doi: 10.1021/acsmedchemlett.6b00125

572. Retraction for Shu et al., Signing at the beginning makes ethics salient and decreases dishonest self-reports in comparison to signing at the end. Proceedings of the National Academy of Sciences. 2021. doi: 10.1073/pnas.2115397118

573. O'Grady C. After honesty researcher's retractions, colleagues expand scrutiny of her work. *Science* 2023. https://www.science.org/content/article/after-honesty-researcher-s-retractions-colleagues-expand-scrutiny-her-work

574. Tolsa L, et al. 'We have guidelines, but we can also be artists': Neurologists discuss prognostic uncertainty, cognitive biases, and scoring tools. *Brain Sci* 2022. doi: 10.3390/brainsci12111591

575. Cloft HJ, et al. Scaling back on scales with a scale of scales. *AJNR Am J Neuroradiol* 2011. doi: 10.3174/ajnr.A2432

576. Uher J. Rating scales institutionalise a network of logical errors and conceptual problems in research practices: A rigorous analysis showing ways to tackle psychology's crises. *Front Psychol* 2022. doi: 10.3389/fpsyg.2022.1009893

577. Cano SJ, et al. The problem with health measurement. *Patient Prefer Adherence* 2011. doi: 10.2147/ppa.S14399

578. Grudniewicz A, et al. Predatory journals: No definition, no defence. *Nature* 2019. doi: 10.1038/d41586-019-03759-y

579. Chawla DS. The undercover academic keeping tabs on 'predatory' publishing. *Nature*. 2018. https://www.nature.com/articles/d41586-018-02921-2

580. Onwuzo C, et al. DASH diet: A review of its scientifically proven hypertension reduction and health benefits. *Cureus* 2023. doi: 10.7759/cureus.44692

581. Saposnik G, et al. Cognitive biases associated with medical decisions: A systematic review. *BMC Med Inform Decis Mak* 2016. doi: 10.1186/s12911-016-0377-1

582. Croskerry P, et al. Cognitive debiasing 1: Origins of bias and theory of debiasing. *BMJ Qual Saf*. 2013. doi: 10.1136/bmjqs-2012-001712

583. Colgrove R. But my white count…. *N Engl J Med* 2024. doi: 10.1056/NEJMp2313303

584. Lee S-F. *Logic: A Complete Introduction*. Philadelphia: Teach Yourself; 2017. ISBN: 9781473608436

585. Bluedorn N, et al. *The Fallacy Detective: Thirty-eight Lessons on How to Recognize Bad Reasoning, 2015 Edition*. 4th Edition. Muscatine: Christian Logic; 2015. ISBN: 9780974531571

586. Casarett D. The science of choosing wisely — Overcoming the therapeutic illusion. *N Engl J Med* 2016. doi: 10.1056/NEJMp1516803

587. Johnson DDP, et al. The evolution of overconfidence. *Nature* 2011. doi: 10.1038/nature10384

588. Cassam Q. Diagnostic error, overconfidence and self-knowledge. *Palgrave Commun* 2017. doi: 10.1057/palcomms.2017.25

589. Tenney ER, et al. Research: When overconfidence is an asset, and when it's a liability. *Harvard Business Review*. 2018. https://hbr.org/2018/12/research-when-overconfidence-is-an-asset-and-when-its-a-liability

590. Goldflam K, et al. Emergency medicine residents consistently rate themselves higher than attending assessments on ACGME milestones. *West J Emerg Med* 2015. doi: 10.5811/westjem.2015.8.27247

591. Knof H, et al. Prevalence of Dunning-Kruger effect in first semester medical students: A correlational study of self-assessment and actual academic performance. *BMC Med Educ* 2024. doi: 10.1186/s12909-024-06121-7

592. Han Y, et al. Metaknowledge of experts versus nonexperts: Do experts know better what they do and do not know? *J Behav Decis Mak* 2024. doi: 10.1002/bdm.2375

593. Harwood J. Social identity theory. *The International Encyclopedia of Media Psychology* 2020. doi: 10.1002/9781119011071.iemp0153

594. Bilgiç B, et al. Functional neural substrates of football fanaticism: Different pattern of brain responses and connectivity in fanatics. *Psychiatry Clin Neurosci* 2020. doi: 10.1111/pcn.13076

595. de Bruin D, et al. Shared neural representations and temporal segmentation of political content predict ideological similarity. *Sci Adv* 2023. doi: 10.1126/sciadv.abq5920

596. Roediger HL, 3rd, et al. Competing national memories of World War II. *Proc Natl Acad Sci USA* 2019. doi: 10.1073/pnas.1907992116

597. Kaplan JT, et al. Neural correlates of maintaining one's political beliefs in the face of counterevidence. *Sci Rep* 2016. doi: 10.1038/srep39589

598. Borinca I, et al. Neural correlates of maintaining one's political beliefs in the face of counterevidence. *Curr Opin Behav Sci* 2023. doi: 10.1016/j.cobeha.2023.101247

599. Howard J. *Cognitive Errors and Diagnostic Mistakes: A Case-Based Guide to Critical Thinking in Medicine*. Cham: Springer International Publishing AG; 2019. ISBN: 9783319932231

600. Encarnacion Ramirez MJ, et al. The importance of social networks in neurosurgery training in low/middle income countries. *Front Surg* 2024. doi: 10.3389/fsurg.2024.1341148

601. D'Souza F, et al. Social media: Medical education's double-edged sword. *Future Healthc J* 2021. doi: 10.7861/fhj.2020-0164

602. What is an Aunt Minnie? 2015. https://www.auntminnie.com/home/article/15557584/what-is-an-aunt-minnie#:~:text=AuntMinnie's%20founder%2C%20radiologist%20Dr.,Radiology%20Decisions%20Start%20HereTM.%22

603. Disinformation Nation: Social Media's Role in Promoting Extremism and Misinformation: Hearing before the House Energy and Commerce (March 25, 2021).

604. National PR. npr. Capitol Hill lawmakers tell tech CEOs that they have failed to protect children. 2024. https://www.npr.org/2024/02/01/1228286342/capitol-hill-lawmakers-tell-tech-ceos-that-they-have-failed-to-protect-children

605. US SG. *Social Media and Youth Mental Health: The U.S. Sugeon General's Advisory*. https://hhs.gov: Dept. of Health and Human Services, 2023

606. Cavanagh SR. No, Smartphones are Not Destroying a Generation: The kids are going to be all right. *Psychology Today*. 2017. https://www.psychologytoday.com/intl/blog/once-more-feeling/201708/no-smartphones-are-not-destroying-generation?amp

607. Cavanagh SR. *Hivemind: The New Science of Tribalism in Our Divided World*. New York City: Grand Central Publishing; 2019. ISBN: 9781538713327

608. Odgers CL. The great rewiring: Is social media really behind an epidemic of teenage mental illness? *Nature* 2024. doi: 10.1038/d41586-024-00902-2

609. Orben A, et al. The association between adolescent well-being and digital technology use. *Nat Hum Behav* 2019. doi: 10.1038/s41562-018-0506-1

610. Lewin KM, et al. Social comparison and problematic social media use: Relationships between five different social media platforms and three different social comparison constructs. *Personal Individ Differ* 2022. doi: 10.1016/j.paid.2022.111865

611. Miller J, et al. Impact of digital screen media activity on functional brain organization in late childhood: Evidence from the ABCD study. *Cortex* 2023. doi: 10.1016/j.cortex.2023.09.009

612. Przybylski AK, et al. A large-scale test of the goldilocks hypothesis: Quantifying the relations between digital-screen use and the mental well-being of adolescents. *Psychol Sci* 2017. doi: 10.1177/0956797616678438

613. Robinson A, et al. Social comparisons, social media addiction, and social interaction: An examination of specific social media behaviors related to major depressive disorder in a millennial population. *J Appl Biobehav Res* 2019. doi: 10.1111/jabr.12158

614. Samra A, et al. Social comparisons: A potential mechanism linking problematic social media use with depression. *J Behav Addict* 2022. doi: 10.1556/2006.2022.00023

615. Steers MN, et al. Seeing everyone else's highlight reels: How facebook usage is linked to depressive symptoms. *J Soc Clin Psychol* 2014. doi: 10.1521/jscp.2014.33.8.701

616. Vuorre M, et al. Estimating the association between Facebook adoption and well-being in 72 countries. *R Soc Open Sci* 2023. doi: 10.1098/rsos.221451

617. Fox S. Accessing health topics on the internet. *Pew Research Center*. 2011. https://www.pewresearch.org/2011/02/01/accessing-health-topics-on-the-internet/

618. Burke M. Ohio doctor fired after anti-Semitic tweets surface, including threat to give Jews 'wrong meds'. *NBC News*, US News. 2019. https://www.nbcnews.com/news/us-news/ohio-doctor-fired-after-anti-semitic-tweets-surface-including-threat-n953916

619. Crump J. Doctors investigated for playing 'Price Is Right' game with patients' organs on Instagram. *Independent*. 2021. https://www.the-independent.com/news/world/americas/doctors-investigated-michigan-price-is-right-b1817446.html

620. Retraction Notice. *J Vasc Surg*. 2020. doi: 10.1016/j.jvs.2020.08.018

621. Hardouin S, et al. RETRACTED: Prevalence of unprofessional social media content among young vascular surgeons. *J Vasc Surg* 2020. doi: 10.1016/j.jvs.2019.10.069

622. Frehse R, et al. Ohio plastic surgeon who livestreamed patient operations on TikTok has state medical license revoked permanently. *CNN US Crime + Justice*. 2023. https://www.cnn.com/2023/07/13/us/ohio-doctor-tiktok-license-revoked/index.html

623. FOX13 MNS. Doctor files lawsuit after losing her job because of a social media post. *FOX 13 News*. 2020. https://www.fox13memphis.com/news/doctor-files-lawsuit-after-losing-her-job-because-of-a-social-media-post/article_274effc0-0aea-581e-ad24-6e7394b596a2.html

624. Bennett KG, et al. When is posting about patients on social media unethical "medutainment"? *AMA J Ethics* 2018. doi: 10.1001/journalofethics.2018.20.4.ecas1-1804

625. Kind T. Professional guidelines for social media use: A starting point. *AMA J Ethics* 2015. doi: 10.1001/journalofethics.2015.17.5.nlit1-1505

626. Ventola CL. Social media and health care professionals: Benefits, risks, and best practices. *Journal* 2014. PMID: 25083128.

627. Bennis W. *On Becoming a Leader*. 4th Edition. New York City: Basic Books; 2009. ISBN: 9780465014088

628. Berry LL, et al. *Management Lessons from Mayo Clinic: Inside One of the World's Most Admired Service Organizations*. New York City: McGraw Hill; 2017. ISBN: 9780071590730

629. Blanchard K, et al. *The One Minute Manager*. New York City: Berkley Books; 1982. ISBN: 9780425098479

630. Burns JM. *Leadership*. New York City: HarperCollins; 1978. ISBN: 9780060105884

631. McRaven WH. *Make Your Bed*. New York City: Grand Central Publishing; 2017. ISBN: 9781455570249

632. Machiavelli N. *The Prince*. New Delhi: Fingerprint Publishing; 2022. ISBN: 9354406688

633. Babiak P, et al. *Snakes in Suits: When Psychopaths Go To Work*. New York City: Harper; 2007. ISBN: 9780061147890

634. Mueller S. A new Apple ad is sparking backlash from viewers who say it hits the wrong note. *CNN Business*. 2024. https://www.cnn.com/2024/05/08/tech/apple-ipad-pro-ad-backlash-cec/index.html

635. Ortiz A. Peloton ad is criticized as sexist and dystopian. *The New York Times*. 2019. https://www.nytimes.com/2019/12/03/business/peloton-bike-ad-stock.html

636. Umoh RJB Mark cuban and elon musk avoid this productivity killer—and you should too. *CNBC Make It*. 2018. https://www.cnbc.com/2018/06/13/jeff-bezos-mark-cuban-and-elon-musk-all-avoid-meetings.html

637. Perlow LA, et al. Stop the meeting madness. *Harvard Business Review*. 2017. https://hbr.org/2017/07/stop-the-meeting-madness

638. Hakim AC, et al. *Working with Difficult People: Handling the Ten Types of Problem People Without Losing Your Mind, Second Revised Edition*. Second Revised Edition ed. New York City: Tarcher Perigree; 2016. ISBN: 9780143111870

639. Minkel JR. Fear review: Critique of forensic psychopathy scale delayed 3 years by threat of lawsuit. *Sci Am*. 2010. https://www.scientificamerican.com/article/critique-of-forensic-psychopathy-scale-delayed-by-lawsuit/

640. Qadar S. Machiavellianism, and the 'dark triad' of personality. 2020. https://www.abc.net.au/listen/programs/allinthemind/machiavellianism/12340352?utm_campaign=related_content&utm_source=HEALTH&utm_medium=communities

641. Stout M. *The Sociopath Next Door*. New York City: Harmony Books; 2005. ISBN: 9780767915823

642. Hare RD. *Without Conscience: The Disturbing World of the Psychopaths Among Us*. New York City: The Guildford Press; 1993. ISBN: 9781572304512

643. Lewis P. 3 steps to manage your office politics during difficult times. *Forbes Leadership Leadership Strategy*. 2020.

644. Llopis G. Hidden agendas disrupt business growth and leadership. *Forbes Leadership Leadership Strategy*. 2011. https://www.forbes.com/sites/glennllopis/2011/11/07/objectives-define-intentions-why-leaders-must-reveal-their-hidden-agendas/?sh=146124be6cd4

645. Mallick M. How to intervene when a manager is gaslighting their employees. *Harvard Business Review Power and Influence*. 2021. https://hbr.org/2021/09/how-to-intervene-when-a-manager-is-gaslighting-their-employees

646. Cassling K, et al. Four lessons to take from athena-without disguising oneself as the mortal, *Mentor J Grad Med Educ* 2022. doi: 10.4300/jgme-d-21-00572.1

647. Koven S. What is a mentor? *N Engl J Med* 2024. doi: 10.1056/NEJMp2313304

648. Hammer B. *15 Lies Women Are Told at Work: …And the Truth We Need to Succeed*. New York City: Simon Element; 2024. ISBN: 9781668027615

649. MacLeod S. The challenge of providing mentorship in primary care. *Postgrad Med J* 2007. doi: 10.1136/pgmj.2006.054155

650. Ibarra H, et al. Why men still get more promotions than women. *Harvard Business Review Career Planning*. 2010. https://hbr.org/2010/09/why-men-still-get-more-promotions-than-women

651. Patton EW, et al. Differences in mentor-mentee sponsorship in male vs female recipients of national institutes of health grants. *JAMA Intern Med* 2017. doi: 10.1001/jamainternmed.2016.9391

652. Warner LL, et al. Impact of mentorship, by gender, on career trajectory in an academic anesthesiology department: A survey study. *J Contin Educ Heal Prof* 2022. doi: 10.1097/ceh.0000000000000378

653. Hughes P, et al. Can we improve on how we select medical students?. *J R Soc Med* 2002. doi: 10.1177/014107680209500106

654. Bradley TR, et al. Academic faculty demonstrate weak agreement in evaluating orthopaedic surgery residents. *JB JS Open Access* 2023. doi: 10.2106/jbjs.Oa.23.00061

655. Ezeh UC, et al. Relationship Between National Residency Matching Program (NRMP) rank order and otolaryngology residency performance. *OTO Open* 2024. doi: 10.1002/oto2.127

656. Ryan JG, et al. The relationship between faculty performance assessment and results on the in-training examination for residents in an emergency medicine training program. *J Grad Med Educ* 2013. doi: 10.4300/jgme-d-12-00240.1

657. Wise S, et al. Assessment of resident knowledge: Subjective assessment versus performance on the ACR in-training examination. *Acad Radiol* 1999. doi: 10.1016/s1076-6332(99)80064-6

658. Zuckerman SL, et al. Predicting resident performance from presidency factors: A systematic review and applicability to neurosurgical training. *World Neurosurg* 2018. doi: 10.1016/j.wneu.2017.11.078

659. McGaghie WC. Mastery learning: It is time for medical education to join the 21st century. *Acad Med* 2015. doi: 10.1097/acm.0000000000000911

660. Smith MM, et al. Clinical experience is not a proxy for competence: Comparing fellow and medical student performance in a breaking bad news simulation-based mastery learning curriculum. *Am J Hosp Palliat Care* 2023. doi: 10.1177/10499091221106176

661. Johnston H, et al. Practical and customizable study strategies for clerkship year success. *Can Med Educ J* 2023. doi: 10.36834/cmej.75072

662. Taking an NBME® Subject Examination. 2024. https://www.nbme.org/examinees/subject-exams

663. Bearman G, et al. Healthcare personnel attire in non-operating-room settings. *Infect Control Hosp Epidemiol* 2014. doi: 10.1086/675066

664. Bad Boss Index: 1,000 Employees Name Worst Manager Behaviors [Infographic]. 2019. https://www.bamboohr.com/blog/bad-boss-index-the-worst-boss-behaviors-according-to-employees-infographic

665. Jones AL, et al. Facial first impressions form two clusters representing approach-avoidance. *Cogn Psychol* 2021. doi: 10.1016/j.cogpsych.2021.101387

666. Hall P, et al. Interdisciplinary education and teamwork: A long and winding road. *Med Educ* 2001. doi: 10.1046/j.1365-2923.2001.00919.x

667. Thibault GE. The future of health professions education: Emerging trends in the United States. *FASEB Bioadv* 2020. doi: 10.1096/fba.2020-00061

668. Samuriwo R. Interprofessional collaboration-time for a new theory of action? *Front Med (Lausanne)* 2022. doi: 10.3389/fmed.2022.876715

669. Whyte S, et al. Misalignments of purpose and power in an early Canadian interprofessional education initiative. *Adv Health Sci Educ Theory Pract* 2017. doi: 10.1007/s10459-016-9746-x

670. Schubach A, et al. To preround or not to preround. *N Engl J Med* 2024. doi: 10.1056/NEJMclde2312601

671. Luks AM, et al. Watch your language!—Misusage and neologisms in clinical communication. *JAMA Intern Med* 2021. doi: 10.1001/jamainternmed.2020.5679

672. Stewart MT, et al. Conceptual models for understanding physician burnout, professional fulfillment, and well-being. *Curr Probl Pediatr Adolesc Health Care* 2019. doi: 10.1016/j.cppeds.2019.100658

673. Camina E, et al. The neuroanatomical, neurophysiological and psychological basis of memory: Current models and their origins. *Front Pharmacol* 2017. doi: 10.3389/fphar.2017.00438

674. Borrell-Carrió F, et al. The biopsychosocial model 25 years later: Principles, practice, and scientific inquiry. *Ann Fam Med* 2004. doi: 10.1370/afm.245

675. Neff J, et al. Structural competency: Curriculum for medical students, residents, and interprofessional teams on the structural factors that produce health disparities. *MedEdPORTAL* 2020. doi: 10.15766/mep_2374-8265.10888

676. Commission on SDoH. *Closing the Gap in a Generation: Health equity through action on the social determinants of health.* https://www.who.int/publications/i/item/WHO-IER-CSDH-08.1 World Health Organization, 2008

677. Dako F, et al. Understanding health-related social risks. *J Am Coll Radiol* 2024. doi: 10.1016/j.jacr.2024.03.004

678. Avvisati F. The measure of socio-economic status in PISA: A review and some suggested improvements. *Large Scale Assessmen Edu* 2020. doi: 10.1186/s40536-020-00086-x

679. Phelan JC, et al. Is racism a fundamental cause of inequalities in health? *Annu Rev Sociol* 2015. doi: 10.1146/annurev-soc-073014-112305

680. Andermann A. Taking action on the social determinants of health in clinical practice: A framework for health professionals. *CMAJ* 2016. doi: 10.1503/cmaj.160177

681. Thimm-Kaiser M, et al. Conceptualizing the mechanisms of social determinants of health: A heuristic framework to inform future directions for mitigation. *Milbank Q* 2023. doi: 10.1111/1468-0009.12642

682. Guidi J, et al. Allostatic load and its impact on health: A systematic review. *Psychother Psychosom* 2020. doi: 10.1159/000510696

683. Sturmberg JP, et al. Beyond multimorbidity: What can we learn from complexity science? *J Eval Clin Pract* 2021. doi: 10.1111/jep.13521

684. Bigrigg A, et al. Use of a staff administered structured questionnaire to identify relevant life-style issues and social-health determinants in a sexual and reproductive health service. *Eur J Contracept Reprod Health Care* 2005. doi: 10.1080/13625180500039191

685. Brcic V, et al. Development of a tool to identify poverty in a family practice setting: A pilot study. *Int J Family Med* 2011. doi: 10.1155/2011/812182

686. Kangovi S, et al. Evidence-based community health worker program addresses unmet social needs and generates positive return on investment. *Health Aff* 2020. doi: 10.1377/hlthaff.2019.00981

687. Yousaf A. The era of the ill-prepared medical student. 2016. https://blogs.jwatch.org/general-medicine/index.php/2016/03/the-era-of-the-ill-prepared-medical-student/

688. Spooner M, et al. "Tell me what is 'better'!" How medical students experience feedback, through the lens of self-regulatory learning. *BMC Med Educ* 2023. doi: 10.1186/s12909-023-04842-9

689. Schwarz R. "The sandwich approach" undermines your feedback. *Harvard Business Review Giving Feedback.* 2013. https://hbr.org/2013/04/the-sandwich-approach-undermin

690. Lee KB, et al. "Making the grade:" Noncognitive predictors of medical students' clinical clerkship grades. *J Natl Med Assoc* 2007. PMID: 17987918.

691. Tran T-V, et al. The relationship between subjectivity in managerial performance evaluation and the three dimensions of justice perception. *J Manag Control* 2021. doi: 10.1007/s00187-021-00319-2

692. Futela D, et al. Accuracy of financial disclosures in radiology journals. *J Am Coll Radiol* 2024. doi: 10.1016/j.jacr.2024.01.027

693. Doo FX, et al. Conflicts of interest in radiology publishing. *J Am Coll Radiol* 2024. doi: 10.1016/j.jacr.2024.03.014

694. Karabel J. *The Chosen: The Hidden History of Admission and Exclusion at Harvard, Yale, and Princeton.* New York City: Harper Paperbacks; 2006. ISBN: 9780618773558

695. Maxfield CM, et al. The influence of extracurricular activities on radiology resident selection decisions. *J Am Coll Radiol* 2024. doi: 10.1016/j.jacr.2023.09.013

696. Hussain A. Sea changes in dermatology residency application processes. *The Dermatologist.* 2024. https://www.hmpgloballearningnetwork.com/site/thederm/cover-story/sea-changes-dermatology-residency-application-processes

697. Holland L, et al. Medical students' perceptions of pathology and the effect of the second-year pathology course. *Hum Pathol* 2006. doi: 10.1016/j.humpath.2005.10.004

698. Johannessen LE. The narrative (re)production of prestige: How neurosurgeons teach medical students to valorise diseases. *Soc Sci Med* 2014. doi: 10.1016/j.socscimed.2014.09.013

699. Darves B. Physicians' career priorities and expectations undergoing shifts. *NEJM Career Center.* 2024. https://resources.nejmcareercenter.org/article/physicians-career-priorities-and-expectations-undergoing-shifts/

700. Thompson C. *Smarter Than You Think: How Technology is Changing Our Minds for the Better.* London: Penguin Press; 2013. ISBN: 9781594204456

701. Huynh A, et al. Fixing a broken clerkship assessment process: Reflections on objectivity and equity following the USMLE step 1 change to pass/fail. *Acad Med* 2023. doi: 10.1097/acm.0000000000005168

702. Alexander EK, et al. Variation and imprecision of clerkship grading in U.S. medical schools. *Acad Med* 2012. doi: 10.1097/ACM.0b013e31825d0a2a

703. Naidich JB, et al. A program director's guide to the medical student performance evaluation (former Dean's letter) with a database. *J Am Coll Radiol* 2014. doi: 10.1016/j.jacr.2013.11.012

704. Diab J, et al. A multicenter study of the family educational rights and privacy act and the standardized letter of recommendation: Impact on emergency medicine residency applicant and faculty behaviors. *J Grad Med Educ* 2014. doi: 10.4300/jgme-d-13-00179.1

705. Hughes P. Can we improve on how we select medical students? *J R Soc Med* 2002. doi: 10.1177/014107680209500106

706. Preparing for Residency. 2025. https://www.ama-assn.org/topics/preparing-residency

707. Wingert AM, et al. Postinterview communication in the diagnostic radiology match and its impact on program directors' ranking of applicants. *J Am Coll Radiol* 2024. doi: 10.1016/j.jacr.2023.05.028

708. Shah AS, et al. Analysis of national resident matching program for radiology fellowships: Factors affecting program fill rates. *J Am Coll Radiol* 2024. doi: 10.1016/j.jacr.2024.04.011

709. Khawar A, et al. What are the characteristics of excellent physicians and residents in the clinical workplace? A systematic review *BMJ Open* 2022. doi: 10.1136/bmjopen-2022-065333

710. Jahoda G. Quetelet and the emergence of the behavioral sciences. *Springerplus* 2015. PMID 26361574.

711. Gleick J. *Chaos: Making a New Science.* New York City: Penguin Books; 2008. ISBN: 9780143113454

712. Arnold M, et al. Dealing with information overload: A comprehensive review. *Front Psychol* 2023. doi: 10.3389/fpsyg.2023.1122200

713. Klerings I, et al. Information overload in healthcare: Too much of a good thing? *Z Evid Fortbild Qual Gesundhwes* 2015. doi: 10.1016/j.zefq.2015.06.005

714. Kumar A, et al. Coping up with the information overload in the medical profession. *J Biosci Med* 2015. doi: 10.4236/jbm.2015.311016

715. Nijor S, et al. Patient safety issues from information overload in electronic medical records. *J Patient Saf* 2022. doi: 10.1097/pts.0000000000001002

716. Ericsson KA. Deliberate practice and the acquisition and maintenance of expert performance in medicine and related domains. *Acad Med* 2004. doi: 10.1097/00001888-200410001-00022

717. Antioxidants and Cancer Prevention. 2017. https://www.cancer.gov/about-cancer/causes-prevention/risk/diet/antioxidants-fact-sheet

718. Berg SH, et al. Exponential growth bias of infectious diseases: Protocol for a systematic review. *JMIR Res Protoc* 2022. doi: 10.2196/37441

719. Chesnaye NC, et al. Non-linear relationships in clinical research. *Nephrol Dial Transplant* 2024. doi: 10.1093/ndt/gfae187

720. Bhaskaran K, et al. Association of BMI with overall and cause-specific mortality: A population-based cohort study of 3.6 million adults in the UK. *Lancet Diabetes Endocrinol.* 2018. doi: 10.1016/S2213-8587(18)30288-2

721. Watts DJ, et al. Collective dynamics of 'small-world' networks. *Nature* 1998. doi: 10.1038/30918

722. Sporns O. *Networks of the Brain*. Cambridge, MA: MIT Press; 2011. ISBN: 978-0-262-01469-4

723. Trpevski D, et al. Model for rumor spreading over networks. *Phys Rev E Stat Nonlinear Soft Matter Phys* 2010. doi: 10.1103/PhysRevE.81.056102

724. Captur G, et al. The fractal heart – Embracing mathematics in the cardiology clinic. *Nat Rev Cardiol* 2017. doi: 10.1038/nrcardio.2016.161

725. Grosu GF, et al. The fractal brain: Scale-invariance in structure and dynamics. *Cereb Cortex* 2023. doi: 10.1093/cercor/bhac363..

726. Suckling J, et al. Unintended consequences: Unknowable and unavoidable, or knowable and unforgivable? *Front Climat* 2021. doi: 10.3389/fclim.2021.737929

727. Stempniak M. Radiology resident thumbs nose at Nobel Prize winner who predicted specialty would become obsolete. *Radiology Business*. 2024. https://radiologybusiness.com/topics/artificial-intelligence/radiology-resident-thumbs-nose-nobel-prize-winner-who-predicted-specialty-would-become-obsolete

728. Weissleder R, et al. Molecular imaging. *Radiology* 2001. doi: 10.1148/radiology.219.2.r01ma19316

729. Dobler CC, et al. Users' guide to medical decision analysis. *Mayo Clin Proc* 2021. doi: 10.1016/j.mayocp.2021.02.003

730. Barile JP, et al. Patterns of chronic conditions and their associations with behaviors and quality of life, 2010. *Prev Chronic Dis* 2015. doi: 10.5888/pcd12.150179

731. Hernández B, et al. Comparisons of disease cluster patterns, prevalence and health factors in the USA, Canada, England and Ireland. *BMC Public Health* 2021. doi: 10.1186/s12889-021-11706-8

732. Schäfer I, et al. Reducing complexity: A visualisation of multimorbidity by combining disease clusters and triads. *BMC Public Health* 2014. doi: 10.1186/1471-2458-14-1285

733. Wallace E, et al. Managing patients with multimorbidity in primary care. *BMJ* 2015. doi: 10.1136/bmj.h176

734. Gordon JE. *Structures: Or Why Things Don't Fall Down*. Burlington: Da Capo Publishing, Inc.; 2003. ISBN: 9780306812835

735. Kuehn R, et al. Overly complex methods may impair pragmatic use of core evidence-based medicine principles. *BMJ Evid Based Med* 2024. doi: 10.1136/bmjebm-2024-112868

736. Gleick J. *The Information*. New York City: Pantheon Books; 2012. ISBN: 978-1400096237

737. Rickles D, et al. A simple guide to chaos and complexity. *J Epidemiol Community Health* 2007. doi: 10.1136/jech.2006.054254

738. Pryor RGL, et al. Applying chaos theory to careers: Attraction and attractors. *J Vocat Behav* 2007. doi: 10.1016/j.jvb.2007.05.002

739. Vogler C. *The Writer's Journey*. Studio City, CA: Michael Wise Productions; 2007. ISBN: 9781932907360

Index

Pages in *italics* refer to figures, pages in **bold** refer to tables, and pages followed by n refer to notes

For Product Safety Concerns and Information please contact our EU
representative GPSR@taylorandfrancis.com
Taylor & Francis Verlag GmbH, Kaufingerstraße 24, 80331 München, Germany